Editors:
Theodore M. Dembroski,
St. Petersburg, Fla.
Thomas H. Schmidt, Cologne
Gerhard Blümchen, Leichlingen

Biobehavioral Bases of Coronary Heart Disease

100 figures and 51 tables, 1983

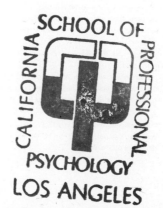

CALIFORNIA SCHOOL OF PROFESSIONAL PSYCHOLOGY LOS ANGELES

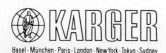 KARGER

Basel · München · Paris · London · New York · Tokyo · Sydney

Karger Biobehavioral Medicine Series

Vol. 1: C.B. Scrignar (New Orleans, La.):
Stress Strategies. The Treatment of the Anxiety Disorders
X + 262 p., 12 fig., 8 tab., 1983. ISBN 3–8055–3605–4

National Library of Medicine, Cataloging in Publication

Biobehavioral bases of coronary heart disease/
Editors, Theodore M. Dembroski, Thomas H. Schmidt, Gerhard Blümchen.–
Basel; New York: Karger, 1983. (Karger biobehavioral medicine series; v.2)
Based on a conference held at Altenberg, West Germany in June 1981.
1. Coronary Disease – psychology – congresses 2. Stress, Psychological – physiopathology – congresses I. Blümchen,
Gerhard II. Dembroski, Theodore M. III. Schmidt, Thomas M. IV. Series
W1 KA812M v.2 [WG 300 B6145 1981]
ISBN 3–8055–3629–1

Drug Dosage

The authors and the publisher have exerted every effort to ensure that drug selection and dosage set forth in this text are in accord with current recommendations and practice at the time of publication. However, in view of ongoing research, changes in government regulations, and the constant flow of information relating to drug therapy and drug reactions, the reader is urged to check the package insert for each drug for any change in indications and dosage and for added warnings and precautions. This is particularly important when the recommended agent is a new and/or infrequently employed drug.

Contents

Association

Assessment

Human Psychophysiology

Contents

T.H. Schmidt

9 Cardiovascular Reactions and Cardiovascular Risk   130

J.E. Dimsdale

10 Wet Holter Monitoring: Techniques for Studying Plasma Responses to Stress in Ambulatory Subjects   175

H. Rüddel, E. Gogolin, G. Friedrich, H. Neus, W. Schulte

11 Coronary-Prone Behavior and Blood Pressure Reactivity in Laboratory and Life Stress   185

W. Langosch, G. Brodner, F. Foerster

12 Psychophysiological Testing of Postinfarction Patients. A Study Determining the Cardiological Importance of Psychophysiolog-ical Variables   197

Contents

Pathophysiology in Animals

Contents

M. Kornitzer, F. Kittel, M. Dramaix, G. De Backer

27 Psychosocial Variables in Relation with Coronary Risk Status

List of Contributors

Appels, A., Department of Medical Psychology, State University of Limburg, Maastricht, The Netherlands

Benson, Herbert, The Charles A. Dana Research Institute and the Thorndike Laboratory, Harvard Medical School, Boston, Mass., USA

Blümchen, Gerhard, Klinik Roderbirken, Leichlingen, FRG

Brodner, G., Benedikt-Kreutz-Rehabilitationszentrum, Bad Krotzingen, FRG

Buell, James C., Department of Preventive and Stress Medicine, University of Nebraska Medical Center, Omaha, Nebr., USA

Chesney, Margaret A., Behavioral Medicine Program, Stanford Research Institute, Menlo Park, Calif., USA

Cottier, Christopher, Department of Medicine, University of Basel, Basel, Switzerland

De Backer, G., Laboratory of Epidemiology and Social Medicine, Free University of Brussels, Brussels, Belgium

Dembroski, Theodore M., Stress and Cardiovascular Research Center, Eckerd College, St. Petersburg, Fla., USA

Dimsdale, Joel E., Department of Psychiatry, Massachusetts General Hospital, Harvard Medical School, Boston, Mass., USA

Dramaix, M., Laboratory of Epidemiology and Social Medicine, Free University of Brussels, Brussels, Belgium

Eliot, Robert S., Department of Preventive and Stress Medicine, University of Nebraska Medical Center, Omaha, Nebr., USA

Engel, Bernard T., National Institute on Aging, National Institutes of Health, Baltimore, Md., USA

Foerster, F., Forschungsgruppe Psychophysiologie, Freiburg, FRG

Fokkema, D. S., Department of Zoology, State University of Groningen, Groningen, The Netherlands

Frankenhaeuser, Department of Psychology, Karolinska Institutet, Stockholm, Sweden

Frantík, E., Institute of Hygiene and Epidemiology, Prague, CSSR

Friedrich, G., Department of Medicine, University of Bonn, Bonn, FRG

Fuchs, E., Lehrstuhl für Tierphysiologie, Universität Bayreuth, Bayreuth, FRG

Gogolin, E., Department of Medicine, University of Bonn, Bonn, FRG

Henry, James P., Department of Physiology and Biophysics, University of Southern California School of Medicine, Los Angeles, Calif., USA

Herd, J. Alan, Sid W. Richardson Institute for Preventive Medicine, Baylor College of Medicine, Houston, Tex., USA

Horváth, M., Institute of Hygiene and Epidemiology, Prague, CSSR

Julius, Stevo, Department of Internal Medicine, University of Michigan Medical School, Ann Arbor, Mich., USA

Kittel, F., Laboratory of Epidemiology and Social Medicine, Free University of Brussels, Brussels, Belgium

Koepke, John P., Department of Psychiatry, University of North Carolina School of Medicine, Chapel Hill, N.C., USA

Koolhaas, J.M., Department of Zoology, State University of Groningen, Groningen, The Netherlands

Kornitzer, Marcel, Laboratory of Epidemiology and Social Medicine, Free University of Brussels, Brussels, Belgium

Lamprecht, F., Department of Psychosomatic Medicine and Psychotherapy, Klinikum Steglitz, Freie Universität Berlin, Berlin, FRG

Langer, Alan W., Department of Psychology, University of North Carolina School of Medicine, Chapel Hill, N.C., USA

Langosch, Wolfgang, Benedikt-Kreutz-Rehabilitationszentrum, Bad Krotzingen, FRG

Light, Kathleen C., Division of Health Affairs, University of North Carolina, Chapel Hill, N.C., USA

MacDougall, James M., Stress and Cardiovascular Research Center, Eckerd College, St. Petersburg, Fla., USA

Matthews, Karen A., Department of Psychiatry, University of Pittsburgh, Pittsburgh, Pa., USA

Neus, H., Department of Medicine, University of Bonn, Bonn, FRG

Obrist, Paul A., Department of Psychiatry, University of North Carolina School of Medicine, Chapel Hill, N.C., USA

Patel, Chandra, Department of Epidemiology, The London School of Hygiene and Tropical Medicine, London, England

Pepping, Georg, Fachbereich Psychologie der Universität, Giessen, FRG

Rosenman, Ray H., Behavioral Medicine Program, Stanford Research Institute, Menlo Park, Calif., USA

Rüddel, Heinz, Department of Medicine, University of Bonn, Bonn, FRG

Schmidt, Thomas H., Psychosomatische Abteilung der Universitätskliniken der Universität zu Köln, Köln, FRG

Schneiderman, Neil, Department of Psychology, University of Miami, Coral Gables, Fla., USA

Schulte, W., Department of Medicine, University of Bonn, Bonn, FRG

Schuurman, T., Tropon Werke, Pharmakologie II, Köln, FRG

Slabý, A., Institute of Hygiene and Epidemiology, Prague, CSSR

Stöhr, W., Lehrstuhl für Tierphysiologie, Universität Bayreuth, Bayreuth, FRG

Vaitl, Dieter, Fachbereich Psychologie der Universität, Giessen, FRG

von Holst, D., Lehrstuhl für Tierphysiologie, Universität Bayreuth, Bayreuth, FRG

Williams, Redford B., Departments of Psychiatry and Medicine, Duke University Medical Center, Durham, N.C., USA

Preface

Coronary-prone behaviors can be divided into two general categories. The first of these includes primarily consumatory behaviors involving intake of substances likely to impact negatively on the cardiovascular system. During the 1970s, public and private agencies devoted enormous effort and resources to educationally based preventive programs designed to alter cigarette smoking, dietary habits, and other health compliance behaviors in large numbers of people. But, during the same decade little attention was devoted to the second category of coronary-prone behaviors, which can be encompassed under the general concept of stress. The reason for this relative neglect of stress-related behaviors in the etiology of coronary heart disease (CHD) can probably be attributed to the fact that the epidemiological evidence in the area had not yet been systematically and critically reviewed by the biomedical and behavioral science communities. In fact, the interface discipline of behavioral medicine was just beginning to emerge.

Yet, during this period the relationship between stress and CHD was not entirely ignored. A number of events in the USA and Europe resulted in increased attention to the stress issue. For example, under the direction of Dr. *M.J. Halhuber* a series of conferences was held at Klinik Höhenried near Munich. The theme of these conferences was psychosocial stress and CHD. The conferences involved international participation of scientists from both the biomedical and behavioral science communities. The meetings promoted lively exchange of ideas and data that found their way into the published *Proceedings* of the conferences. With the generous support of the firm of Pharma Schwarz, several of these conferences helped, in part, to form the foundation for the present volume.

A parallel series of conferences in the USA during the late 1970s also partly layed the groundwork for the present volume. In June 1977, with the support of the National Heart, Lung, and Blood Institute, Eckerd College sponsored the first National Forum on Coronary-Prone Behavior, which was held in St. Petersburg, Florida. The purpose of the Forum was to organize in one place the evidence for the association of the type A coronary-prone behavior pattern with CHD; to examine how the pattern is assessed; to explore the physiological mechanisms linking behavior with disease; to inspect the developmental origins of and cultural influences on the coronary-prone behavior pattern; and to review extant efforts at intervention aimed at altering the type A coronary-prone behavior pattern. The book *Coronary-Prone Behavior* was an outgrowth of the Forum and was used as the major information source for a subsequent conference held at Amelia Island, Florida, in December 1978.

With support again from the National Heart, Lung, and Blood Institute, the Amelia Island conference provided the opportunity to assemble a panel of experts who were not directly associated with nor who held a vested interest in research on the coronary-prone behavior pattern, but clearly possessed the necessary expertise to systematically and critically evaluate the evidence for the validity of coronary-prone behavior as a risk factor for CHD. The results of the conference were published in the June 1981 issue of *Circulation.* The following is a quote from the Panel's final report: 'The Review Panel accepts the available body of scientific evidence as demonstrating that type A behavior... is associated with an increased risk of clinically apparent CHD in employed, middle-aged US citizens. This increased risk is over and above that imposed by age, systolic blood pressure, serum cholesterol, and smoking and appears to be of the same order of magnitude as the relative risk associated with any of these other factors.' Thus, a critical consensus of behavioral and biomedical scientists of diverse backgrounds who were not directly involved in the area had concluded for the first time that the type A pattern, originally conceptualized by Drs. *Friedman* and *Rosenman,* is a legitimate risk factor for CHD. At the same time, parallel acceptance of the validity of coronary-prone behavior was also growing in Europe.

Although the concept that a behavior pattern not related to consumatory activity could play a role in the etiology of CHD was gaining international recognition, perhaps the most frequently asked question concerned the mechanisms through which behavior is translated into hypertension, atherosclerosis, and sudden cardiac death. In fact, study of this issue was the major recommendation of the Amelia Review Panel. Clearly, the question regarding the relationship between behavior and disease requires physiologically oriented answers and few having a sound data base were available. Said differently, much research in the 1970s was directed at linking 'stress'-related behavior to the prevalence and incidence of CHD. Thus, a clear need existed for more physiological-based research. This is illustrated by the paucity of articles in precursor volumes of the present series that were directed toward a physiological analysis of coronary-prone behaviors. For example, in *Coronary-Prone Behavior*, only about 20% of the chapters had such a focus. In the present volume approximately 80% of the chapters address primarily physiologically oriented issues. There are chapters devoted to epidemiological findings, behavioral assessment, methodological issues and the like, but the bulk of the book clearly reflects the theme of the title: *Biobehavioral Bases of Coronary Heart Disease.*

The volume is divided into six sections. (1) *Association.* This section primarily deals with epidemiological issues concerning the relationship between behavior and CHD. (2) *Assessment.* Here, the focus is on methodological issues involved in the measurement of stress-related behaviors and examination of the implications of various sorts of behavior. (3) *Psychophysiology.* The chapters in this section deal with methods and findings in the area of research involving the relationship between human behavior and physiologic responses in various environments both in the laboratory and in naturalistic settings. (4) *Pathophysiology in Humans.* The primary focus here is on the basic human pathophysiologic mechanisms that mediate the relationships between behavior-physiological response and hypertension, atherosclerosis, and sudden cardiac death. (5) *Pathophysiology in Animals.* The intent of this section is identical to the latter except that animal research is the primary focus. (6) *Intervention.* The intent of this section is to examine the alteration of potentially damaging physiological states primarily through behavioral intervention methods.

This volume, like *Coronary-Prone Behavior* and the volumes edited by Prof. *Halhuber* and co-workers, is based upon a conference. The title of the conference was 'Biological Basis of Coronary-Prone Behavior: Behavioral Approaches to a 20th Century Epidemic'. The conference was held in June 1981 in Altenberg, West Germany. Even a cursory inspection of the list of contributors will reveal a truly international assemblage. Both the conference and this volume were made possible by the humanitarian concern and most generous financial support of the firm of Pharma Schwarz which, as mentioned earlier, historically has played a very significant role in the advancement of scientific study of stress and CHD. All of the contributors to this volume join us in extending our deepest gratitude to the firm for its generosity. As with the conferences before it, the data and ideas presented engendered exciting debate and discussion, which significantly influenced the content of many chapters in this book. In fact, we believe that the closing remarks of the conference at Altenberg given by Dr. *Robert S. Eliot* serve as a most appropriate basis for the introduction to the present volume. Finally, we gratefully acknowledge the splendid work of Stans Dembroski, which significantly contributed to the preparation of this volume for publication.

Theodore M. Dembroski
Thomas H. Schmidt
Gerhard Blümchen

Introduction

Robert S. Eliot

The contributions which comprise this volume provide clear evidence that this field is developing an increasingly sound scientific base. There is now a need to communicate this new information so that the field and its potential benefits become incorporated into the substance and practice of medicine. It is equally important to continue to build more information upon this established research base. To be sound and enduring, each of these steps must of necessity be based upon the development and communication of data derived from questions that have been soundly posed and answered in a rigorous and rational manner.

The first question is: 'What is the supportive evidence that life-style, behavior, and stress can induce, enhance, or perpetrate cardiovascular disorders?' The evidence for this ranges from superficial environmental studies indicating that 26% of those who drop dead do so on Monday, to clear evidence that myofibrillar necrosis can be directly induced by boluses of catecholamines, prevented by beta blockade, and that these features are histopathologically identical with those found in 80% of the 400,000 victims of sudden cardiac death per annum in the USA.

Furthermore, there is evidence that the central nervous system through the pituitary adrenocortical axis can lead to an acceleration of atherosclerosis and hypertension in much the same fashion demonstrated by the more extreme experiment of nature, Cushing's syndrome. Indeed, a myriad of neuroendocrine pathways have been identified that contribute to and/or control such critical and diverse cardiovascular phenomena as the synthesis of cholesterol, an increase in platelet adhesiveness, injury to the intimal wall, susceptibility and lability of blood pressure response, the lowering of ventricular fibrillatory thresholds, the induction of coronary spasm and, as mentioned above, the 'rupture' of myofibrills by direct catecholamine assault. Although these phenomena cannot be isolated in a simplistic fashion and obviously are multi-faceted in character, it is clear that the gamut of cardiovascular disorders is influenced through central nervous system mechanisms in direct relationship to life-style, behavior, and the perception and management of stress.

Animal experiments have led the way to these observations and continue to supplement them. Highlights of this volume range from the social hierarchal data D. *Henry* presented demonstrating cardiovascular disasters in mice and the potential relationship of these phenomena to those in men, to the fascinating studies of Prof. *von Holst* who demonstrated hypertensive deaths in submissive tree shrews exposed without physical contact to more dominant males. It is indeed unfortunate that *Wilhelm Raab* could not contribute to this volume to be rewarded and reinforced by the above observations, which he sought and predicted many years ago. Viewed from the perspective of *Raab, Henry, von Holst,* and others, it is clear that the many similarities between animals and man are more important than their differences. Thus, it is now well established – through both animal and human experimentation – that there is a series of pathophysiologic events and pathways that definitely link lifestyle, behavior, and stress to hypertension, coronary heart disease, and sudden cardiac death. Indeed, these phenomena are not separate and distinct, but appear to be deeply interwoven with the basic mechanisms and established risk factors as outlined above. From this it is reasonable to infer that the control of risks associated with the cardiovascular epidemics of the industrialized world will require an understanding of the behavioral mechanisms involved. Required also will be the implementation of appropriate behavioral modification methods and systems to facilitate successful change toward healthful life-style.

A second major question is dependent upon the first; that is, if it is clear that behavioral factors are contributing to cardiovascular disorders, then what accurate means of detection and measurement of risk are available or must be sought? The first link between behavior and coronary disease which has been formally accepted by the medical profession is that of type A behavior. The Western Collaborative Group Study [1] demonstrated that type A behavior was a population risk factor, and a recent report published in *Circulation* concludes that type A behavior was a risk factor 'equal to if not greater than' other established risk factors in coronary heart disease. Thus, for the first time a behavioral link with coronary heart disease – or for that matter, any cardiovascular disorder – is now an accepted part of medical science.

It is important, however, to know the specificity and selectivity of this behavioral factor. It is well understood that type A behavior does not inevitably lead to coronary heart disease; equally type B behavior does not inevitably exclude it. Thus, one of the challenges to clinical investigators in the detection of individuals at risk is the development of a more selective means of identifying coronary-prone behavior. *One* component of coronary-prone behavior is type A behavior. However, the multifactorial dimensions of the type A pattern need further elaboration. The question remains: 'Why is type A behavior a coronary risk factor?'

In cooperation with Drs. *Dembroski, MacDougall, Buell,* and other members of my department, we have been steadily working toward an understanding of what is meant by physiologic arousal in response to mental tasks and challenges. To be valid and relevant in clinical medicine, these responses must be measured against standardised tests. We employ the *Cold pressor test, Tilt table,* and *Treadmill stress tests* as baseline studies. Against these known standards, individuals are challenged with a spectrum of psychomotor and mental tasks to determine potential physiologic overreactivity and cardiovascular vulnerability. We employ instrumentation capable of delivering complex hemodynamic answers. It has been suggested in much of the literature that physiologic arousal is more common among type A than among type B individuals, but it is also clear that the relationship is far from uniform. Thus, a better understanding of the facility with which physiologic arousal takes place may lead toward the next step in detection, which is greater specificity. Our preference for physiologic measurements over stylistic behavioral measurements is the difference between the subjective and objective or the overt and covert. The ability to place numbers on sociobiological events may allow us to test further the validity of our initial observations concerning physiologically overreactive individuals, termed 'hot reactors', who subsequently experienced early cardiovascular disasters. The next decade should see much activity in this area.

The third major question must ask, 'What are the prudent and scientifically based management principles and techniques?' In separate studies, Drs. *Patel, Benson, Engel,* and many others have made important steps in this direction. Their individual efforts have begun to demonstrate that behavior can be modified provided that custom tailored reward systems are clearly identified, their mechanisms understood, and their utilization including positive forms of feedback to reinforce healthful rather than self-destructive behavior.

From our experience, and many others, it is becoming apparent that the orchestration of many behavioral facets appears more fruitful and fulfilling than a series of solo performances. Systematic admixtures of biofeedback, cognitive restructuring, deep-muscle relaxation, noncultist yoga techniques, and other approaches can be demonstrated to improve psychological and, indeed, physiological states.

Simplistic approaches developed by cults often have counter-productive or even destructive influences on individuals, corporations, and society in general. For this reason, it seems prudent that responsible and scientifically based researchers and practitioners must assume the responsibility for public education. Where proof is not available, prudence is warranted. We are reminded of *Neil Miller's* statement, 'We must be bold about what we attempt and cautious about what we claim.'

With the opportunity and chemistry that has been provided by the present group of authors, it is clear that further interdisciplinary work is important and some of this should be stimulated by this important volume. From it will emanate state-of-the-art papers that can lead toward a more clear understanding of the complexities within the field. It will be of added importance to continue piecing together practical elements necessary for clinical implementation. This also will involve that which is represented by this group of authors; namely, an assemblage of those with different backgrounds working toward a common goal.

In 1623, *William Harvey* stated, 'Every affection of the mind that is attended with either pain or pleasure, hope or fear, is the cause of an agitation, whose influence extends to the heart.' He set the stage for this volume and for the continuing efforts that will develop from it. That *Harvey's* statement is leading to established pathophysiologic meaning, early objective testing systems, and prudent behavioral management is clear from the outcome of this volume. The challenge that remains ahead by further development of these three dimensions will be that of substituting scientifically based preventive, behavioral, and self-regulatory mechanisms for the expensive, highly technical, and extremely limited practices of interventive contemporary medicine and cardiology. Everyone has a stake in this group's continued success.

Reference

1   Rosenman, R.H.; Friedman, M.; Straus, R.; Wurm, M.; Kositchek, R.; Mann, W.; Werthessen, N.: A predictive study of coronary heart disease: the Western Collaborative Group Study. J. Am. med. Ass. *189:* 15 (1964).

1 Current Status of Risk Factors and Type A Behavior Pattern in the Pathogenesis of Ischemic Heart Disease

Ray H. Rosenman

Industrialized societies have suffered a variably increased rate of is-chemic heart disease (IHD) in the 20th century. As *White* [94] emphasized, this cannot be simply ascribed to a larger population of older subjects, improved diagnosis, or any improbable rapid change of genetic factors. Coronary atherosclerosis (CAD) and IHD have multifactorial etiologies whose pathogenetic links are still imperfectly understood, but it has become clear that environmental factors must play a dominant role in the 20th cen-tury incidence of IHD. It is generally believed that dietary fat intake, physical inactivity, cigarette smoking and risk factors such as the blood pressure and serum lipid-lipoprotein levels are most relevant. However, it has become clear that such variables fall far short of fully explaining the new incidence of IHD [10, 13].

The compelling reasons to implicate dietary fat intake have been re-viewed far too often [47, 87] to require restatement here. However, there are many inconsistencies in the correlations of saturated fat intake and either serum lipid levels or rates of IHD in different populations. Indeed, no rela-tionship has been found within populations between diet and either lipids or occurrence of IHD in any prospective study, despite the wide variance of both dietary fat and serum lipids, as for example in Framingham [46].

The study of Irish siblings found that those remaining in Ireland had lower serum cholesterols and lower IHD incidence compared to those who had migrated to Boston, despite the former's higher intake of calories and percentage of dietary saturated fats [90]. Serum cholesterols and IHD rates are higher in East than West Finland [48], despite closely similar dietary intakes [75]. Bedouin Arabs with little IHD in their nomadic existence begin to acquire IHD when they migrate to Israeli cities, despite ingesting a diet higher in polyunsaturated fats, confirmed by analysis of their subcutaneous fat composition [67]. From North to South Italy there is a decrease of serum cholesterol and rate of IHD that cannot be ascribed to dietary differences or other risk factors [74], and the recent decline of IHD mortality in Italy occurred in the face of marked increase of dietary meat intake [32]. The low rate of IHD in France [15] can hardly be ascribed to low intake of saturated fats. For many decades in the USA the lowest IHD rates occur in the farm belt region where habitual intake of saturated fats in meat and dairy products must be at least as high as in the densely populated, industrialized regions with much higher rates of IHD. The small secular change of serum cholesterol in the USA from 1960 to 1971–74 cannot be correlated with dietary changes, and the changes of serum cholesterol associated with dietary changes from 1910 to 1965 were minor, hardly supporting a major role of the diet for the marked rise of IHD that was observed during these decades [43, 71]. IHD mortality continues to fall in Japan despite marked increase of dietary saturated fat and of smoking. Nor do dietary differences explain the higher rates of IHD in Japanese-Americans in Hawaii and California compared to Japan [63, 64]. Moreover, neither the increase of IHD in the 20th century in the USA, nor the decline of IHD mortality that began in the 1940s can be explained by parallel dietary changes [60, 89].

The rarity of IHD in the 19th century cannot be explained either by lower dietary saturated fat intake of by greater indulgence in aerobic activity by millions of upper class subjects at risk for IHD. Physical activity does appear to afford some protection against IHD [70]. It favorably influences other risk factors, reduces fatigue, improves endurance, diminishes emotional anxiety and depression, and induces a sense of well-being. However, there is little evidence that aerobic conditioning enlarges coronary arteries, promotes collateral circulation, dissolves atheromatous plaques, improves myocardial blood flow, or reduces rates of either IHD or reinfarction. It would seem that physical conditioning promotes well-being at all ages and enables subjects with IHD to tolerate their disease far better, but that the effects are largely if not entirely of functional nature [16].

A large body of evidence relates conventional risk factors to IHD incidence in all prospective studies. They offer the possibility of identifying high and low risk groups and of predicting their actual rates of IHD with considerable accuracy [29]. However, the Framingham findings do not prevail in other population groups. For example, after full adjustment for all conventional risk factors is made, the incidence of IHD in males at Framingham is 2–3 times higher than those observed in Puerto Rico and Honolulu [28], Yugoslavia [51], Paris [15] or Japan [63]. Thus, the conventional risk factors predict the relative IHD risk, but fail to predict either the absolute risk of IHD or to identify the specific future victims of IHD [29]. Indeed, even when full account is taken of all conventional risk factors, they fail to account for well over half of the numerical incidence of IHD in prospective studies [47].

Moreover, they are poor predictors of either the distribution or severity of CAD [35, 92, 93], or the rate of its progression [52]. In view of the lack of quantitative relationship between the anatomic lesions and either the clinical incidence or symptoms of IHD [7], it is not surprising that prevalence of CAD far exceeds that of IHD.

Burch [8] has provided a lucid analysis of the role of risk factors from considerations of their mortality ratios. The secular increase and age dependence of recorded IHD mortality rates cannot plausibly be reconciled with the view that risk factors actually *cause* CAD. *Burch* [8] emphasizes that increased rates of IHD must be explained by some precipitating factor acting in conjunction with diet and other risk factors. Accordingly, intervention programs that do not involve such precipitating factors may be doomed to disappointment, and his prediction appears to be confirmed by the failure of most such programs to demonstrate any clear-cut reductions of either primary or secondary IHD rates. Although attempts to alter risk factors are very plausible [27, 50, 72], they are difficult to accomplish in large population groups [76]. Moreover, the evidence that such attempts are associated with reduction of IHD is still lacking [75].

A decline of IHD *mortality* has occurred more recently in some countries, with no change or increased rates in others. The decline may in part be ascribed to altered diet and risk factors, but careful scrutiny fails to identify any clear relationships. In large part it may be due to decreased case-fatality rates. Thus, a decline of IHD mortality also occurred at Framingham despite no change of IHD morbidity [45]. In Malmö, a significant decline of IHD mortality occurred from 1963 to 1972 despite increased IHD morbidity [36]. International differences in rates of IHD as well as changing rates of mortality from IHD in the USA over time appear to correlate most closely with intakes of alcohol [55]. In prospective studies, alcohol consistently shows an inverse relationship with IHD incidence [34, 55].

Considerable interest has accrued to high-density lipoprotein (HDL) cholesterol levels, since these are inversely related to CAD and to prevalence and incidence of IHD. HDL has a unique function that is subserved by its ability to bind to cell surface receptors. After attachment, unesterified cholesterol within the cell moves into the HDL, followed by its detachment, thereby reducing the total sterol burden within the cell. However, it appears that the binding activity of both HDL and low-density lipoproteins (LDL) to surface receptors cannot simplistically explain atherosclerosis. The receptor-mediated process is self-regulating, with a feedback system that allows fibroblasts and smooth muscles cells only a limited amount of cholesterol uptake before the availability of cell surface receptors is repressed. Smooth muscle and fibroblast cells will not normally accumulate large amount of cholesterol, regardless of which lipoproteins are exposed to the cell, and they will not load themselves with fat and become the loaded foam cells observed in the atheroma [59]. CAD is initiated by intimal damage, followed by intimal smooth muscle proliferation, with lipid desposition into the hyperplastic bed. It is reasonable to believe that any factor that enhances rates of intimal damage or of lipid deposition will accelerate progression of CAD [83].

Ongoing cell proliferation occurs in response to recurrent injury and fibrous plaques become atheromas only when influx of circulating lipids exceeds the cellular metabolic capacity for their degradation and elimination. Lipid deposition then stimulates growth of atheromatous plaques. Atherogenesis is not passive and progressive, but is a dynamic interaction of smooth muscle tone activity, proliferation and connective tissue synthesis in equilibrium with the bathing milieu, neurogenic inputs, hemodynamic stresses, and circulating platelets [4]. It is plausible that some factor, as inferred by *Burch* [8], has interrupted the normal feedback system that prevents smooth muscle cells from accumulating excess lipid [5], and that this factor does this by increasing the rate of intimal damage and its smooth muscle-fibroblast proliferating response. Decreased presence of such a factor might then explain the infrequency of IHD in the 19th century in populations with plethoric diets, untreated hypertension, etc. Differences in such a factor might explain the wide variance of IHD rates in many populations at similar levels of conventional risk factors [15, 22], the association of increased IHD with urbanization [62], and why rates of IHD have not increased in certain populations despite increased dietary saturated fat, cigarette smoking, hypertension, etc. [15]. For example, the Maoris are Polynesians who migrated to New Zealand long ago. They have a much higher rate of IHD than their counterparts who remained behind on small Pacific islands, in whom IHD is rare despite their higher dietary saturated fat intake [1]. It is of interest that the only risk factor that correlates with IHD in the Maoris is the systolic blood pressure [67]. Yemenites with low rates of IHD prior to migration to Israel continue to exhibit low rates compared to other Israeli groups, the differences not being explained by the risk factors. Increase of IHD with urbanization in Puerto Rico is not explained by the risk factors, and it is significant that higher rates of IHD are observed in migrants to urban areas than in established urban dwellers [22].

The studies of Japanese are particularly illuminating [12]. The IHD rate remains low in Japan and increases in Japanese-Americans in Hawaii and

California. The differences are explained only in part by diet and risk factors and are much more strongly related to social and cultural factors [12, 62–64] that appear to act as the precipitating factor inferred by *Burch* [8].

There is considerable evidence to suggest that this factor lies in psycho-social variables [37, 38]. Possible roles are held for demographic, socioeco-nomic, psychological and emotional factors that include social class and status, education, religion, ethnicity, marital status, occupation, job respon-sibilities, social and geographic mobility, status incongruities, life events, life dissatisfactions, and emotional deprivation and loss. The strongest evidence is found in the relationships of type A behavior pattern (TABP) to CAD and IHD. TABP appears to be the common denominator for the interaction of such variables, other risk factors and IHD. Conventional risk factors show only small causal relationship to the risk of IHD in the absence of the coping methodology used by subjects with TABP. The type A individual appears to have an enhanced rate of intimal damage, that becomes the precipitating fac-tor suggested by *Burch* [8], that explains the inconsistent relationships between risk factors and IHD, and that appears to operate via adrenergic mechanisms that were suspected by *Osler* [69] and *Raab* [73].

TABP is an action-emotion complex exhibited by increasing numbers of individuals in their interaction with others and against opposition of time, persons, and things [78, 83]. It is not a personality typology but is a behavioral syndrome that is correlated with enhanced neuro-hormonal responses.

It includes behavioral dispositions such as ambitiousness, aggressive-ness, competitiveness, and impatience; specific behaviors, such as muscle tenseness, mental alertness, rapid and emphatic speech stylistics, and rapid pace of most activities; and emotional responses such as irritation, hostility and anger that is usually covert. TABP is neither a stressor situation nor a dis-tressed response, but is a behavioral syndrome with characteristic values, thoughts, interpersonal relationships, gestures, facial expressions, motor activity and pace, stylistics of speech and other mannerisms [78, 81]. The con-verse type B individual is more relaxed, unhurried, more easily satisfied, and uses an alternative method of coping in daily living that does not often lead to time urgency or competitive hostility.

TABP is thus an integrated pattern of behaviors that differs in its psycho-logical dimensions from those of anxiety, depression, distress, neurosis, and psychopathology [11]. Its prevalence is increased by urbanization and by technological progress that present uniquely new milieu challenges not experienced by previous generations and simpler societies. It stems in part from certain personality and behavioral predispositions, but emerges when the environmental challenges elicit the particular set of type A behaviors. Thus, TABP responses typically involve both an intrinsic and an environmental component [81].

Many investigators have confirmed these observations, giving TABP a strong construct validity [81]. Most type A behaviors are overt, but the hostility characteristic of type As can be suppressed and not evident to the untrained observer, but becomes overt when such persons perceive frustration in their achievement-orientation. Type As exhibit an increased drive to succeed, an increased pace of activity and manifest hostility particularly when stressor stimuli are perceived as uncontrollable and when others are perceived as impeding their aims and work [23–26].

Stress is regarded by some as a nonspecific reaction to any stressor, and by others as a nonspecific physiological response that varies with the particular type of stressor and surrounding context. However, psychophysiological responses to stressful events may depend upon the failure or success of coping mechanisms as well as upon the manner in which events are perceived. TABP is a characteristic style of response to environmental stressors and is enhanced when the stressors threaten the individual with a perceived loss of control over his milieu [23].

TABP is best assessed by the Structured Interview (SI) that was designed for this purpose [78, 84]. The SI takes into account the stylistics of speech, the content of answers to the questions asked, and the overt psychomotor and other nonverbal behaviors that subjects exhibit during the interview. An array of psychometric questionnaires has been tested for assessment of TABP, including those patterned after the SI, but they fall significantly short of accurate assessment compared to the SI [11, 40, 81, 85], probably because of the hurry, poor insight, and inaccuracy of self-appraisal particularly by type As [81].

TABP is strongly related to the prevalence, incidence, and mortality rates of IHD [19, 30, 42, 82]. The relationship of TABP to IHD prevalence has been widely confirmed in studies that also provide cross-cultural validation [33, 37, 38, 68, 81]. Its association with the incidence of IHD [79] also has been confirmed in the Framingham Study [31], in the Japanese-American Study [63], and in the Minnesota Study [6] in which a significant positive association was found between the major type A attributes and the IHD incidence, using the Thurstone Activity Scale that correlates well with TABP [85]. Associations of TABP and IHD continue to be affirmed by all studies of this relationship [37, 81]. The data suggest that there is a synergistic pattern for

IHD risk in which TABP operates with nearly a constant multiplicative effect applied to whatever background level results from other risk factors [3]. In these relationships, TABP appears to double the risk of IHD at all levels of other risk factors [81]. The observed associations cannot be ascribed to chance fluctuations since both adjusted and nonadjusted risk ratios for type A/B subjects in these studies achieve high statistical significance and are, moreover, closely similar in California and Framingham [3]. The risk associated with TABP is direct in that it is independent of other risk factors and does not diminish with age [80].

The association of TABP and IHD prevails for the incidence of both symptomatic and silent myocardial infarction as well as for IHD initially manifest as angina pectoris without infarction [39, 79], and prevails for the risk of reinfarction [41]. TABP also is strongly related to the severity of basic CAD [2, 17, 20, 96] and to its rate of progression [54] in associations that are also independent of other risk factors.

TABP was originally conceived as having the described behavioral components [78]. In all studies that have examined the relationship of TABP to the components associated with coronary-proneness, it is the pace and time urgency and the competitive hostility behaviors that are particularly related to the risk of IHD and to the severity of basic CAD [66, 95].

TABP is a response style that leads to more or chronic performance at near maximum capacity, with an hyperresponsiveness to actual or perceived challenges. Therefore, as might be anticipated, type As respond to challenges, particularly those considered as salient, with enhanced secretion of norepinephrine (NE) [18] that appears to occur throughout the working day milieu [21]. A host of studies have confirmed that type As, compared to type Bs, exhibit enhanced secretion of NE, with associated greater rise of blood pressure and heart rate in response to many cognitive and physical performance tasks and to cold pressor testing. The enhanced response is generally greater in males than females, in response to high- than low-order challenge, and is greatest in type A subjects who exhibit the same type A components that are most strongly associated with the incidence of IHD and the severity of CAD [58, 81]. Recent studies have confirmed [23, 91] the earlier investigations of these responses [18, 21].

Although there is some evidence of an intrinsic hyperreactivity in type A subjects [44], the results of most studies suggest that type As do not possess any constitutional hyperreactivity but only augmented adrenergic responses due to their heightened perception of most milieu stressors as being salient challenges [18]. Type B behavior is not merely the absence of type A response styles, but is a different set of coping behaviors. Type As report more stressful life events and more life events as stressful [9, 53]. Active coping with stressors increases NE secretion [14] and coronary-prone subjects appear to suffer greater distress in response to life events [9]. Normal physiologic response to stress must be distinguished from excess and inappropriate adrenergic response, and laboratory stressors only approximate real life situations. However, in TABP the responses consistently observed in the laboratory are also found throughout the working milieu [21]. Humans adapt better to acute than to chronic stress, but cardiovascular responsiveness to challenge appears to be reproducible in most subjects [61]. It is important to note that the baseline systolic blood pressure is closely related to plasma NE level. It is relevant that the response to cold pressor testing was a strong predictor of IHD in the Minnesota Study [6] and that the systolic is a stronger predictor of IHD than is the diastolic blood pressure in most prospective studies [86, 88], confirming actuarial data.

Catecholamines affect hemodynamics and platelet aggregation, enhance intimal damage, can trigger plaque rupture with either intramural hemorrhage or intraluminal thrombosis [77], and play a dominant role in sudden coronary death from ventricular fibrillation [57, 65]. It is now well recognized that endothelial injury with plaque ulcerations, erosions, and disruption underly most occlusive coronary thrombosis that causes myocardial infarction, although acute coronary events have no linear relationship to the severity of CAD [7]. Catecholamines are related to most risk factors for IHD, including cigarette smoking, hypertension, TABP, physical inactivity, and diet in relation to obesity [77], and are related to serum cholesterol and LDL levels. They thus appear to have a special significance for CAD as well as for morbidity and mortality from IHD [56, 77]. There is increasing reason to believe that the behavioral responses to type A subjects that are related both to the severity of basic coronary atherosclerosis and to the incidence of IHD are mediated by their enhanced secretion of NE in response to the daily life milieu [21, 77].

References

1   Beaglehole, R.; Foulkes, M.A.; Orior, I.A.M.; et al.: Cholesterol and mortality in New Zealand Maoris. Br. med. J. *1:* 285–288 (1980).
2   Blumenthal, J.A.; Williams, R.; Kong, Y.; Schanberg, S.M.; Thompson, L.W.: Type A behavior and angiographically documented coronary disease. Circulation *58:* 634–639 (1978).

3   Brand, R.J.; Rosenman, R.H.; Sholtz, R.I.; Friedman, M.: Multivariate prediction of coronary heart disease in the Western Collaborative Group study compared to the findings of the Framingham study. Circulation *53:* 348–355 (1976).
4   Brown, H.G.: Coronary vasospasm. Observations linking the clinical spectrum of ischemic heart disease to the dynamic pathology of coronary atherosclerosis. Archs. intern. Med. *141:* 716–721 (1981).
5   Brown, M.S.; Kovanen, P.T.; Goldstein, J.L.: Regulation of lipoprotein cholesterol by lipoprotein receptors. Science *212:* 628–635 (1981).
6   Brozek, J.; Keys, A.; Blackburn, H.: Personality differences between potential coronary and noncoronary subjects. Ann. N.Y. Acad. Sci. *134:* 1057–1064 (1966).
7   Buja, L.M.; Willerson, J.T.: Cliniopathologic correlates of acute ischemic heart disease syndromes. Am. J. Cardiol. *47:* 343–349 (1981).
8   Burch, P.R.J.: Coronary disease: risk factors, age and time. Editorial. Am. Heart J. *97:* 415–419 (1979).
9   Byrne, D.G.; Whyte, H.M.: Life events and myocardial infarction revisited. The role of measures of individual impact. Psychosom. Med. *42:* 1–10 (1980).
10   Can I avoid a heart attack? Editorial. Lancet *i* (1974).
11   Chesney, M.A.; Black, G.W.; Chadwick, J.H.; Rosenman, R.H.: Psychological correlates of the coronary-prone behavior pattern. J. behav. Med. *4:* 217–229 (1981).
12   Cohen, J.B.; Syme, S.L.; Jenkins, C.D.; Dagan, A.; Zyzanski, S.J.: The cultural context of type A behavior and the risk of CHD. Am. J. Epidem. *102:* 434 (1975).
13   Corday, E.; Corday, S.R.: Prevention of heart disease by control of risk factors. The time has come to face the facts. Editorial. Am. J. Cardiol. *35:* 330–334 (1975).
14   Davidson, D.M.; Winchester, M.A.; Taylor, C.B.; et al.: Effects of relaxation therapy on cardiac performance and sympathetic activity in patients with organic heart disease. Psychosom. Med. *41:* 303–306 (1979).
15   Ducimetiere, P.; Cambien, F.; Richard, J.L.; Rakotovao, R.; Claude, J.R.: Coronary heart disease in middle-aged Frenchmen. Lancet *i:* 1346–1349 (1980).
16   Fischell, T.: Running and the primary prevention of coronary heart disease. Cardiovasc. Rev. Rep. *2:* 238–244 (1981).
17   Frank, K.A.; Heller, S.S.; Kornfield, D.S.; Sporn, A.A.; Weiss, M.B.: Type A behavior and coronary heart disease. Angiographic confirmation. J. Am. med. Ass. *240:* 761–763 (1978).
18   Friedman, M.; Byers, S.O.; Diamant, J.; Rosenman, R.H.: Plasma catecholamine response of coronary-prone subjects (type A) to a specific challenge. Metabolism *4:* 205–210 (1975).
19   Friedman, M.; Rosenman, R.H.: Association of specific overt behavior pattern with blood and cardiovascular findings. J. Am. med. Ass. *169:* 1286–1296 (1959).
20   Friedman, M.; Rosenman, R.H.; Straus, R.; Wurm, M.; Kositchek, R.: The relationship of behavior pattern A to the state of the coronary vasculature. A study of fifty-one autopsy subjects. Am. J. Med. *44:* 525–537 (1968).
21   Friedman, M.; St. George, S.; Byers, S.O.: Excretion of catecholamines, 17-ketosteroids, 17-hydroxycorticoids, and 5-hydroxyindole in men exhibiting a particular behavior pattern (A) associated with high incidence of clinical coronary artery disease. J. clin. Invest. *39:* 758–764 (1960).
22   Garcia-Palmieri, M.R.; Costas, R.; Cruz-Vidal, M.; et al.: Urban-rural differences in coronary heart disease in a low incidence area. Am. J. Epidem. *107:* 206–215 (1978).
23   Glass, D.C.: Behavior patterns, stress and coronary disease (Erlbaum, Hillsdale 1977).

24 Glass, D.C.; Carver, C.S.: Environmental stress and the type A response; in Baum, Singer, Valins, Advances in environmental psychology, vol. 2 (Erlbaum, Hillsdale 1980).

25 Glass, D.C.; Krakoff, L.W.; Contrada R.; et al.: Effect of harassment and competition on cardiovascular and plasma catecholamine responses in type A and type B individuals. Psychophysiology *17:* 453–454 (1980).

26 Glass, D.C.; Krakoff, L.R.; Finkelman, J.; et al.: Effect of task overload upon cardiovascular and plasma catecholamine responses in type A and B individuals. Basic appl. soc. Psychol. *1:* 199–218 (1960).

27 Goldberg, S.J.; Allen, H.D.; Friedman, G.; et al.: Use health education to modify atherosclerotic risk factors. Am. J. clin. Nutr. *33:* 1272–1278 (1980).

28 Gordon, T.; Garcia-Palmieri, M.R.; Kagan, A.; Kannel, W.B.; Schiffman, J.: Differences in coronary heart disease in Framingham, Honolulu and Puerto Rico. J. chron. Dis. *27:* 329–337 (1974).

29 Gordon, T.; Kannel, W.G.; Halperin, M.: Predictability of coronary heart disease. J. chron. Dis. *32:* 427–434 (1979).

30 Haynes, S.G.; Feinleib, M.: Women, work and coronary heart disease. Prospective findings from the Framingham Heart Study. Am. J. publ. Hlth *70:* 133–141 (1980).

31 Haynes, S.G.; Feinleib, M.; Kannel, W.B.: The relationship of psychosocial factors to coronary heart disease in the Framingham study. III. 8-year incidence of CHD. Am. J. Epidem. *3:* 37–58 (1980).

32 Hegyeli, R.J.: Measurement and control of cardiovascular risk factors. Atherosclerosis reviews, vol. 7 (Raven Press, New York 1980).

33 Heller, R.F.: Type A behaviour and coronary heart disease. Br. med. J. *2:* 368–369 (1979).

34 Hennekens, C.H.; Willett, W.; Rosener, B.; et al.: Effects of beer, wine, and liquour in coronary deaths. J. Am. med. Ass. *242:* 1973–1974 (1979).

35 Holmes, D.R.; Elveback, L.R.; Frye, R.L.; et al.: Association of risk factor variables and coronary artery disease documented with angiography. Circulation *63:* 293–249 (1981).

36 Isaacson, S.O.; Johansson, B.W.: Myocardial infarction in Malmö during the ten-year period 1963–1972. Acta med. scand. *206:* 293–298 (1979).

37 Jenkins, C.D.: Psychological and social precursors of coronary disease. New Engl. J. Med. *284:* 244–255, 307–317 (1971).

38 Jenkins, C.D.: Recent evidence supporting psychologic and social risk factors for coronary disease. New Engl. J. Med. *294:* 987–994, 1033–1038 (1976).

39 Jenkins, C.D.; Rosenman, R.H.; Friedman, M.: Components of the coronary-prone behavior pattern. J. chron. Dis. *19:* 599–609 (1966).

40 Jenkins, C.D.; Rosenman, R.H.; Zyzanski, S.J.: Jenkins Activity Survey (Psychological Corporation, New York 1979).

41 Jenkins, C.D.; Zyzanski, S.J.; Rosenman, R.H.: Risk of new myocardial infarction in middle-aged men with manifest coronary heart disease. Circulation *53:* 342–347 (1976).

42 Jouve, A.; Drivet-Perrin, J.; Bernet, A.; et al.: Conditions socio-professionelles et personnalité du coronarien. Ann. cardiol. angelol. *29:* 223–230 (1980).

43 Kahn, H.A.: Change in serum cholesterol associated with changes in the United States civilian diet, 1909–1965. Am. J. clin. Nutr. *23:* 879–882 (1970).

44 Kahn, J.P.; Kornfeld, M.D.; Frank, K.A.; Heller, S.S.; Hoar, P.F.: Type A behavior and blood pressure during coronary artery bypass surgery. Psychosom. Med. *42:* 407–414 (1980).

45 Kannel, W.B.: Implications of the recent decline in cardiovascular mortality. Cardiovasc. Med. *September* (1979).

46 Kannel, W.B.; et al.: The Framingham Study. Section 24 – The Framingham Diet Study. DHEW Publication of National Heart and Lung Institute (US Government Printing Office, Washington 1970).

47 Keys, A.; Aravanis, C.; Blackburn, H.; Vanbuchem, F.S.P.; Buzina, R.; Djordjenic, B.S.; Fidanza, F.; Karvonen, M.J.; Menotti, A.; Puddu, V.; Taylor, H.L.: Probability of middle-aged men developing coronary heart disease in 5 years. Circulation *45:* 815–828 (1972).

48 Keys, A.; Karvonen, M.J.; Fidanza, F.: Serum cholesterol studies in Finland. Lancet *ii:* 175–178 (1970).

49 Keys, A.; Taylor, H.L.; Blackburn, H.; Brozek, J.; Anderson, J.T.: Mortality and coronary heart disease among men studied for 23 years. Ann. intern. Med. *128:* 201–205 (1971).

50 Kornitzer, M.; De Backer, G.; Dramaix, M.; et al.: The Belgian Heart Disease Prevention Project: Modification of the coronary risk profile in an industrial population. Circulation *61:* 18–25 (1980).

51 Kozarevic, D.; Pirc, B.; Ravic, Z.; Dawber, T.R.; Gordon, T.; Zukel, W.J.: The Yugoslavia cardiovascular disease study. II. Factors in the incidence of coronary heart disease. Am. J. Epidem. *104:* 133–140 (1976).

52 Kramer, J.R.; Matsuda, Y.; Mulligan, J.C.; et al.: Progression of coronary atherosclerosis. Circulation *63:* 519–527 (1981).

53 Krantz, D.S.: Cognitive process and recovery from heart attack. A review and theoretical analysis. J. hum. Stress *6:* 27–38 (1980).

54 Krantz, D.S.; Sanmarco, M.I.; Selvester, R.H.; Mathews, K.: Psychological correlates of progression of atherosclerosis in man. Psychosom. Med. *41:* 467–475 (1975).

55 LaPorte, R.E.; Cresanta, J.L.; Kuller, L.H.: The relationship of alcohol consumption to atherosclerotic heart disease. Prev. Med. *9:* 22–40 (1980).

56 Lee, J.A.: Ischaemic heart disease and the autonomic nervous system. Letter to Editor. Lancet *ii:* 747 (1980).

57 Lown, B.; Verrier, R.L.: Neural activity and ventricular fibrillation. New Engl. J. Med. *294:* 1165–1170 (1976).

58 MacDougall, J.M.; Dembroski, T.M.; Krantz, D.S.: Effects of types of challenge on pressor and heart rate responses in type A and B women. Psychophysiology *18:* 1–5 (1981).

59 Mahley, R.W.: The role of dietary fat and cholesterol in atherosclerosis and lipoprotein metabolism. Medical Staff Conference, University of California. West. J. Med. *134:* 34–42 (1981).

60 Mann, G.V.: Diet-heart: end of an era. New Engl. J. Med. *297:* 644–650 (1977).

61 Manuck, S.G.; Garland, F.N.: Stability of individual differences in cardiovascular reactivity: a thirteen-month follow-up. Physiol. Behav. *24:* 621–624 (1980).

62 Marmot, M.G.; Kagan, A.; Kato, H.: Hypertension and heart disease in the Ni-Hon-San study; in Kesteloot, Joossens, Epidemiology of arterial disease (Nijhoff, The Hague 1980).

63 Marmot, M.G.; Syme, S.L.: Acculturation and coronary heart disease in Japanese-Americans. Am. J. Epidem. *104:* 225–247 (1976).

64 Marmot, M.G.; Syme, S.L.; Sacks, S.T.; et al.: Japanese culture and coronary heart disease; in Orimo, Shimada, Iriki, Maeda, Recent advances in gerontology (Excerpta Medica, Amsterdam 1979).

65   Maseri, A.; Chierchia, P.: Coronary vasospasm in ischemic heart disease. Chest *78:* 210–214 (1980).
66   Matthews, K.A.; Glass, D.C.; Rosenman, R.H.; Bortner, R.W.: Competitive drive, pattern A, and coronary heart disease: a further analysis of some data from the Western Collaborative Group Study. J. chron. Dis. *30:* 489–498 (1977).
67   McMichael, J.: Fats and arterial disease. Am. Heart J. *98:* 409–412 (1979).
68   Orth-Gomer, K.; Ahlbom, A.; Theorell, T.: Impact of pattern A behavior on ischemic heart disease when controlling for conventional risk indicators. J. hum. Stress *6:* 7–13 (1980).
69   Osler, W.: The Lumleian lectures on angina pectoris. Lancet *i:* 829–844 (1892).
70   Paffenbarger, R.D.; Wing, A.L.; Hyde, R.T.: Physical activity as an index of heart attack risk in college alumni. Am. J. Epidem. *108:* 161–175 (1978).
71   Page, L.; Friend, B.: The changing United States diet. Bioscience *28:* 192–199 (1978).
72   Puska, P.; Tuomilehro, J.; Salonen, J.; et al.: Changes in coronary risk factors during comprehensive five-year community programme to control cardiovascular diseases (North Karelia project). Br. med. J. *2:* 1173–1178 (1979).
73   Raab, W.: Hormonal and neurogenic cardiovascular disorders (Williams & Wilkins, Baltimore 1953), and Prevention of ischemic heart disease (Thomas, Springfield 1966).
74   Research Group ATS-RF2 of the Italian National Research Council. Distribution of some risk factors for atherosclerosis in nine Italian population samples. Am. J. Epidem. *113:* 338–346 (1981).
75   Roine, P.; et al.: Diet and cardiovascular disease in Finland. Lancet *ii:* 173–175 (1958).
76   Rose, G.; Heller, R.F.; Pedoe, H.T.; et al.: Heart disease prevention project. A randomized controlled trial in industry. Br. med. J. *March 15:* 1272–1278 (1980).
77   Rosenman, R.H.: The role of the type A behavior pattern in ischemic heart disease. Modification of its effects by beta-blocking agents. Br. J. clin. Pract. *32:* suppl. 1, pp. 58–65 (1978).
78   Rosenman, R.H.: The interview method of assessment of the coronary prone behavior pattern; in Dembroski, Weiss, Shields, Haynes, Feinleib, Coronary-prone behavior (Springer, New York 1978).
79   Rosenman, R.H.; Brand, R.J.; Jenkins, C.D.; Friedman, M.; Straus, R.; Wurm, M.: Coronary heart disease in the Western Collaborative Group Study: final follow-up of 8½ years. J. Am. med. Ass. *233:* 872–877 (1975).
80   Rosenman, R.H.; Brand, R.J.; Sholtz, R.I.; Friedman, M.: Multivariate prediction of coronary heart disease during 8.5-year follow-up in the Western Collaborative Group Study. Am. J. Cardiol. *37:* 903–910 (1976).
81   Rosenman, R.H.; Chesney, M.A.: The relationship of type A behavior pattern to coronary heart disease. Activitas nerv. sup. *22:* 1–45 (1980).
82   Rosenman, R.H.; Friedman, M.: Association of specific behavior pattern in women with blood and cardiovascular findings. J. Am. med. Ass. *24:* 1173–1184 (1961).
83   Rosenman, R.H.; Friedman, M.: Neurogenic factors in pathogenesis of coronary heart disease. Med. Clins N. Am. *58:* 269–279 (1974).
84   Rosenman, R.H.; Friedman, M.; Straus, R.; Wurm, M.; Kositchek, R.; Hahn, W.; Werthessen, N.T.: A predictive study of coronary heart disease. The Western Collaborative Group Study. J. Am. med. Ass. *189:* 15–22 (1964).
85   Rosenman, R.H.; Rahe, R.H.; Borhani, N.O.; Feinleib, M.: Heritability of personality and

behavior. Proc. 1st Int. Congr. of Twin Studies, Rome 1974. Acta Genet. med. Gemell. *25:* 221–224 (1976).

86   Rosenman, R.H.; Sholtz, R.I.; Brand, R.J.: Study of comparative blood pressure in predicting risk of coronary heart disease. Circulation *54:* 51–58 (1976).

87   Stamler, J.: The established relationship among diet, serum cholesterol and coronary heart disease. Acta med. scand. *207:* 433–446 (1980).

88   Thomas, C.B.: Psychobiological characteristics in youth as predictors of five disease states. Johns Hopkins med. J. *132:* 16–43 (1973).

89   Trulson, F.F.: The American diet: past and present. Am. J. clin. Nutr. *7:* 91–97 (1959).

90   Trulson, M.F.; Clancy, D.E.; Jessor, W.J.E.; et al.: Comparison of siblings in Boston and Ireland. J. Am. diet. Ass. *45:* 225–229 (1964).

91   VanEgeren, L.F.: Social interactions, communications, and the coronary-prone behavior pattern. A psychophysiologic study. Psychosom. Med. *41:* 2–18 (1979).

92   Vanhaecke, J.; Piessens, J.; Willems, J.L.; et al.: Coronary arterial lesions in young men who survived a first myocardial infarction. Clinical and electrocardiographic predictors of multivessel disease. Am. J. Cardiol. *47:* 810–817 (1981).

93   Vliestra, R.E.; Frye, R.L.; Kronmal, R.A.; et al.: III. Risk factors and angiographic coronary artery disease. A report from the Coronary Artery Surgery Study (CASS). Circulation *62:* 254–261 (1980).

94   White, P.D.: The historical background of angina pectoris. Modern Concepts cardiovasc. Dis. *43:* 109–112 (1974).

95   Williams, R.B.; Thomas, T.L.; Lee, K.L.; Kong, Y.; Blumenthal, J.A.; Whalen, R.E.: Type A behavior, hostility, and coronary atherosclerosis. Psychosom. Med. *42:* 539–549 (1980).

96   Zyzanski, S.J.; Jenkins, C.D.; Ryan, T.J.; Flessas, A.; Everist, M.: Psychological correlates of coronary angiographic findings. Archs intern. Med. *136:* 1234–1237 (1976).

2 The Year before Myocardial Infarction

A. Appels

One of the major problems of preventive cardiology is formed by the fact that more than half of those who suffer a myocardial infarction (MI) or die suddenly have visited a medical doctor in the 4 weeks prior to the coronary event [9, 40]. Since the symptoms, presented by the patient during that contact are mostly vague and often difficult to interpret, their significance is often not recognized at that contact, which causes much chagrin for both the doctor and his patient.

Several investigators have studied retrospectively which type of complaints or feelings coronary patients had experienced in the months preceding their disease or death. Table I presents their major findings.

Within the list of prodromal complaints the cluster formed by feelings of fatigue – emotional changes – general malaise is most often noted. In general it can be said that the more recent a study is, the more those types of feelings are noted [19]. These studies are retrospective and therefore open to a series of factors which might influence the reliability of the data in a negative way. As a WHO working group stated in 1971 [49]: 'Useful though retrospective studies are their value as guides to prediction is open to doubt, firstly because hindsight assists in the interpretation of atypical symptoms, and secondly because they do not supply information on how often "prodromal" symptoms are not followed by heart attacks.' Given the importance of the issue, it seems worthwhile to also study the complex of tiredness-general malaise with behavioral methods in order to describe them more precisely, to make them measurable and to test to what extent they are able to predict the onset of cardiovascular disease.

The first opportunity to approach these problems was offered by the Imminent Myocardial Infarction Rotterdam (IMIR) study. This IMIR project was a joint project of the departments of general practice and cardiology of the Erasmus University in Rotterdam. Its main aim was to study the problem of how a general practitioner can recognize an imminent MI (IMI) [15]. The psychological part of this study has been described in detail elsewhere. It consisted of two parts. The first part of the study investigated whether those

Table I. Premonitory symptoms of MI and sudden death in three studies (percentage)

	Alonzo et al. [2]		Rissanen et al. [35]	Kuller et al. [27]
	myocardial infarction	sudden death	sudden death	sudden death
Chest pain	67	35		37
Discomfort in the chest			24	
Changed angina pectoris			15	
Recent angina pectoris			6	
Dyspnea	36	39	15	42
Dizziness-syncope-fainting	10	8		14
Heaviness of arms	14	10	3	
Fatigue-weakness	38	42	32	56
Emotional changes	14	20		
Nervousness-depression			3	
Difficulty-sleeping				28
General malaise	16	17	5	
Anorexia-nausea	14	17	4	
Dysrhythmia			5	
Sweating			3	
Coughing				31
Palpitation				11
Ankle edema-ascites	1	7		

who visited their general practitioners because of complaints of possible cardiac origin and who got a new coronary event (sudden death, MI or serious deterioration of cardiac status) had a higher mean score at intake on a specially designed questionnaire compared to those who visited their general practitioner for the same reason but did not get a new coronary event within the 10-month follow-up period. In the second part of this study the group which got a new coronary event was compared with a healthy control group. Because the cases from this second part of the study were the same as those of the prospective study and answered the questionnaire before the occurrence of the new coronary event, a major bias of retrospective case-control studies could be avoided. It was found that the questionnaire had a predictive power in the cohort study and strongly discriminated between cases and controls in the second part of this study. The questionnaire received the name Maastricht Questionnaire (MQ) according to the place where it was developed [3].

The second step in the construction of the MQ was formed by a case-control study in which both the structured type A interview and the Jenkins Activity Survey (JAS) were included. A discriminant analysis showed that the MQ discriminated between cases and controls independently of the type A behavior pattern [46].

After these studies the MQ was revised. Nondiscriminating items were dropped and others (mainly obtained from clinical interviews) were added. To study the construct measured by the MQ, 10 persons who had elevated scores, but who did not have cardiovascular complaints, were interviewed by an experienced psychotherapist. According to her judgment, these people were all characterized by feelings of vital exhaustion and depression (VED). Because this description of the construct measured by the MQ fitted nicely into the results of a hierarchical cluster analysis of the discriminating items, this description of the content will be used further on.

The validity of the revised questionnaire has actually been studied in a new prospective study among 4,000 city employees of Rotterdam. The data, obtained from screening the first half of the study population, allow testing of the hypothesis that those who, at intake, are placed by the cardiologists into the diagnostic category 'IMI' have elevated scores on the MQ.

Material and Methods

In 1978 the municipal health center of Rotterdam started a voluntary health checkup service for the city employees of Rotterdam. This checkup consists of a general examination, with special emphasis upon the cardiovascular system. For the latter, the Rose Questionnaire for the assessment of angina pectoris (AP) [36], and some additional questions were used.

The city employees were invited by age and branch groups which resulted in a sample formed by two distinct age groups. Because only a relatively small number of women participated in the health checkup, females were excluded from the data analyses. Furthermore, those subjects who possibly had experienced a MI in the past were excluded, in order to avoid the possibility that their scores on the MQ could be caused by their disease. Finally, those who did not answer four or more MQ questions were also excluded. Table II shows the final composition of the two samples.

The Maastricht Questionnaire

The current form of the MQ consists of 50 items. In this form, the questionnaire is more or less an item pool which has to be shortened when sufficient information about each item has been obtained. Each question has

Table II. Composition of the study population

	Age 40–45	Age 55–65
Participants	895	1,244
Possible or probable MI in the past	17	89
Incomplete questionnaire	26	14
Study population	852	1,141

Table III. MQ items which discriminate between those with normal ECG and those whose ECG indicates ischemia (odds ratios)

Do you feel more listless lately than before?	2.10
Do you often worry about your health?	2.34
Do you have to take more time to solve a difficult problem lately than a year ago?	4.40
Does the feeling of being a failure ever come upon you?	3.38
Are you becoming less satisfied with yourself?	2.60
Have you had the feeling lately of not achieving enough, that you could achieve more if only you were healthier and not so weak?	3.36
Do you feel downcast?	3.36
Do you want to be dead at times?	4.68
Can you bring yourself less and less to leave the house and go somewhere for a visit?	1.93
Do you feel dejected?	3.99
Do you feel unhappy because of ill health?	2.62
Recently, do you shrink from your regular work as if it were a mountain to climb?	2.40
When you have done something, do you check more often than before whether you did it right?	2.94
Have you become more quiet lately?	2.42

three response categories: 'yes', 'don't know', 'no'. The confirmation of a complaint is coded as 3, the question mark as 2, and the negation as 1. The questions ask for feelings of tiredness, loss of vitality, depression, feelings of helplessness or hopelessness, hypochondriac feelings, irritation, and sleep disturbance. The items presented in table III illustrate the content of the questionnaire.

The internal consistency of the questionnaire is respectively 0.91 and 0.93 in both age groups (Crombach's alpha). A principal component analysis shows that the questionnaire measures essentially one dimension. These features of the MQ justify summation of the answers to all questions.

Table IV. Product-moment correlations between MQ and three somatic risk factors

	Age group	
	40–45 (n = 852)	55–65 (n = 1,141)
Cholesterol	0.00	0.00
Systolic blood pressure	– 0.03 (n.s.)	– 0.12 (p = 0.001)
Diastolic blood pressure	– 0.03	– 0.06 (p = 0.02)

Table V. Association between MQ and smoking

	Age 40–45		Age 55–65	
	n	mean MQ	n	mean MQ
Never smoked	143	67	112	75
Stopped more than 5 years ago	152	68	287	76
Stopped less than 5 years ago	87	70	108	82
Pipe or cigars only	41	70	74	75
1–4 cigarettes daily	27	69	43	76
5–9 cigarettes daily	66	67	95	75
10–24 cigarettes daily	284	70	357	76
25–39 cigarettes daily	39	77	54	79
40– cigarettes daily	13	73	11	73
N	852		1,141	
Mean and SD	69 (13.89)		76 (18.33)	
Univariate F	2.81 (p = 0.04)		1.73 (n.s.)	
Deviation from linearity	2.03 (p = 0.04)		1.93 (n.s.)	

MQ and Somatic Risk Factors

Table IV presents the product-moment correlations between the MQ and cholesterol/blood pressure in both groups. As can be seen no correlation was found between MQ and cholesterol. Close inspection of the differences in mean MQ scores across the deciles of the risk factors did not show any curvilinear association. The correlation with blood pressure, especially with systolic blood pressure is negative. Although the correlations between MQ and systolic blood pressure are not high the negative association fits into the clinical appearance of the VED syndrome: a general decrease of social, intellectual and physical functioning. In the younger group, a small but significant

association was found between MQ and smoking (table V). This may indicate
that smoking contributes to the origin of feelings of vital exhaustion and
depression or that people who feel deeply tired and helpless smoke more to
activate themselves. But whatever the explanation might be (and the association is so small that there is not much to be explained) it means that smoking
might be a confounding factor which could possibly explain the association
between MQ and IMI.

MQ and Imminent Myocardial Infarction

The protocol defines IMI as: AP which is recent and/or increasing
and/or more frequent. The prevalence of IMI was 5 per thousand in the
younger age group, and 14 per thousand in the older group. These figures are
relatively high and are probably due to the fact that an assessment of chest
complaints by means of a structured interview causes an overestimation of
the prevalence of AP. The association between MQ and IMI was computed
by splitting both age groups, at the median of the MQ, into a vital and an
exhausted-depressive group. In the younger age group, all those receiving the
diagnosis IMI had MQ scores above the median. In the older group 1 out of
575 scoring below the median had an IMI compared to 15 persons out of the
566 people scoring above the median. The rate ratio in the older group is
15.59. That means that the chance to be diagnosed as having an IMI is more
than 15 times as high in the group scoring above the median of the MQ compared to those who score below the median (fig. 1). These findings corrobo-
rate the hypothesis formulated above.

MQ and Abnormalities in the ECG

Although the ECG taken during rest has little to contribute to the diagnosis of IMI, an analysis of the relation between MQ and ECG abnormalities
gives some additional information about the relation between VED and
coronary heart disease.

The ECG of the participants was coded according to the Minnesota
code. Five classifications were used: no deviations, aspecific ST deviations,
possible ischaemia, probable ischaemia, other deviations, pacemaker. To
study the associations between each item of the MQ and ECG abnormalities,
those who had no ECG deviations were compared with those with possible
or probable ischemia. Table III presents those items which had a positive
association with ECG deviations, indicating ischemia in the younger age
group. Each item is followed by the relative odds ratio. That ratio gives an
indication of the strength of the association (the computational procedure is

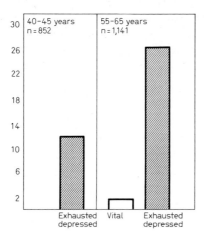

Fig. 1. Prevalence of IMI per thousand subjects; scoring below or above the median of the MQ in two cohorts.

explained in appendix I, p. 38). More items than would be epected by chance were found to be associated with ECG deviations in the younger age group. In the older age group, however, no single item had a positive association. The latter result is puzzling.

Discussion

The self reports of many coronary patients or their relatives indicate that, although unexpected, MI does not afflict people like a bolt from the blue. Coronary events take place in a sky which is darkly clouded by feelings of tiredness and general malaise. The precise delineation of these feelings and the tests of their predictive power are confronted with a series of major questions. What is the exact nature of these emotional changes? What is the empirical evidence which supports the belief that vital exhaustion and depression belong to the prodromata of MI and sudden death? What are the major methodological problems? What is the direction of the association between VED and IMI? What are the psychophysiological and neurohormonal correlates of that syndrome? What can be said about its specificity and sensitivity?

In medicine the clinic is the mother of science. Therefore, the following four case reports illustrate how coronary patients may present their experiences during the year before MI.

Case History 1

Mr. B. is 61 years old. He is married, but has lost his emotional ties to his wife. When she leaves home she never wants to tell him where she goes. He knows that she always goes with another woman to do some shopping and window-shopping but he cannot tolerate the fact that she does not tell him. He had worked as a foreman in a carpenter's yard. He explains that he was famous for his accuracy, his sense of responsibility, and his job involvement. He is very punctual. Each morning he left his home at precisely 7.14 a.m. to catch his bus.

When he was 59 years old he had an accident and had to stop working. This disability was hard to accept as reflected in such comments as: 'Somebody who does not work has lost his respectability.' He struggles with that feeling for almost 1 year. During that year he left his home each day at 7.14 a.m. and took his bus. But after 1 year he started to realize that taking a bus to nowhere was merely self-deception. He became depressed, and often found himself silently crying in his chair. He had the feeling that his energy was slowly ebbing away. Some months after the onset of these feelings he suffered a MI.

Case History 2

Mr. P. is 44 years old. He is married and has 3 sons, who are all very good high school students. When he was 16 years old he secured a job working in the harbor. Later, he decided to work on his own and started a garage. He worked 17h daily in that garage. After 3 years he began to suffer from back pain and was forced to close the garage. He was unemployed for 6 months. After 7 months he started a cafeteria. He worked 70–80h weekly. 2 years later the neighborhood he lived in was reconstructed. Old appartment buildings were demolished to be replaced by new ones. During that time he lost a large number of customers. He asked his bank to give him a loan but the bank refused. For this reason he had to close the cafeteria. Becoming more and more disabled by his back pain, he decided to look for an administrative job. He sought this work for 2 years. After 2 years he got a job as a custodian in a high school. This high school is located in three provisional buildings at different locations in the town. After he had worked there for 1 year, the high school received permission from the government to build a new high school. At this new high school there is room for only two custodians. This means that 1 out of the 3 custodians who are working in the provisional buildings has to leave his job. Again he enters another period of uncertainty. He cannot control the decision as to which custodian has to loose his position. He becomes tired, sleeps badly and often wakes up during the night. He then goes to his living room to smoke cigarettes. He gets a feeling of hopelessness. He becomes easily irritated and does not feel well. Sometimes he experiences unusual chest pains. But he does not tell anyone. When he watches the TV news at 8.00 p.m. he often falls into a sleep which is so deep that his wife cannot wake him. After discovering that he selected an uncomfortable chair from the kitchen to watch television. During this period his dog ate something in a nearby field. He recalls that several dogs from his neighborhood died there. He accuses the hunters in a local newspaper of poisoning dogs. He asks the police to help him. The police respond that there is absolutely no proof and that he should take care to avoid a libel suit. After that reaction he feels completely helpless. 5 days later he has a heart attack.

Case History 3

Mr. V. is 31 years old. He is married and has 2 young children. He is a former swimming champion. He works as a cook in a tourist hotel. During the season he works 15–16h daily. 6 years ago he was overworked. He once got so angry at a waiter who did not take the dishes out of the kitchen in time that he put him on the cooking-range for a full minute. He was fired for

that reason. A general practitioner said that he was overworked and prescribed rest and seda-
tives.

After 6 months he started working again at another tourist restaurant. During the season
he worked 70–80h weekly. At the end of the third season he became listless and tired. He
avoided company and no longer joined his colleagues during coffee breaks. He wanted peace,
quiet, and rest. He became depressed and observed that he was often thinking about his father
who died a year and a half earlier. He read the obituaries in the local newspaper, something
that he had never done before.

He had many animals at home, which he started to sell one after another. When he had
sold all his birds, dogs, rabbits, and guinea pigs, he told his wife that he wanted a divorce. His
wife organized a meeting with a psychiatrist. The first question the psychiatrist asked was why
he wanted a divorce. Mr. V., however, could not give an answer to that question. He just wanted
it. 1 week later he suffered a large MI.

Case History 4

Mr. B. (59 years old) is a well-known actor. He is married and has 3 children, who no longer
live at home. In World War II he was a district leader in the underground resistance organization.
For the past 12 years he has suffered from hypertension. His manner of speaking exhibits all
the characteristics of the type A behavior pattern. Shortly before his infarction, he was engaged
in the translation of a stage play. He had received the commission for that piece of work a long
time before the play. But he did not start working on it until the last 3 weeks before the play
was to go on. He reported: 'I could not start working until I was under pressure.'

His friends noticed that he had grown quieter during the last year. He began to retire from
company. He had also disposed of his TV ('The only thing you see on that screen is naked
womenfolk.'). He has all but stopped reading. He felt too listless, too apathic to read. 'What I
felt is what the poet *J. Engelman* called "ironic laziness": doing nothing any more because
everything is just too relative, nothing is worth your while.'

'I used to depend on crowds for my living. Now I avoid them. Once, the applause tickled
my vanity. Now I just grin and think: where can I get a good glass of wine? I get more out of
that. Why am I standing here anyway?'

He is inclined to go to bed early. 'That is a form of withdrawing. Why stay up if the evening
has nothing to offer for you?' It is against this background that his irritation arises. 'One has been
warned that nothing is valuable. By nature, I am a perfectionist. In the past I became over-
strained twice because I made too many high demands on myself and others. Now I can get furi-
ous if a clock does not run properly. A clock should function properly. If it doesn't, it confirms
to the world that it is of no value. To me, the cardiac infarction is a refuge. Society cannot call
on me any more. I now have a certificate in my pocket, my legalized excuse for not having to
be active any more. What I would like best is to retire, and take a sleeping pill on the pretense
of having a headache. If there is nothing to stay awake for, there is nothing as wonderful as sleeping. I do not long for death, either. My problems are not great enough for me to do so. I am
in the gray area in between, no violent emotions any more, no profound sadness. It is the domain
of "l'ennuie" in the sense meant by *Bernanos*. What's the meaning of it all, the theatre company,
the performances, the resistance during the War? Where is the sting, the enthusiasm? The heyday
is past. All that is left for me to do is to become a decent old grandpa. I am too rational to enter
into new human relations. But it would be wonderful to fall in love once more. I feel as if I am
in a small boat passing by the harbor. It is an age-bound depression. One has no more
experiences that make life worthwhile. Sometimes I get terribly annoyed by my wife's patroniz-

ing remarks like: "Wouldn't it be wiser for you to take tonic instead of beer?" I have no real grit any more, either. Sometimes, when I have done a small job, like repairing a clock, I can lie deadbeat on the couch for an hour. I also checked up to five times to see if I had made no mistakes in doing something. When I went out I walked back as often as three times to check if the door was properly locked. That's a symptom of insecurity. One doesn't have oneself under control any more. My wife said: "You've become so uncertain".'

Early descriptions of the nature of the emotional changes before the onset of MI and sudden death are given by *Wolf* [48] and by *Bruhn* et al. [12] who spoke about 'emotional drain' preceding death from MI. They defined 'emotional drain' as: 'A frustrating, long-term involvement of the individual's mental processes in his attempt to live with, or cope with, some life facts or conflict which involved some deeply ingrained aspect of the individual, such as his values, beliefs, self-concept, or interpersonal relationships.' In their view, 'emotional drain is felt to begin early in the life of an individual and to accumulate in intensity if no mitigating variables intervene. It is perceived by the individual to be unalterable or unsolvable, regardless of whether it is a conscious or unconscious conflict. Emotional drain implies a nearly constant state of mental preparedness on the part of the individual to cope with his conflict. If additional traumatic incidents arise they become superimposed on an already mobilized organism. Depending upon the meaning to the individual of subsequent events and their duration, they can further drain the energy resources of the body to the point where the total organism is left in a state of physical and mental exhaustion. Emotional drain implies the lack of supportive and meaningful relationships with others. The full impact of emotional drain comes to be realized as a personal burden. Thus, the life-long conflicts that are perceived to be unsolvable to an individual whose mental resources are continually mobilized as if he were attempting to solve them may eventually leave him in a state of mental and physical exhaustion. It is this stage that may set the stage for a MI and sudden death' [12].

The emotional changes which characterize the year before MI are, in the opinion of these authors, the final end stage of a long-term process. That final stage is not yet described by them in much detail. *Nixon* [30] should be credited for being the first who has attempted to give a detailed description of this end stage. According to him 'the symptoms are bad temper, continual grumbling, long hours worked but less achieved, repeated minor sickness and preoccupation, together with insecurity about health and the future, procrastination, losing sight of long-term aims in preoccupation with minor matters, feelings of frustration and persecution by colleagues, with complaints of lack of cooperation, technical jargon and catch-phases replacing original thought. Previously acceptable mannerisms become neurotic and disrupt peace of mind of others. Sleep becomes inadequate, increasing the exhaustion and promoting another vicious circle of deterioration. The qualities required for success disappear. The mind becomes set against change and adaptability is lost. Leadership becomes to depend upon tradition and seniority instead of ability. Eating, drinking, smoking and talking increase and a competitive drive for stimulating circumstances may dominate life.' 'In exhaustion and ill health there are two main emotional responses. One is rage and frustration, and the other is insecurity with despair and hopelessness. Both are accepted as precipitants of heart failure. They probably correspond to the final common pathway of fruitless activity or giving up that are followed when the individual loses his ability to predict and maintain control over his environment.' 'In predicting whether an individual under hardship might break down it is more useful to assess his reserves from his position and stability on his own function curve than to weigh the changes that are pressing upon him. The most important cause of a morbid level of arousal seems to be the threatened actual loss of ability to understand and to control the environment and this affects highly aggressive individuals more than the passive. The commonest examples seen in cardiovascular practice are "people poisoning" (mind-battering, recurrent anxiety created by a person or persons whom yout cannot escape), unacceptable time pressure, high levels of resentment about changes imposed by others in hierarchies and families, and the fruitless hyperactivity responses to anxiety' [30].

The description of *Nixon* [30] is vivid and colorful. We would paint that picture with less brilliant colors. In the year before their MI people are no dying heroes but bakers, cooks, and foremen who have worked too many hours to make a living; farmers and bookkeepers who met depressing problems, which they could no longer solve. But *Nixon's* [30] description corresponds essentially with the impression we have derived from our clinical interviews. The empirical evidence which supports the claim that the VED syndrome precedes MI is still scarce. The major findings regarding the MQ are presented above. They are completed by two case-control studies which both showed that the mean scores on the retrospective form of the MQ (i.e. the form which asks 'How did you feel?' instead of 'How do you feel?') of MI patients differed more than one standard deviation from the mean score of a healthy control group [4, 5]. There is a series of other studies which give some indirect evidence by showing relationships between depression and several forms of CHD. *Shekelle and Ostfeld* [39] found in a prospective study that nonsurvivors of MI had a higher mean score on the MMPI depression scale than survivors did. *Jenkins* et al. [24] studied male patients undergoing coronary angiography and found a positive association between depression as measured by the Dempsy depression scale and the amount of vessel obstruction. Sleep disturbances, a well-known element of depression, was found to be predictive both of future AP and MI in four different studies [10, 20, 44, 45].

A positive association between depression and premature ventricular beats has been demonstrated by *Orth-Gomer* [31]. *Dreyfuss* et al. [16] reported that patients treated in a mental hospital for some form of depression have a significantly higher incidence of MI than those with nondepressive symptoms. That finding has been confirmed in Holland [7] (the lower incidence in other groups of mental patients can, however, be due to an underreporting of bodily complaints by schizophrenic patients). On an ecological level *Eastwood* [17] and *Hagnell* [22] have found that mental illness and cardiovascular disease tend to cluster together. The combined evidence of these very different studies gives an indication that some elements of emotional drain/ depression can have a positive association with CHD.

The major methodological problem regarding the measurement of the syndrome of VED is probably not the retrospective bias of case-control studies. We do not believe that the MI and the hospitalization causes feelings of VED. The depression which one may observe in the coronary care or the coming-home depression are extensions of a status which already existed before the onset of MI. The experience of such a life-threatening event and the need to rethink the future may evoke feelings of anxienty and depression and, therefore, influence the answers to a questionnaire or interview, but does not generally cause deep changes in the personality structure. In our clinical experience many coronary patients feel much better and vital after their attack, which in many cases can simply be explained by the fact that they finally got the rest they badly needed. This statement, however, still waits for an empirical test.

The major methodological problem is formed by the fact that any instrument to measure this syndrome, and especially a questionnaire, presents a list of complaints and belongs by that quality to the broad category of neuroticism tests. Neuroticism is nothing but the willingness to complain on invitation. Any neuroticism test therefore correlates with AP because the diagnosis AP is mainly based upon the subjective complaints of a person. In prevalence or cross-sectional studies, this tendency to complain is a confounding factor. It leads not only to an overestimation of the prevalence of AP in the population under study, but also to an overestimation of the relationship between VED and AP. To correct the data for that confounding factor would require a test which measures that tendency without asking for complaints which do belong to the domain of VED of neuroticism. Such a test is not available, at least not in Holland.

The data presented above concerning the association VED-IMI may also have been confounded by that underlying response set. The definition of IMI used in that study is a specification of AP. The evidence that the association is not accounted for by that hidden factor is only indirect. It is given by the association between the MQ and the objective ECG criterion (table III) and by the positive association between the MQ and those chest complaints which are not general complaints, but very specific for AP: pain occurring during transition from a warm to a cold place ($F = 14.23$ in the younger group and 8.01 in the older group); pain is experienced during effort ($F = 14.14$ and 5.24) and after a meal ($F = 0.10$ and 5.96).

Another important issue concerns the direction of the association VED-IMI. Does the deteriorated health status cause feelings of vital exhaustion and depression, do these feelings precede and contribute to the onset of MI, or are both mutually reinforcing elements of the same process?

Many clinicians understand these feelings as a side effect of a diseased heart. *Friedman* et al. [20] followed that tradition in analyzing the data from the Kaiser-Permanente Study. They compared 330 infarct patients who had participated in a multiphasic health checkup with a control group from the same study. They found that a list of neuromental questions (included in the checkup to detect people with mental problems) also discriminated between cases and controls. Most of the discriminating items are similar or equal to some MQ questions. Are these complaints symptoms of already existing heart disease or are they psychological traits? To *Friedman* et al. [20] this was an either-or question and, therefore, he recomputed the data after removing those 'with coronary symptoms and diagnosis at the time of testing'. As a result of this, the items lost their discriminating power.

Aside from the loss in statistical power when smaller groups are compared, the question should be asked whether their analysis makes sense. Is the assumption correct that these feelings represent a psychological trait or should one say that they reflect a (transitory) state? Is it wise to remove a phase from a developmental process [20]?

2 years after the publication of *Friedman* et al. [20], *Klatsky* et al. [25] reported on the same study. Their data are based on a larger number of cases and on a slightly different questionnaire. They compared the infarction

patients with a healthy control group matched on ECG deviations, smoking, cholesterol, blood pressure, glucose intolerance and Quetelet index. *Klatsky* et al. [25] found that the following items discriminated between the groups: 'In the past 6 months have you had a serious loss of your sexual ability or nature?' 'In the past year did you have spells of shaking and trembling all over?' 'In the past year did little things get on your nerves and wear you out?' 'In the past year did your health make you miserable most of the time?' This set of items, which belongs to the syndrome of vital exhaustion and depression, proved to have a predictive power which is unconfounded by the major risk factors or ECG deviations. But they do not solve the question about the direction of the association. The data of *Klatsky* et al. [25] prove that these feelings foreshadow the onset of MI, but the items can be interpreted as symptoms of a deteriorating health status. Their findings also do not solve the question about the origin of these feelings, but show that regardless of the interpretation, these items might be useful in identifying infarction-prone persons.

If one approaches the question about the origin of these feelings as an either-or question, the discussion between those who favor a more psychological interpretation and those who advocate the position of *Friedman* et al. [20] becomes a stalemate. The 'somaticists' cannot indicate a clear pathophysiological basis for these emotions. Pathoanatomical studies could not establish any relation between findings at autopsy and the premonitory symptoms [28, 29, 35]. Furthermore, ballistocardiographic study by *Theorell* et al. [43] suggests that feelings of passivity and being defeated precede a decrease in cardiac output. On the other hand one cannot deny that feelings of anginal pain may evoke hypochondriacal and depressive reactions.

One could stop at this point and say that we need more data. But it would be more fruitful to ask whether we really are confronted with an either-or question. The psychological symptoms reflect more a state than a stable personality trait and that suggests that we are confronted with a phase of a process in which both the somatic and emotional conditions can mutually influence each other. The mental state forms one side of a coin. Because it seems unlikely that the syndrome of VED can be completely explained as a side effect of a decreasing health status, the question should be asked how the development of VED can be explained in a more psychological way. Both the idea of learned helplessness and the idea of symbolic or real object loss can give some insight. But first of all, one should look at the number of hours worked during a number of years. Mental and social conflicts may result in exhaustion and the life histories of many coronary patients are filled with a highly energy-consuming conflict. The fatigue, however, caused by working too long or too much (and type As tend to deny or suppress feelings of fatigue!), is so obvious that one runs the risk not to notice it. During the last two decades much attention has been given to the type A behavior pattern. There were a number of good reasons to do so. However, it has put some important, older findings in the background. *Russek and Zohman* [37] noticed already in 1958 that 25% of the coronary patients held a second job in addition to a regular, full-time job and an additional 46% had worked 60 h or more a week for long periods preceding attack. *Buell and Breslow* [13] found an excess of coronary mortality among light workers who are on the job more than 48 h a week, especially before age 45. In Sweden also, one of the differences between coronary cases and healthy controls proved to be the amount of overwork [42]. To make a living and to have access to the wealth and benefits of an industrialized world, especially the lower educated groups have to work hard and long. The description of type A behavior, especially when done by the questionnaires, catches only a part of that job effort. The fact that the type A coronary-prone behavior is positively associated with socioeconomical status, while the gradient between SES and CHD in most countries is either zero or negative, could be caused by the fact that questions about a second job or number of hours worked per week are not included in any of the assessments.

The syndrome of VED has, in many cases, an obvious physical origin: too many hours worked. The depressive component of VED shows that something additional has happened: a real or symbolic object loss, or a series of negative experiences which form the basis of what is called 'learned helplessness'.

Behavioristic psychology teaches that depression is learned behavior, learned in those situations in which there is no contingency between effort and result [1]. In this approach depression equals the chronic frustration which is caused by the inability to control one's environment, by loss of control. The person feels helpless and may try to get the gratifications, which he is unable to obtain in his daily life, through privileges which are connected with being sick. Learned helplessness is a behavior pattern characterized by the inability to start initiatives to escape traumatic events, and by the inability to learn that one's own behavior is an instrument to end negative stimuli. The negative expectation regarding the effectiveness of one's own efforts to get control of one's situation leads to passivity and to a decrease in initiative. One does one's best, but (again) one does not succeed. The efforts are never rewarded, however much one does one's best. It is not the passivity which is the central characteristic of depression, but the absence of positive reinforcement of those behaviors which are intended to solve a problem.

In this approach, the type A person can be perceived as somebody who has a strong need for control. This need leads to a hyperresponsive reaction to a new task. He mobilizes a lot of energy to solve a new problem or to master a new task. If these efforts are unsuccessful, the type A person might show hyporesponsive behavior. When confronted with salient uncontrollable events, type As increase their initial efforts to assert control. However, extended exposure to uncontrollability leads to greater helplessness in type As than in type Bs [21, 26]. After a series of these uncontrollable events, one stops one's action, feels 'dead' tired and helpless. By way of their life-style, type As do not only meet more stressful life events, but they experience these life events as more distressing than type Bs do [41]. This may lead to a gradually built up, subclinical form of depression, which is masked by the general activity level so characteristic for the type A. From this perspective, the prodromal state of VED is a renewal and/or deepening of earlier phases of helplessness. An argument which supports this view is formed by the finding that more than half of the coronary patients say that they have been overtrained one or more times in their life [4]. Two studies have found a significant positive correlation between the Jenkins Activity Survey for the assessment of type A behavior and the score on the MQ [6, 18].

A second approach to the genesis of the syndrome of vital exhaustion and depression could be based on classical psychoanalysis, specifically the ego-analytical theory. In this approach, the striking awareness of the ego that it is helpless regarding its aspirations forms the nucleus of normal and neurotic depression [11]. Feelings of helplessness and hopelessness arise when the ego realizes that it is unable to reach its goals. The depressive person, disappointed by himself and others, does not urge himself anymore and gives up. He does not give up his ideals, but gives up his attempts to realize them, because he feels that these attempts are useless. He feels tired, unable to develop new initiatives, and depressive. Vitality is lowered or even completely inhibited. This situation often occurs after a loss experience. This loss may be a real one, as for example the loss of one's wife, or a symbolic loss, as for example the loss of identity and selfesteem after involuntary discharge by invalidity, or the close down of an industry. The first reaction to this object loss is often formed by an increased level of activities to get the lost object back. Because this effort is bound to fail, the object becomes more intense. The depression becomes deeper and now includes inactivity, doing nothing, withdrawal from company, listlessness, loss of sexual interest, which often shows up as impotence. The syndrome is an attempt to save energy. The threshold for new stimuli is heightened. The tiredness is a warning signal not to exert oneself anymore. It becomes hard to tolerate noises or minor inconveniences. Irritability is increased. There is a strong need for rest. People may sleep deeply at very unusual times. Ordinary sleep, however, is often disturbed.

This psychoanalytic approach of object loss is supported by the well-documented relation between bereavement and heart disease [14, 32, 34]. An unreported finding from the IMIR study, illustrating declined tolerance, can also be mentioned here. In that study, it was found that the incidence of new coronary events among women who consulted their general practitioner for complaints of possible cardiac origin was twice as high among those women who had answered 'yes' to the question whether it had become hard for them during the last few months to have small children around them than among those who visited their doctor for the same reason but gave a negative answer to that question.

Both approaches, the behavioral and the psychoanalytic, have their own merit. Both illustrate that during the year before MI vicious circles may develop. The increasing distance between aspiration and activity evokes a series of negative feelings, especially among those who are very active by nature. If one starts to feel helpless, one might direct one's energy in a last effort towards the solution of one's problem. If no relief is experienced, the feelings of helplessness and hopelessness may be deepened. One feels tired and ill. One lacks the reserves to tolerate new frustrations, which leads to an increase in irritability. These irritations stimulate the excretion of norepinephrine which may reinforce anginal pain. Anginal pain may evoke feelings of anxiety or uncertainty, making the chance to regain one's self-confidence smaller and, thus, depression with its hypochondriac elements is reinforced.

It is beyond my competence to address the question of which psycho-physiological or neurohormonal mechanisms might link the syndrome of VED with MI and sudden death. Some interesting suggestions are given by *Raab* [33], *Henry and Stephens* [23], and *Selye* [38]. It is possible that some people smoke more, or drink more coffee during this mental and physical state to stimulate themselves, while some others may eat more or drink more alcohol [47]. It is likely that these harmful habits per se, or in interaction with neurohormonal concomitants of VED, contribute to the pathogenesis of CHD.

The final question addresses the specificity and sensitivity of the syndrome. Is VED a precursor of other diseases too? How many people who have elevated scores on the MQ do not get some form of CHD. These questions cannot yet be answered, because of lack of data. We believe that the syndrome is neither a necessary nor a sufficient cause of MI. The frequency distributions of the MQ as answered by MI patients seems to have a bimodal distribution. About one third has no or only a few signs of VED in the year before MI. Two thirds has elevated scores. This is a preliminary picture which can still change after final item selection. The syndrome is not a sufficient cause. Without a somatic predisposition one would pass a difficult mental period during a state of VED but not become ill.

Acknowledgements

We express our gratitude to Dr. *M. Ceha* for the interviews she did and to Dr. *van der Meer*, director, and *A. Molendijk* and *A. Dubbeldam-Marree* of the Department of Occupational Health of the municipal health centre in Rotterdam for the opportunity they provided to do the study among the city employees.

References

1   Abramson, L.Y.; Seligman, M.E.: Learned helplessness in humans: critique and reformulation. J. abnorm. Psychol. *87:* 49–74 (1978).
2   Alonzo, A.A.; Simon, A.B.; Feinleib, M.: Prodromata of myocardial infarction and sudden death. Circulation *52:* 1056–1062 (1975).
3   Appels, A.: Psychological prodromata of myocardial infarction and sudden death. Psychother. Psychosom. *34:* 187–195 (1980).
4   Appels, A.: Vitale Erschöpfung und Depression als Vorboten des Herzinfarkts; in Langosch, Psychosoziale Probleme und psychotherapeutische Interventionsmöglichkeiten bei Herzinfarktpatienten (Minerva, München 1980).
5   Appels, A.: Vital exhaustion and depression as precursor of myocardial infarction; in Spielberger, Defares, Stress and anxiety, vol. 10 (in press).
6   Appels, A.: The syndrome of vital exhaustion and depression and its relationship to coronary heart disease; in Siegrist, Halhuber, Myocardial infarction and psychosocial risks (Springer, Berlin 1981).
7   Appels, A.: Myocardial infarction and depression. A cross-validation of Dreyfuss' findings. Activitas nerv. sup. *21:* 65–66 (1979).
8   Appels, A.; Bressers, I.: Pre-coronary ill health. Proc. 13th Conf. of the European Society for Psychosomatic Research, Instanbul 1980 (in press).
9   Bekker, B.V.: Interim verslag resultaten WHO registratie projekt, ischaemische hartziekten, Nijmegen 1972.
10   Bengtsson C.; Hällstrom, T.; Tibblin, G.: Social factors, stress experience and personality

traits in women with ischaemic heart disease, compared to a population sample of women. Acta med. scand. suppl. *549:* 82–92 (1973).

11 Bibring, E.: The mechanism of depression; in Greenacre, Affective disorders (International University Press, New York 1968).

12 Bruhn, J.G.; McCrady, K.E.; Plessis, A.: Evidence of 'emotional drain' preceding death from myocardial infarction. Psychiat. Dig. *29:* 34–40 (1968).

13 Buell, P.; Breslow, L.: Mortality from coronary heart disease in California men who work long hours. J. chron. Dis. *11:* 615–626 (1960).

14 Cottington, E.; Mattheus, K.; Talbott, E.; Kuller, L.: Environmental events preceding sudden death in women. Psychosom. Med. *42:* 567–574 (1980).

15 Does, E. Van der; Lubsen, J.: Acute coronary events in general practice: the imminent myocardial infarction. Rotterdam Study, Rotterdam 1978.

16 Dreyfuss, F.; Dasberg, H.; Assael, M.I.: The relationship of myocardial infarction to depressive illness. Psychother. Psychosom. *17:* 73–81 (1969).

17 Eastwood, M.R.: The relation between physical and mental illness (University of Toronto Press, Toronto 1975).

18 Falger, P.: Life changes in middle adulthood, coronary prone behavior and vital exhaustion depression; in Spielberger, Sarason, Defares, Stress and anxiety, vol. IX (in press).

19 Feinleib, M.; Simon, A.; Gillum, R.F.; Margolis, J.R.: Prodromal symptoms and signs of sudden death. Circulation *51/52:* suppl., pp. 155–159 (1975).

20 Friedman, G.D.; Ury, H.K.; Klatsky, A.L.; Siegelaub, A.R.: A psychological questionnaire predictive of myocardial infarction. Psychosom. Med. *36:* 327–343 (1974).

21 Glass, D.C.: Behavior patterns, stress and coronary disease (Erlbaum, Hillsdale 1977).

22 Hagnell, O.: A prospective study of the incidence of mental disorders (Scandinavian University Books, Stockholm 1966).

23 Henry, J.P.; Stephens, P.M.: Stress, health and the social environment (Springer, New York 1977).

24 Jenkins, C.D.; Zyzanski, S.; Ryann, T.; Flessas, A.; Tannerbaum, S.: Social insecurity and coronary prone type A responses as identifiers of severe atherosclerosis. J. consult. clin. Psychol. *45:* 1060–1067 (1977).

25 Klatsky, A.; Friedman, G.; Siegelaub, A.: Medical history questions predictive of myocardial infarction. J. chron. Dis. *29:* 683–696 (1976).

26 Krantz, D.C.; Glass, D.C.; Snyder, M.L.: Helplessness, stress level and the coronary-prone behavior pattern. J. exp. soc. Psychol. *10:* 284–300 (1974).

27 Kuller, L.; Cooper, M.; Perper, J.: Epidemiology of sudden death. Archs intern. Med. *129:* 724–719 (1972).

28 Kuller, L.H.: Prodromata of sudden death and myocardial infarction. Adv. Cardiol. *25:* 61–72 (1978).

29 Meyers, A.; Dewar, H.A.: Circumstances attending 100 sudden deaths from coronary artery disease with coroners autopsies. Br. Heart J. *37:* 1133–1143 (1975).

30 Nixon, P.G.F.: The human function curve. Practitioner *217:* 765–770, 935–944 (1976).

31 Orth-Gomer, K.: Relation between ventricular arrhythmias and psychological profile. Acta med. scand. *207:* 31–36 (1980).

32 Parkes, C.M.; Benjamin, B.; Fitzgerald, R.G.: Broken heart: a statistical study of increased mortality among widowers. Br. med. J. *i:* 740–743 (1969).

33 Raab, W.: Emotional and sensory stress factors in myocardial pathology. Am. Heart J. *72:* 538–564 (1966).

34   Rees, W.D.; Luthius, S.G.: Mortality of bereavement. Br. med. J. *iv:* 13–16 (1967).

35   Rissanen, V.; Romo, M.; Siltanen, P.: Premonitory symptoms and stress factors preceding sudden death from ischaemic heart disease. Acta med. scand. *204:* 389–396 (1978).

36   Rose, G.A.; Blackburn, H.: Cardiovascular survey methods (World Health Organization, Genève 1969).

37   Russek, H.; Zohman, B.L.: Relative significance of heredity, diet and occupational stress in coronary heart disease in young adults. Am. J. M.S. *235:* 266–272 (1958).

38   Selye, H.: Conditioning by cortisol for the production of acute massive myocardial necroses during neuromuscular exertion. Circulation Res. *6:* 168–171 (1958).

39   Shekelle, R.B.; Ostfeld, A.M.: Psychometric evaluations in cardiovascular epidemiology. Ann. N.Y. Acad. Sci. *126:* 696–705 (1965).

40   Solomon, H.; Edwards, A.L.; Killip, T.: Prodromata in acute myocardial infarction. Circulation *40:* 463–471 (1969).

41   Suls, J.; Gastdorf, J.W.; Witenberg, S.M.: Life events, psychological distress and the type A coronary prone behavior pattern. J. psychosom. Med. *23:* 315–319 (1979).

42   Theorell, T.; Rahe, R.H.: Behavior and life satisfactions characteristics of Swedish subjects with myocardial infarction. J. chron. Dis. *25:* 139–147 (1972).

43   Theorell, T.; Blunk, D.; Wolf, S.: Emotions and cardiac contractility as reflected in ballistocardiographic recordings. Pavlov J. biol. Sci. *9:* 65–75 (1974).

44   Thiel, H.; Parker, D.; Bruce, T.: Stress factors and the risk of myocardial infarction. J. psychosom. Res. *17:* 43–57 (1973).

45   Thomas, B.C.: Psychobiological characteristics in youth as predictors of five disease states. Johns Hopkins med. J. *132:* 16–43 (1973).

46   Verhagen, F.; Nass, C.; Appels, A.; van Bastelaer, A.; Winnubst, J.: Cross-validation of the A/B typology in the Netherlands. Psychother. Psychosom. *34:* 178–186 (1980).

47   Wilhelmsen, L.: Coffee consumption and coronary heart disease in middle-aged Swedish men. Acta med. scand. *201:* 547–552 (1977).

48   Wolf, S.: Psychosocial forces in myocardial infarction and sudden death. Circulation *40:* suppl. IV, pp. 74–83 (1969).

49   World Health Organization, Regional Office for Europe: The prodromal symptoms of myocardial infarction and sudden death. Report of a working group, Copenhagen 1971.

(*Appendix* see following page.)

Appendix I. Computation of the odds ratio

	Question	
	positive	negative
Disease present	a	b
Disease absent	c	d

If a certain characteristic (response to a question; exposure to a toxic agent, etc.) has an association with the occurrence of a disease, there will be more persons in the cells a and d. The larger the association between characteristic and diseace, the larger the ratio between a-d and b-c, which is expressed by the formula ad/bc. If there is no association the ratio equals 1.00. In other words: the odds ratio expresses the probability that a diseased and a nondiseased person have a certain characteristic. A major advantage of the odds ratio is that its absolute magnitude is independent of the number of observations within the cells.

3 Behavioral Correlates of Angiographic Findings[1]

Redford B. Williams, Jr.

Since the formulation of the type A behavior pattern (TABP) concept by *Rosenman* et al. [11] a considerable body of research has been carried out [3; *Rosenman*, this volume] culminating in the general acceptance of TABP as a risk factor, at least among middle-aged males, for developing clinical manifestations of coronary heart disease (CHD). While the prospective association of TABP with subsequent CHD events is undisputed, the question remains: Is TABP involved only in the precipitation of acute clinical events, or is it also involved in the process of atherogenesis? If TABP can be implicated in atherogenesis, not only would the case for its role in the pathogenesis be strengthened, but important additional evidence would be provided concerning mechanisms whereby that pathogenetic influence is exerted. That is, rather than postulating simply that once coronary atherosclerosis (CAD) is present, cardiovascular and/or neuroendocrine hyperresponsivity among type A persons is responsible for precipitating acute episodes of myocardial ischemia, it would be necessary to hypothesize as well that such hyperresponsivity is also occurring for decades prior to the acute event and playing a role in promoting the endothelial injury and lipid accumulation which have been proposed [12] as the principal etiologic events in atherogenesis. This second hypothesis has important implications for the kinds of research needed to unravel the mystery of why only some type As develop clinical CHD-studies of psychophysiologic and psychoneuroendocrine mechanisms would need to be carried out not only among subjects in the age range where clinical manifestations of CHD begin to appear; such studies would be appropriate among younger subjects as well.

In this paper I shall critically review the evidence concerning the role of TABP in atherogenesis and then consider briefly some of the evidence recently obtained in our laboratories at Duke University relating to potential mechanisms for the putative increased rate of atherogenesis among type A persons.

[1] Preparation of this paper was supported in part by Grants HL-18589 and HL-22740 from the National Heart, Lung and Blood Institute and a Research Scientist Development Award, MH-70482, from the National Institute of Mental Health.

TABP and Atherogenesis

At the time of the Forum on Coronary-Prone Behavior [3], there were three studies of TABP among patients undergoing diagnostic coronary arteriography, all providing positive evidence for involvement of TABP in atherogenesis. *Zyzanski* et al. [17] found in a study of 94 men, that those with two or more major coronary arteries with luminal narrowing of 50% or more scored higher on all four scales of the Jenkins Activity Survey (JAS) than did patients with zero or one artery with 50% narrowing. Multivariate analysis of their data showed only the JAS A scale to be associated with increased CAD, independently of degree of angina pain, age, prior experience of myocardial infarction and various anxiety and neuroticism scales derived from the MMPI. In addition to JAS A score, low levels of denial and high levels of anxiety and depression were also found independently and significantly related to increased CAD.

Frank et al. [6] reported an association between TABP and increased severity (assessed in terms of number of major coronary arteries with a greater than 50% occlusion) of CAD among a sample of 124 men and 23 women undergoing angiography. This study extended the findings of the *Zyzanski* et al. [17] study in several important respects. First, the sample included women, and the relationship between TABP and CAD was found to be equally strong in women compared to men. Second, the traditional physical risk factors of age, sex, cholesterol, smoking history and hypertension were all evaluated with regard to CAD severity and entered first in a multiple regression analysis prior to entry of TABP; despite adjustment for all these physical risk factors, TABP was found to still account for a significant proportion of disease, above and beyond the cumulative effects of the physical risk factors. Third, the means of assessing TABP was the structured interview (SI) [10], instead of the JAS, which was not employed in this study. An additional methodological consideration, which may assume greater importance as we turn to other studies was that a subset of 20 taped SIs was rated by *Rosenman* [10] and an agreement rate of 90% was found with the TABP ratings on the same tapes by the investigators.

The third study in this 'pre-Forum' era was that of *Blumenthal* et al. [1], which in many respects replicated the *Frank* et al. [6] findings, and contained some further refinements, as well. Like the *Frank* et al. [6] study, this sample of 142 patients included both men and women, though a greater proportion (44%) were women. This study also evaluated traditional physical risk factors and found cholesterol and history of cigarette smoking to be associated with

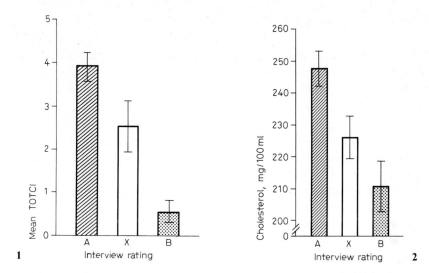

Fig. 1. Relationship between TOTCI scores (see text for definition) and TABP as assessed using the structured interview [based on data from ref. 1].

Fig. 2. Relationship between serum cholesterol level and TABP [based on data from ref. 1].

increased CAD severity. Rather than presence or absence or number of arteries with 50% or greater occlusions, the *Blumenthal* et al. [1] study employed a more refined measure of CAD severity – TOTCI – an index made up of a score given to each of the four major coronary arteries based on the following scoring system: '0' if no obstruction, '1' if less than 75% obstruction, '2' if between 75 and 95% obstruction, and '3' if 100% obstructed. As can be seen in figure 1, there was a striking progression in TOTCI scores, from less than one among type Bs, to 2.5 among intermediate type Xs, to 4 among type As. This association between TABP (assessed by the SI) and increased CAD severity was highly significant ($p < 0.001$); moreover, this association was not altered even after simultaneous statistical adjustment for traditional physical risk factors: age, sex, cigarette smoking, blood pressure and cholesterol level – even though the latter was found (fig. 2) to be increased among type As. Thus, the *Blumenthal* et al. [1] study essentially replicated all the important findings of the *Frank* et al. [6] study: TABP was associated with increased CAD, independently of physical risk factors and among women was well as men. In addition, the *Blumenthal* et al. [1] study went beyond the *Frank* et al. [6] study in several important respects. First, it employed the JAS in addition to the SI as a measure of TABP. It was noteworthy that whereas SI-determined TABP was found to be strongly related to CAD levels, JAS-determined TABP did not relate significantly to CAD level, despite a moderate correlation between JAS scores and SI results. A second aspect of this study involved the measurement of an index of genetically determined sympathetic nervous system (SNS) activity levels – serum levels of the norepinephrine synthesizing enzyme dopamine-β-hydroxylase (DBH) in a subset of 83 patients. No relationship was found between DBH levels and CAD severity, suggesting that with respect to genetically determined chronic levels of SNS activity, increased SNS activity is not involved in atherogenesis. It should be noted, however, that this only pertains to genetically determined, chronic SNS activity, not acute behaviorally or situationally induced increases. While the reasons for the failure to replicate the JAS results of *Zyzanski* et al. [17] may never be conclusively resolved, it appears likely that the presence of a substantial proportion of women and patients from rural, rather than urban backgrounds may have been factors.

In contrast to the above series of studies which found a relationship between TABP and CAD severity, one study employing only the SI as a measure of TABP, one using only the JAS and one using both, *Dimsdale* et al. [4, 5] at the Massachusetts General Hospital, have found no relationship between CAD and TABP, whether assessed by the JAS [4] or the SI [5]. Since these negative findings have been widely cited as weakening the case provided by the first three studies for a role of TABP in atherogenesis, they deserve special attention in order to attempt to achieve some perspective regarding how they should weigh in the balance of evidence with the other studies. First of all, there is no disagreement between the *Dimsdale* et al. [4] finding of no relationship between JAS-determined TABP and CAD and the similar finding in the *Blumenthal* et al. [1] study. Since this study employed both the SI and the JAS, it might be possible to conclude that when both are used, the SI will relate better to CAD, especially in populations different from that in which the JAS was developed and standardized. However, the *Dimsdale* et al. [5] study did use the SI and still found no relationship of TABP to CAD. We must ask how this failure to replicate the *Frank* et al. [6] and the *Blumenthal* et al. [1] studies came about. First of all, it may be simply a chance failure to replicate – a phenomenon that is to be expected even with a significant and real relationship when that relationship is subjected to test a number of times – one time out of 20 would be the rate of failure to replicate a real finding by chance alone. A similar argument is currently raging concerning the studies of β-blockers in the prevention of recurrent myocardial infarction. Some studies are positive and some are negative, and the question is asked:

which results are those due to chance – the positive or negative ones? Another possibility is that the patient population in Boston is sufficiently different from that in New York City and Durham that the relationship between TABP and CAD simply does not hold there as it does in the other sites; perhaps religious or ethnic differences between the samples are involved.

Another area where possible explanations for the failure of *Dimsdale's* group to replicate the *Frank* et al. [6] and *Blumenthal* et al. [1] findings may be found concerns various aspects of the methodologies employed in the various studies. First, both of the latter two studies employed samples (147 and 142) that were nearly 40% larger than that studied by *Dimsdale* et al. [5]. While not highly likely, it is still possible that with a larger sample, *Dimsdale* and his coworkers would find a more positive relationship. Another difference concerns the means of assessing extent of CAD. Both *Dimsdale* et al. and *Frank* et al. employed a 50% occlusion as the cutoff point between diseased and nondiseased vessels. In contrast, *Blumenthal* et al. [1] employed a more information-containing index, the TOTCI. While *Dimsdale* et al. [5] analyzed their data in a manner similar to *Frank* et al. [6] – proportion of type As in groups with one, two and three-four arteries with 50% occlusion or greater – and found no relationship between CAD and TABP, perhaps if they had employed an index like the TOTCI, a more positive relationship would have been found. An additional, and perhaps more likely source of error in the *Dimsdale* et al. [5] study relates to the reliability of the SI assessment procedures employed. While it is indicated that both interviewers were trained and certified at the Harold Brunn Institute, it is also indicated that no systematic validation of the SI assessments, such as that described above for the *Frank* et al. [6] study, were undertaken – only that those interviews 'that were regarded as technically questionable or those on which the two raters could not agree were sent for arbitration to the Harold Brunn Institute' [5]. It is possible that there could have been systematic errors made by the interviewers with regard to the bulk of the interviews on which they agreed (e.g. assigning patients to the type B group on the basis of content, while a more careful evaluation of voice stylistics – tendency to interrupt the interviewer – would have resulted in their being termed type A), and which were not sent for auditing in terms of the 'gold standard' at Harold Brunn Institute. As will be described below, in our ongoing studies at Duke University, we have taken care to send a random sample of 100 SIs to Harold Brunn Institute for auditing, with the result that we are confident that our SI assessments are in substantial agreement (85%) with the only gold standard currently available. Until the SI of *Dimsdale* et al. [4, 5] is subjected to similar validation, there

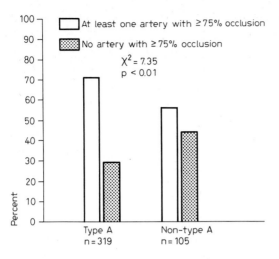

Fig. 3. Relationship between TABP and presence/absence of significant coronary athero-sclerosis [from ref. 15].

must remain some question as to the validity of their assessment procedures and, hence, the reality of their failure to find a relationship between TABP and CAD.

Based on our earlier finding [1] of a relationship between SI-determined TABP and CAD, we have been collecting in a more systematic manner a wide gamut of psychological, social and behavioral information on all patients undergoing coronary arteriography at Duke University since 1976. The overall study design is shown in table I. All the behavioral/psychosocial as well as clinical and catheterization variables are stored in the Cardiology Data Bank, thus greatly facilitating the simultaneous evaluation of relation-ships between behavioral/psychosocial variables and indices of CAD out-comes. At the present time we have complete behavioral/psychosocial data sets on over 2,000 patients who have undergone coronary arteriography, and I shall describe some of our further findings concerning the relationship of TABP and other psychological characteristics to coronary angiographic indices.

One of our first analyses addressed the question of the relationship between SI-determined TABP and CAD in a far larger sample (424) of patients than had previously been reported [15]. As shown in figure 3, we again found a significant relationship between TABP and CAD: over 70% of the 319 type As studied had at least one artery with a clinically significant

Table I. Study design for ongoing collection of behavioral and psychosocial data among patients referred to Duke University Medical Center for diagnostic coronary angiography [from ref. 15]

Days −2, −1	Day 0	Day +1	Day +2 and later

Admission
History and P.E.
Exercise ECG
Echocardiogram
Blood chemistries
	Coronary
	arteriogram
		a.m.
		Behavioral assessment
		1 Structured Interview
		   (type A_1, A_2, X or B)
		2 JAS
		3 MMPI (566 items)
		4 Zung Self-Rating
		   Depression Scale
		5 Zung Self-Rating
		   Anxiety Scale
		6 Life Change
		   Questionnaire
		7 Functional Status
		   Questionnaire
		8 Social Support
		   Networks
		   Questionnaire
		p.m.
		Patient learns results of
		arteriogram
			Subsequent treatment
			1 Coronary bypass
			   surgery
			2 Discharge to medical
			   management
			Follow-up annually
			re outcomes
			A. Physical
			   1 Mortality
			   2 Pain status
			   3 Myocardial infarction
			   4 Functional status
			B. Psychological
			   1 Type A (JAS)
			   2 Life change
			   3 Anxiety
			   4 Depression
			   5 Social supports

(greater than or equal to 75%) occlusion, in comparison to only 56% with significant occlusions among the 105 type Bs. Based upon earlier work [9] showing potential for hostility to be associated with increased risk of CHD events in the WCGS, we scored the MMPI protocols on these 424 patients for *Cook and Medley's* [2] Hostility (Ho) scale. An interesting, nonlinear relationship was found (fig. 4) between Ho score and presence of significant CAD: among those patients who scored in a very low range on the Ho scale – 10 or less, reflecting an essential absence of distrust for and dislike of people in general – there was observed only a 48% rate of significant disease; in contrast, among patient groups scoring anything higher than 10 there was observed a 70% rate of significant disease. Further documenting this relationship between very low Ho score and relative absence of CAD, we found that TOTCI scores were also significantly lower in the group scoring 10 or less compared to the group scoring in the high Ho range (greater than 30) (fig. 5). As an additional check of the possible validity of the Ho score, we evaluated its relationship to TABP (fig. 6) and found a clear and systematic increase in Ho score proceeding from

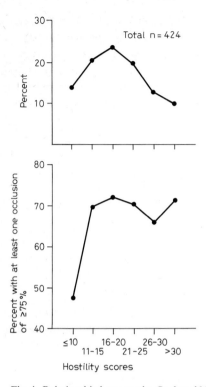

Fig. 4. Relationship between the *Cook and Medley* [2] Hostility (Ho) Scale from the MMPI and presence of significant coronary atherosclerosis [from ref. 15].

Bs to Xs to A2s to A1s. We next evaluated the joint relationship between TABP and Ho score and CAD (controlling for sex, since females are less type A and have lower Ho scores on average). As shown in figure 7, there is a striking progression in the proportion with significant CAD, ranging from only 12.5% among type B women with Ho scores less than 10, to 44% among type A women with Ho scores greater than 10, all the way up to 82% among type A men with Ho scores greater than 10. Despite the clear relationship between TABP and Ho score (fig. 6), both low Ho score and TABP were independently related to presence of significant CAD – a result, no doubt, of the fact that Ho scores of 10 or less were present equally in the type A and non-type A groups.

These findings indicate that it is possible to identify psychometrically determined individual difference measures that relate to CAD independently of the behaviorally determined (via the SI) type A characteristic. We

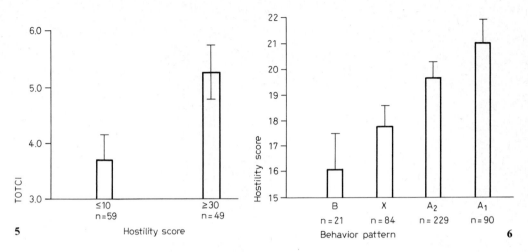

Fig. 5. Relationship between hostility score and TOTCI index of coronary atherosclerosis [based on data from ref. 15].

Fig. 6. Relationship between hostility score and TABP (assessed using the SI) [based on data from ref. 15].

have suggested [15] that this reluctance to endorse items reflective of dislike and distrust of others may also help to explain the relative absence of CHD in Japan, despite the very high prevalence of another risk factor – hypertension – in that country. In addition, it appears that this protective effect of low Ho scoring with regard to CAD in a clinical population referred for diagnostic angiography may also extend to protect free-living populations with regard to CHD mortality. Very recently available and preliminary analyses suggest that among healthy persons at intake in a large-scale prospective study who score in the very low range on the Ho scale there is a significantly lower long-term CHD mortality in comparison to individuals scoring in the higher range of Ho scores.

Perhaps related to this apparent protective effect of very low Ho levels is the finding of *Krantz* et al. [8] that, whereas patients showing progression of disease on repeat coronary angiography do not differ significantly in terms of TABP, there does appear to be a protective effect of absence of type A behavior, such that extreme type B patients were significantly less likely to show progression.

What can we conclude from the findings reviewed thus far? First, the weight of evidence available favors the hypothesized relationship between TABP and atherogenesis. While one group has failed to find a relationship

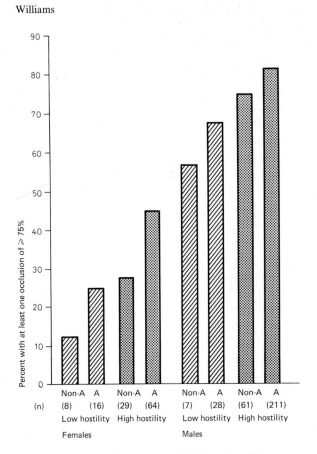

Fig. 7. Joint relationship of gender, TABP and hostility score to presence of significant coronary atherosclerosis [from ref. 15].

between TABP and CAD, there are unresolved questions regarding various aspects of their methodology which suggest that judgment must be withheld regarding the ultimate validity of their failure to replicate the findings of at least three other studies, two of which had moderately (40%) and one markedly (300%) larger samples.

Second, it appears that hostility, measured in a variety of ways, is related to CAD, perhaps independently of TABP. Moreover, it appears that the relation of hostility as indexed by the MMPI Ho scale may also predict mortality in a large-scale prospective study.

Based on the above findings, what directions suggest themselves for further research regarding correlates of angiographic findings?

Future Lines of Research

Three general lines of future research suggest themselves.

1. Evaluate TABP and Atherosclerosis in Groups Other Than Those Referred for Diagnostic Angiography. Obviously, coronary angiography is not so benign a procedure that one can obtain a sample of healthy people and subject them to it. Perhaps the closest approximation to this ideal sort of study is now in progress at San Antonio, where Air Force personnel who develop symptoms or ECG changes suggestive of CAD are sent for medical evaluation prior to being cleared to remain on flight duty. These previously asymptomatic young and middle-aged men often undergo coronary angiography as part of the medical workup, and TABP assessment has been carried out among this sample for a number of years. While no reports have yet been published regarding the observed relationship in this sample between CAD and TABP, hopefully reports will be forthcoming in the not too distant future which could help to further clarify the nature of the relationship between TABP and CAD. An additional approach involves the recently developed technique of radionuclide angiography as a tool in the evaluation of CAD. Compared to coronary angiography, this test is basically noninvasive (a simple intravenous injection) and without appreciable risk, making it appropriate for screening samples of apparently normal individuals. Supporting the utility of such an approach, *Kahn* et al. [7] have recently reported a positive association between SI, TABP and radionuclide angiography-determined coronary insufficiency.

2. Further Refine Our Understanding of Those Psychological Characteristics of Type As which Are Truly Predisposing Them To Develop CAD. One approach that was described earlier is embodied in our recent finding [15] that low scores on an MMPI Ho scale appear to protect against development of significant CAD. We are currently attempting to extend this finding through an empirically based analysis of the MMPI protocols we now have on over 2,000 patients who have undergone coronary angiography at Duke University over the past 5 years. In collaboration with Dr. *Grant Dahlstrom* of the University of North Carolina, we plan to randomly split this sample into two halves, taking care to ensure that each half is matched to contain equal range of CAD severity. We shall then carry out an item analysis on one of the halves, to identify items which reliably discriminate among patients with varying levels of atherosclerosis. Next, we shall perform a factor analysis on the resultant item pool, to identify correlated groups or clusters of items which might then serve as new 'CAD scales'. To evaluate the utility of such item clusters in this regard, we shall compute factor scores for each group of items emerging from the factor analysis in the second half of the original sample. Those item clusters which significantly discriminate among CAD levels we shall consider as having been cross-validated and worthy of further study. For example, interpretation of the content of the items in a given cluster may provide some clues as to the specific nature of the underlying psychological characteristics which predispose to CAD. If covarying such clusters in a multiple regression analysis with type A entered last results in the relationship between TABP and CAD becoming insignificant, we would be in a position to conclude that the variance in CAD accounted for by TABP is more efficiently measured through the MMPI item clusters. The further validity of such clusters could be assessed by scoring MMPI protocols collected on various populations over the past 15–30 years for these item clusters and then seeing if subsequent CHD events are reliably predicted. The already emerging suggestion that the Ho scale is effective in this regard is very encouraging to us, leading us to believe that the approach outlined above will prove fruitful. If so, then we would have obtained a much more precise definition than that provided by the global TABP of just what it is about the psychological makeup of some individuals that predisposes them to develop CAD. In contrast to TABP, which is present in about 50–75% of the normal population, if high scores on these newly developed CAD scales prove to be much less prevalent, we might be in a position to identify much more accurately and precisely those individuals truly at risk, and then proceed with preventive efforts to forestall or prevent the eventual expression of clinical CHD among them. Such MMPI-based CAD scales could be subjected to analysis using sophisticated statistical techniques to evaluate, for example, genetic influences and cross-cultural differences (i.e. the low CHD rates in Japan).

3. Identify Psychophysiological and Psychoneuroendocrine Characteristics which Account not only for the Increased CHD and CAD Rates among Type As as a Group, but which also Help To Subgroup Type As so that Those Truly at Risk Can Be Reliably Identified. This is an exciting area and one in which much research activity is currently going on. Other papers [by *Dembroski, Schmidt, Rüddel, Slaby* and *Langosch*] address this issue in this volume, and I shall not attempt to review this important area here. I shall, however, briefly review recent work in my laboratory which speaks to this issue. I have proposed [14] that the generic behaviors of mental problem solv-

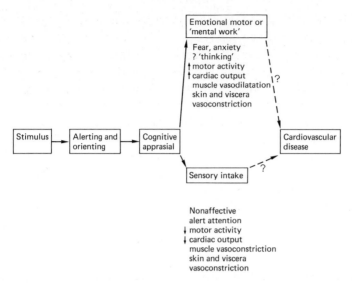

Fig. 8. Proposed theoretical model whereby varying environmental stimuli can produce qualitatively different patterns of arousal.

ing and attending to frequently presented visual stimuli are associated with qualitatively different patterns of cardiovascular response (fig. 8). We have recently subjected a sample of 31 young male undergraduates to both a mental arithmetic task and a sensory intake task, while monitoring both cardiovascular parameters (heart rate, blood pressure, forearm blood flow, and forearm vascular resistance – a measure of skeletal muscle vasomotor tone) and obtaining blood using a continuous exfusion pump to be later assayed for a variety of hormones which may be implicated in the pathogenesis of CAD. Thus far, two major findings are emerging which have relevance for pathogenetic mechanisms.

First, during the mental arithmetic task, a characteristic cardiovascular response pattern is observed – increased heart rate, blood pressure and forearm blood flow, with a decrease in forearm vascular resistance indicating a muscle vasodilatation. In addition, a characteristic neuroendocrine response pattern is also observed – increased plasma levels of epinephrine, norepinephrine, cortisol, and prolactin [16]. Despite only a moderate challenge (a case of beer at the end of the study to the subject making the most correct subtractions in the serial subtraction task employed), the 13 type A subjects showed a significantly greater muscle vasodilatation (decreased forearm vascular resistance) and significantly greater increases in plasma epinephrine, norepinephrine, and cortisol, but not prolactin, during mental arithmetic performance. It is interesting that type As were hyperresponsive in terms of both peripheral sympathetic nerve activity (norepinephrine) and adrenal medullary activity (epinephrine), as well as one parameter of anterior pituitary activity (ACTH) which presumably underlies the observed increased adrenal cortical activitiy (cortisol). In contrast, another parameter reflective of anterior pituitary activity – prolactin – was secreted to exactly the same degree during mental arithmetic performance by both As and Bs. While the epinephrine and norepinephrine hyperresponsivity among type As have obvious physiological and metabolic effects relevant to atherogenesis, the cortisol hyperresponsivity may eventually prove even more interesting. For example, it is known that cortisol can act to potentiate metabolic and physiological effects of catecholamines via two mechanisms: (1) it stimulates activity of catecholamine-synthesizing enzymes, DBH and PNMT, and (2) it inhibits activity of a major catecholamine-degrading enzyme, COMT. In support of the participation of cortisol hyperresponsivity in atherogenesis, *Troxler* et al. [13] found elevated serial a.m. cortisols during an oral glucose tolerance test to be predictive of increased angiographically documented CAD in the Air Force sample.

The second major finding to emerge from our recent research relates to cardiovascular and neuroendocrine response to the sensory intake task, as a function of both TABP and family history of cardiovascular disease. While the entire group of type As did not differ in terms of either cardiovascular or neuroendocrine response to the sensory intake task, when family history (FH) of cardiovascular disease was also taken into account, several significant FH×type A interactions were found. Whereas type As with a +FH showed a greater diastolic BP increase during the task compared to type Bs with +FH, among those subjects with −FH, type As were hyporesponsive compared to Bs in terms of diastolic BP response. Paralleling this cardiovascular hyperresponsivity among type As with +FH, we also found that type As with +FH were also hyperresponsive in terms of cortisol response to the sensory intake task. In contrast, among subjects with −FH, type As were again hyporesponsive relative to Bs with −FH. This suggests that during sensory intake behaviors type As show cardiovascular and neuroendocrine hyperresponsivity relative to Bs only in the presence of a genetic predisposition to cardiovascular disease. In contrast, among persons without such a genetic predisposition, type As are, if anything, hyporesponsive. For males, at least, this FH×type A interaction is not acting during mental arithmetic performance. We have now replicated this FH×type A interaction effect with regard to cardiovascular response in an additional study employing a different sensory intake task. In addition, we have completed one study of female subjects and found that in contrast to males they do not vasodilate during mental arithmetic, but show increases in heart rate, blood pressure and forearm blood flow, without a decrease in FVR. Moreover, for females there is no difference in cardiovascular response between the global type A and type B groups; however, a FH × type A interaction is found, such that type As with a +FH are hyperresponsive relative to Bs with +FH and, again, As with −FH are hyporesponsive.

Our future studies will attempt to extend these findings to samples of older males, additional female samples (both young and older), and patients with varying levels of angiographically documented CAD. If we can eventually show that it is only As who are hyperresponsive in terms of cardiovascular and neuroendocrine parameters to the various tasks we are studying who display significant CAD, then the case for the participation of such hyperresponsivity in atherogenesis will be considerably strengthened.

Conclusions

The efforts currently under way and planned to identify both psychological and biological correlates of angiographic findings clearly represent the most exciting area of research related to TABP at the present time. By defining with greater precision than that permitted by the global assessment of TABP those specific characteristics which truly increase risk of developing CHD, this research will not only document the indisputable scientific basis for the now-recognized association of TABP with clinical CHD, it will also point the way to rational interventions – pharmacologic as well as behavioral – by which the TABP-CAD/CHD linkage can eventually be decoupled.

References

1   Blumenthal, J.A.; Williams, R.B.; Kong, Y.; Schanberg, S.M.; Thompson, L.W.: Type A behavior pattern and coronary atherosclerosis. Circulation *58:* 634–639 (1978).
2   Cook, W.W.; Medley, D.M.: Proposed hostility and pharisaic-virtue scales for the MMPI. J. appl. Psychol. *38:* 414–418 (1954).
3   Dembroski, T.M.; Weiss, S.M.; Shields, J.L.; et al. (eds): Coronary-prone behavior (Springer, New York 1978).

4   Dimsdale, J.E.; Hackett, T.P.; Hutter, A.M.; Block, P.C.; Catanzano, D.M.: Type A perso-
    nality and extent of coronary atherosclerosis. Am J. Cardiol. *42:* 583–586 (1978).
5   Dimsdale, J.E.; Hackett, T.P.; Hutter, A.M.; Block, P.C.; Catanzano, D.M.: Type A
    behavior and angiographic findings. J. psychosom. Res. *23:* 273–276 (1979).
6   Frank, K.A.; Heller, S.S.; Kornfeld, D.S.; Sporn, A.A.; Weiss, M.D.: Type A behavior pat-
    tern and coronary atherosclerosis. J. Am. med. Ass. *240:* 761–763 (1978).
7   Kahn, J.P.; Kornfeld, D.S.; Blood, D.K.; Lynn, R.; Heller, S.S.; Frank, K.A.: Type A
    behavior and Thallium Stress Test. Proc. American Psychosomatic Society Annual Meet-
    ing, 1981.
8   Krantz, D.S.; Sanmario, M.I.; Selvester, R.H.; Matthews, K.A.: Psychological correlates
    of progression of atherosclerosis in men. Psychosom. Med. *41:* 467–475 (1979).
9   Matthews, K.A.; Glass, D.C.; Rosenman, R.H.; et al.: Competitive drive, pattern A and
    coronary heart disease. A further analysis of some data from the Western Collaborative
    Group Study. J. chron. Dis. *30:* 489–498 (1977).
10 Rosenman, R.H.: The interview method of assessment of the coronary-prone behavior
    pattern; in Dembroski, Weiss, Shields, et al., Coronary-prone behavior (Springer, New
    York 1978).
11 Rosenman, R.H.; Friedman, M.; Strauss, R.; et al.: A predictive study of coronary heart
    disease. The Western Collaborative Group Study. J. Am. med. Ass. *189:* 15–22 (1964).
12 Ross, R.; Glomset, J.A.: The pathogenesis of atherosclerosis. New Engl. J. Med. *295:* 295–
    302 (1976).
13 Troxler, R.G.; Sprague, E.A.; Albonese, R.A.; et al.: The association of elevated plasma
    cortisol and early atherosclerosis as demonstrated by coronary angiography. Athero-
    sclerosis *26:* 151–162 (1977).
14 Williams, R.B.: Psychophysiological processes, the coronary-prone behavior pattern, and
    coronary heart disease; in Dembroski, Weiss, Shields, et al., Coronary-prone behavior
    (Springer, New York 1978).
15 Williams, R.B.; Haney, T.L., Lee, K.L.; Kong, Y.; Blumenthal, J.A.; Whalen, R.E.: Type
    A behavior, hostility, and coronary atherosclerosis. Psychosom. Med. *42:* 539–549 (1980).
16 Williams, R.B.; Lane, J.D.; Kuhn, C.M.; Melosh, W.; White, A.D.; Schanberg, S.M.: Type
    A behavior and elevated physiological and neuroendocrine responses to cognitive tasks.
    Science *218:* 483–485 (1982).
17 Zyzanski, S.J.; Jenkins, C.D.; Ryan, T.J.; Flessas, A.; Everist, M.: Psychological correlates
    of coronary angiographic findings. Archs intern. Med. *136:* 1234–1237 (1976).

4 Causal Modeling: A Tool in Epidemiology[1]

Georg Pepping, Dieter Vaitl

We are reporting on a cross-section study, in which medical, psychological, and sociological data on patients with myocardial infarction were collected. Thereby we would like to talk about a method that makes it possible to examine causal relationships between variables by mathematical means.

The Study

Questionnaires were used as instruments of the study. Information on job stress, coping attitudes, and medical risk conditions was gathered on 100 male heart patients and, as a control group, on 100 patients with spinal complaints. 50% of the subjects were blue-collar workers, the others were white-collar workers.

The purpose of the study was to examine psychological and sociological variables within the context of research on coronary heart disease. Through a regression analysis, in which the myocardial infarction diagnosis served as criterion, about 50% of the variance could be explained. The traditional risk conditions such as cigarette smoking and serum cholesterol level received the highest regression weights. Their predictive power overlapped with that of the psychosocial variables. These did not essentially improve the regression equation [for more details see ref. 7]. One might jump to the conclusion that psychological and social factors lack relevance and can be neglected. It is, however, necessary to disentangle the complex causal network of traditional, psychological, and sociological risk factors.

[1] This study was carried out with Dr. *L. v. Ferber*. It was financially supported by a grant from the Deutsche Forschungsgemeinschaft.

The Method

Causal modeling is a method which uses information from correlative data to test causal models empirically. Since causal modeling is not yet often used in psychosomatic and epidemiological research, a few comments on the method may prove useful:

The basic idea of causal modeling is as follows: if causal relationships between variables exist, then the covariance matrix of these variables is structured by certain restrictions; the covariances cannot vary any more freely than if they were calculated from random numbers. Whether the empirical covariance matrix conforms to the supposition of such restrictions can be tested. This can be taken as a test of the model built from the single theoretical statements. A wrong model – or wrong parts of a model – can be falsified.

The model has to be based on substantive theoretical knowledge [10]. This pertains to the causal relationships between variables (the so-called structural model) as well as to the operational definition of latent variables (the so-called measurement model). With the computer program LISREL (linear structural relationships) [5] it is possible to specify theoretical suppositions and to test them with respect to data [for details see 1, 2, 4–6].

Application of Causal Modeling

Figure 1 shows the measurement and structural relationships of several variables in a sample of blue-collar workers (model 1). The ovals represent latent variables. They 'cause' the values of their indicators. As an example, the variable 'blood lipids' is manifested by cholesterol and triglycerides; job involvement is operationalized by items like: 'My work fulfills me completely' or 'I would rather work less'.

Rectangles represent directly measured variables. Variables on the left side of the diagram (working hours per week; job involvement; social stress) are exogenous variables, i.e. they are only causes. The variables in the middle and on the right side are endogenous, i.e. they may be caused by other variables.

The fixing of the variables as manifest/latent or as exogen/endogen is part of the a priori assumptions. These imply that psychosocial risk conditions precede the traditional risks in the causal chain. The myocardial infarction is specified as the last link in the causal chain. It cannot thus be seen as a cause for any other variable. Working hours, job involvement and personal conflicts potentially affect cigarette consumption, blood pressure and blood lipids; the reverse causation is not possible according to the model. This specification reflects the idea that the association between coronary heart disease and social conditions or specific behavior patterns is mediated by adaptive physiological mechanisms. This assumption can often be found in the literature [3, 9].

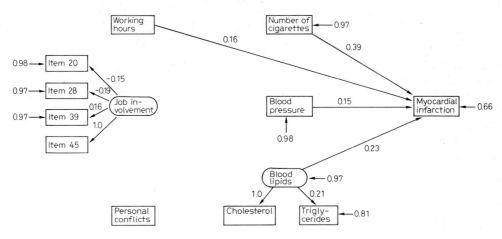

Fig. 1. Causal model (1) of myocardial infarction (blue-collar workers). $\chi^2 = 59.91$; 43 d.f.; p = 0.05; n = 100.

The causal relationships allowed by the model are estimated as free parameters with maximum likelihood. They are included in the diagram as arrows between variables only if they are significant. The interpretation of their numerical values corresponds to that of standardized regression coefficients (beta coefficients), i.e. the increase of the causal variable by one unit leads to an increase of the effect variable by x units, if x stands for the value of the coefficient. The arrows having no defined variable as origin, which point to some of the variables in the system, indicate the variance not explained by the model.

The null hypothesis that the model is compatible with the data is tested by an approximate χ^2 test. A significantly small probability indicates a discrepancy between model and data structure. In our example the value of the χ^2 test just reaches the critical 5% significance level. The model is only just compatible with the data. It has to be kept in mind that the distribution characteristics of these tests are not yet well known for small samples [2, 8].

Results from Causal Modeling

Among the traditional risk conditions, hypertension and blood lipids show a clear influence; cigarette smoking manifests the strongest effect on myocardial infarction. Among the psychological and sociological variables

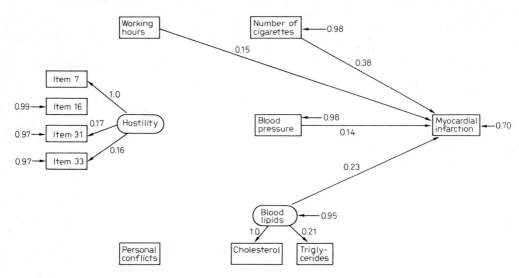

Fig. 2. Causal model (2) of myocardial infarction (blue collar workers). $\chi^2 = 35.11$; 33 d.f.; p = 0.37; n = 100.

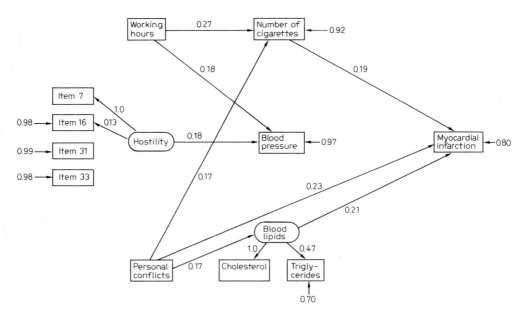

Fig. 3. Causal model (2) of myocardial infarction (white-collar workers). $\chi^2 = 34.46$; 33 d.f.; p = 0.40; n = 100.

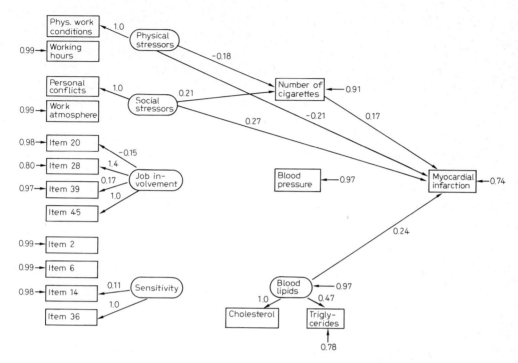

Fig. 4. Causal model (3) of myocardial infarction (white-collar workers). $\chi^2 = 170.14$; 102 d.f.; $p < 0.001$.

only the number of weekly working hours plays a role. Job involvement and personal conflicts remain without a direct or indirect influence on myocardial infarction (fig. 1).

The same model applied to a sample of white-collar workers did not attain adequate conformity to the data.

In a different model (fig. 2) the construct 'Job involvement' has been substituted by 'Hostility'. This is operationalized by items such as 'It's your own fault if you get upset' or 'I think most people are pretty stupid'. This model proved to be compatible with the data of blue- und white-collar workers. The parameter estimates do, however, differ for the two subsamples.

For blue-collar workers (fig. 2) the construct 'Hostility' had no direct influence on other risk conditions or on the heart disease. The role of the other variables essentially corresponds to that shown by the first model.

For white-collar workers (fig. 3) an influence of 'Hostility' on blood pressure is visible. However, no significant effect of blood pressure on myocardial infarction can be found, something for which I have no explanation for the moment. What claims our attention is that personal conflicts for white-collar workers, as opposed to blue-collar workers, affect three different variables: cigarette consumption, blood lipids, and myocardial infarction.

Since I do not want to make too much out of these positive results, for my third example I will show a more complex model (fig. 3), which did not prove acceptable (fig. 4). The interdependency of the traditional risk conditions is as before, but the psychological and sociological conditions are represented by four latent variables: (1) physical stress, indicated by physical working conditions and weekly working hours; (2) social stress, indicated by personal conflicts and work atmosphere; (3) job involvement, defined as before, and (4) sensitivity to bodily processes, indicated by items such as: 'I watch my body carefully to notice as soon as possible, when something is the matter.'

The extremely small probability of the χ^2 value shows that the extended assumptions of the model are not supported by the data. A detailed analysis of the results leads to the conclusion that probably the specified measurement model is not adequate.

Discussion

As far as the application of causal modeling is concerned, one can say that it is appropriate for this kind of problem. The models discussed are, however, somewhat daring since the 'causal distance' between social conditions and coronary heart disease is fairly large. If they have still proved compatible with the data, it is probably because they were weak, i.e. few restrictions have been specified. We lacked the more sophisticated biochemical data such as lipoprotein fractions (LDL/HDL) or catecholamines in order to obtain a more exact picture of the pathogenic mechanisms. The low path coefficients in some of the measurement models show that the selection and operationalization of the psychological constructs should be improved. This could well be done by the analysis of covariance structures.

Taking into consideration these limitations we still can say: (a) The traditional risk conditions retain their place as potential risk factors. By the introduction of psychological and sociological conditions they may become intervening variables. (b) Psychological and social conditions play different roles in different groups. Future should allow for accordingly differential problem formulations.

The further application of causal modeling should concentrate on small, experimentally researched sections of the problem area. This would then offer the possibility of bringing together causal relationships which have been individually experimentally established. The resultant models could epidemiologically, i.e. in the field, be proven valid.

References

1   Bentler, P.M.: The interdependence of theory, methodology, and empirical data: causal modeling as an approach to construct validation; in Kandel, Longitudinal research on drug use: empirical findings and methodological issues, pp. 267–302 (New York 1978).
2   Bentler, P.M.; Bonett, D.G.: Significance tests and goodness of fit in the analysis of covariance structures. Psychol. Bull. *88:* 588–606 (1980).
3   Henry, J.P.; Stephens, P.M.: Stress, health, and the social environment (New York 1977).
4   Jöreskog, K.G.: Structural analysis of covariance and correlation matrices. Psychometrika *43:* 443–477 (1978).
5   Jöreskog, K.G.; Sörbom, D.: LISREL IV user's guide (Chicago 1978).
6   Kenny, D.A.: Correlation and causality (New York 1979).
7   Pepping, G.: Different patterns of stress in patients with internal diseases; in Siegrist, Halhuber, Myocardial infarction and psychosocial risks, pp. 127–132 (Springer, Berlin 1981).
8   Steiger, J.H.: Testing pattern hypotheses on correlation matrices: alternative statistics and some empirical results. Multivar. Behav. Res. *15:* 335–352 (1980).
9   Williams, R.B.; Friedman, M.; Glass, D.C.; Herd, A.; Schneiderman, N.: Mechanisms linking behavioral and pathophysiological processes; in Dembroski, et al., Coronary-prone behavior, pp. 119–128 (Springer, New York 1978).
10   Young, J.W.: The function of theory in a dilemma of path analysis. J. appl. Psychol. *62:* 108–110 (1977).

5 Assessment Issues in Coronary-Prone Behavior

Karen A. Matthews

This paper discusses: (a) status of current knowledge about assessment of the type A coronary-prone behavior pattern; (b) measurement difficulties that have become apparent, and (c) three promising directions for measurement research to take. It is suggested that perhaps the greatest impedence to progress in understanding type A behavior and its associated coronary proneness has arisen by virtue of the way pattern A has been measured. It is hoped that in making explicit some of the assessment issues in coronary-prone behavior, refinements in the type A construct will be promoted and interest in coronary-prone behaviors will be broadened.

Description and Assessment of Pattern A

Pattern A is defined as a 'chronic, incessant struggle to achieve more and more in less and less time, and if required to do so, against the opposing efforts of other things or other persons' [15, p. 67]. The major facets or 'core' elements of this behavior pattern are extremes of aggressiveness, easily aroused hostility, a sense of time urgency, and competitive achievement striving [55]. Strictly speaking, the type A pattern is not considered to be a trait. Rather, it is a set of overt behaviors that is elicited from susceptible individuals by the appropriately challenging environment. Neither is the type A pattern considered to be a typology. Rather it is thought to be a continuum of behaviors ranging from extreme type A to extreme non-type A, or type B.

Assessment of pattern A has been accomplished by three measures, all of which are related prospectively to coronary heart disease in American samples: the Structured Interview (SI) [56]; the Jenkins Activity Survey (JAS) [28, 29]; and the Framingham Type A Scale [22]. While other scales purport to measure type A (Bortner Rating Scale [2]; Bortner Test Battery [3]; Sales Type A Measure [59]; and Vickers adaptation of the Sales Measure [68]), they have not been related to incidence of coronary heart disease and cannot be considered as measures of coronary-prone behavior at present. (At the conference meetings for which this paper was prepared, Dr. *M. Kornitzer* reported that the Bortner Rating Scale has been related to incidence of coronary heart disease in the Belgium Heart Disease Prevention Project. Thus, it appears that future research should focus on what this scale measures and should include it in the test battery of type A coronary-prone behaviors.) Therefore, they are not discussed here.

Structured Interview

The SI contains approximately 25 questions in which individuals are asked about their characteristic way of responding to a variety of situations that should elicit impatience, hostility, and competitiveness from type A individuals [55]. For example, individuals are asked about their reactions to working with a slow partner and to waiting in long lines. Another illustration is that they are asked if a spouse or close friend would describe them as hard-driving and competitive. More importantly, some of the questions are deliberately delivered in such a way as to elicit speech stylistics considered indicative of behavior pattern A. For example, a question with an obvious answer may be asked in a hesitant and slow manner. A type A person typically interrupts and answers the intended question prior to the question being fully asked. Or the interviewer may question the accuracy of an answer, in an attempt to arouse annoyance in a susceptible individual. Behavior pattern classificiation is based both on self-reports of type A behaviors and on speech behaviors observed during the interview itself, although the latter is considered to be more important in reaching a final judgment. The classification is essentially a clinical judgment whereby individuals are classified into one of four categories: A1, or fully developed type A; A2, or incompletely developed type A; Type X, or an equal representation of type A or type B characteristics; type B or an absence of type A characteristics. Judgments by two raters into the four categories and into A-B binary categories agree in 64 and 84% of subjects, respectively, while 80% of a sample of men had the same A-B binary classification at two points in time separated by 12–20 months [27].

In addition to the interview yielding an overall type A judgment, it can be scored reliably for answers to individual type A questions and for type A behaviors that are displayed during the interview [10, 46]. Factor analyses of these ratings in independent samples of male undergraduate and employed working men have yielded four independent factors: clinical ratings (of speech behaviors), and self-reports of pressured drive, anger, and competitiveness [48].

Jenkins Activity Survey

A second technique for pattern A assessment, the JAS, is a self-report measure. It contains 50+ questions similar to those used in the SI. Scoring of the items is based on optimal weights generated by a series of discriminant function analyses predicting the SI classification of large groups of middle-aged men [29]. *21* of the *50+* items contributed to the overall A-B score: 1 on hostility when younger; 5 on harddriving competitiveness; 8 on immediate, quick action; and 7 on a pressured style of working. The JAS A-B scores were normally distributed in the validation sample. Consequently, the JAS scores are standardized so that the mean of the A-B scores is zero with a standard deviation of 10. Positive scores indicate the pattern A direction; negative scores indicate the pattern B direction. Test-retest correlations across 1- to 4-year intervals fall between 0.60 and 0.70 [26].

In addition to yielding an overall A-B score, the JAS can yield three other scores based on repeated factor analyses of *all 50+* JAS items. These are H or hard-driving competitiveness, S or speed and impatience, and J or job involvement [71]. Each factor score has a mean of 0.0 and a standard deviation of 10.0 and is modestly related to the total type A score. None has been related prospectively to coronary heart disease [28].

Framingham Type A Scale

The third operational definition of pattern A, the Framingham Type A Scale, is a self-report measure that contains 10 items assessing the individual's competitive drive, sense of time urgency, and perceptions of job pressures [23]. These items were chosen from a 300-item inventory by a panel of experts as representing aspects of pattern A. Each item is unit weighted and summed to yield a total type A scale. Those scoring above the sample median are considered type A, whereas those who score below are considered type B. The scale has an internal reliability of 0.70.

Comparisons among Measures

The associations among the three operational definitions of type A, which purport to measure the same construct, are lower than one would expect. The JAS and the Framingham Type A Scale agree with the A-B classification made from the SI in about 60–70% of middle-aged white-collar and undergraduate men [22, 26, 37, 48]. By chance, agreement rates should be 50%, if one presumes that 50% of the population is type A. Thus, another way to view the above agreement rates is that the JAS and the Framingham type A measures agree with the SI classification in middle-class men

10–20% above chance levels. For women, the SI and the Framingham Type A Scale were related in an undergraduate sample [37], but not in an adult sample drawn from a predominantly blue-collar community [22]. Thus, it is incorrect to assume that the three type A measures assess the same aspects of pattern A. In brief, the type A measures only have the slimmest margin of overlap. Some of the reasons for this independence will be made apparent later.

What Do the Operational Definitions of Type A Measure?

Having described the three operational definitions of type A, we are now adequately prepared to review what is known presently about what they, in fact, do measure. As was made evident in the previous section, the assessment devices do not overlap substantially. Thus, it is necessary to review the evidence separately for each measure of type A. Because a detailed review of this literature is available elsewhere [42], only the major findings are discussed here.

Structured Interview
The SI has been used to assess type A primarily in psychophysiological and questionnaire studies of men. There have been few investigations of the behaviors of either men or women identified by the SI. The available few concur in showing that type As speak quickly, loudly, and explosively either when reading an exciting paragraph out loud or during the SI itself [14, 48, 60, 63]. Moreover, these speech behaviors are highly related to interview assessment and modestly related to other self-reported type A behaviors during the interview. Similarly, in several questionnaire studies, overall type A assessment was modestly related to self-reports of the basic descriptive elements of type A, e.g. aggressiveness, dominance [4, 7, 54]. These surprisingly low associations between overall type A and self-reported type A behaviors can be attributed to the fact that speech behaviors, which are highly related to overall type A assessment, do not relate highly to other type A behavioral characteristics. Also pertinent is that classification of a person as type A is based on a simple preponderance of type A characteristics. Thus, it is possible for one type A to interrupt the interviewer frequently and report being impatient, whereas another type A may never interrupt the interviewer but express his/her annoyance with an interviewer questioning the accuracy of his/her answers. Thus, psychometric imprecision may result because persons may be

classified as type As for different reasons. Consequently, it may be naive to expect strong associations between overall measures of type A and individual type A behaviors.

The emphasis in the SI on speech behaviors takes on added significance when viewed in light of recent data [12; 36, experiment 2]: the hemodynamic responses of type As to challenging psychomotor tasks [19, 40], which are suspected of playing a role in type As' coronary-risk, also occur during the SI itself [61]. Thus, it appears that the SI simultaneously predicts speech behaviors and cardiovascular changes of type A persons. This fact suggests that the SI may be measuring a general hyperreactivity to challenging events, including a provocative interview style.

In support of this notion is an impressive series of studies by *Matarazzo and Wiens* [41]. They report a strong 'synchrony effect' in which interviewees mimic an interviewer's speed of speech, length of utterance, and response latency. This synchrony effect probably occurs during the SI to some degree such that individuals most likely to be classified as type A are those who respond in kind to the interviewer's challenges.

If the SI does measure a general hyperreactivity, it would be useful to develop continuous measures of reactivity more refined and direct than the SI, which can yield only crude categorical assessments. Some investigators, in fact, are moving in that direction by coding continuous measures of component type A characteristics, including a number of speech behaviors (e.g. explosive, loud speech), which emerge collectively as an independent factor in two separate factor analyses and are highly related to overall assessment [48]. Other investigators are considering continuous measures of autonomic reactivity as the independent predictor variable [38]. It may be fruitful to join these two approaches in developing continuous reactivity measures.

Jenkins Activity Survey

The JAS has been used to assess type A primarily in psychophysiological and survey studies and experimental investigations of the overt behaviors of type A persons. Studies that fall in the last category clearly show that type As are competitive, achievement-oriented, and prefer a rapid pace of living. For example, type As persist in spite of fatigue or the possibility of failure [5, 17], ignore distractions that could interfere with task performance [44], and are aggressive in competitive interactions [6, 66]. Thus, it is not surprising that type As report rapid career advancement [52, 69] and receive more rewards from their work [17, 47].

What is not clear from the experimental studies is whether type A persons are more hostile. Several behavioral studies find no A-B differences in
hostility [20, experiment 2; 66] and, in addition, there are no self-report
studies of A-B hostility. Perhaps the JAS does not measure hostility because
it includes no items measuring either present hostility or other emotional correlates of type A. This is unfortunate as several emotional qualities, e.g. free-
floating hostility and life dissatisfaction, are directly implicated in the
etiology of coronary artery and heart disease and are included among the
behavioral descriptors of pattern A [22, 46, 51, 70].

It should also be noted that not only do the JAS items fail to assess anger,
but that they reflect white-collar, upwardly mobile values, and the Protestant
work ethic. It is possible that these items, while adequately measuring coronary-prone behaviors in white-collar men, may be less sensitive measures in
samples that do not share the above values [8].

A final point relevant here is that like the SI, the JAS does appear to
measure somewhat cardiovascular reactivity in men. Typically, however, the
JAS has less predictive strength than the SI and has little predictive value for
women [11, 36, 39, 67].

Framingham Type A Scale

The Framingham Type A Scale has been used in several survey studies.
This scale and 22 others had been constructed from a 300-item inventory
administered to members of the Framingham Heart Study. Correlations
between the Framingham Type A and remaining scales showed that type A
persons reported emotional lability, marital disagreements, aging and personal worries, daily stress, tension, anxiety, and experiencing many bodily
sensations when angry [23]. In another sample of middle-class men, the type
A scale was related to depression, neuroticism, and anxiety [7]. Taken,
together, these findings suggest that the Framingham Type A Scale uniquely
measures negative affect and adverse symptoms that are associated with a
competitive, pressured life-style.

It is of interest to note that unlike the Framingham measure, the SI and
JAS scores are not related strongly to anxiety measures [7, 53, 69; cf. 35], and
anxiety is related to incidence of coronary heart disease, particularly angina
[24, 25, 51].

Summary. The purpose of this section was to summarize precisely what
is known at present about the operational definitions of type A measure.
Because the SI, JAS, and Framingham type A Scale have only the slimmest

margin of overlap, it was necessary to review what each scale measures separately. This review reveals that the predominant characteristic assessed by the SI may be a general hyperreactivity to challenging environmental events. This reactivity takes the form of rapid, loud, and explosive speech as well as cardiovascular changes, indicative of sympathetic arousal. Type As assessed by the JAS can be characterized as rapid achievement-strivers, who can be aggressive and competitive. Men, but not women, show some indication of cardiovascular changes during difficult and moderately competitive events. Finally, type As assessed by the Framingham Type Scale can be characterized as dissatisfied and uncomfortable with life that has a competitive orientation and job pressures.

The above findings make it apparent why there is a lack of overlap among the three type A measures. The measures assess different characteristics and share little common method variance. Furthermore, they have been employed in different kinds of studies. Nonetheless, all are related to incidence of coronary heart disease and assess some of the behaviors collectively called the type A behavior pattern.

Assessment Problems in Type A

Perhaps the greatest impedence to progress in understanding type A behavior has been the tendency to use only one measure of type A in studies. This has been the case for at least two reasons. First, it was not recognized until recently that only the slimmest margin of overlap existed among the type A measures and the present paper has reviewed why: the measures assess different characteristics within the type A construct. This impedence to progress has been heightened by the fact that the measures have been used in different types of studies. In consequence, it has not been possible to find similar predictive relationships among the three measures and other variables. Nor has it been possible to integrate evidence concerning type A behavioral characteristics across measures.

The second reason for the failure to measure type A in a comprehensive manner is that the multidimensional nature of the type A construct has not been appreciated. As noted earlier, global measures of pattern A give little information about an individual's type A behaviors. An individual might be assessed as type A because she/he shows signs of hostility, although she/he is relatively slow to respond to questions. Another type A might show little hostility, but be very quick in responding. This psychometric imprecision renders interpretation of findings somewhat ambiguous because it is not known which aspects of type A are accounting for the results. In order to rectify this state of affairs, it is imperative that measures of individual type A behaviors [for scoring procedures see *Dembroski and MacDougall,* this volume; 10, 48] and several overall type A measures be included in future research.

A second assessment issue concerns measurement of type A on a continuum. While type A has been defined as a continuum, it has, for the most part, been treated as a typology. For example, the SI yields categorical assessments of A1, A2, X, and B. Because of the increasing preponderance of SI type As in at least American society [32], recent studies have tended to report differences between As and non-As and not even use the crude continuum available from the SI assessment. The JAS, which does yield a normal distribution of scores, is also typically treated as a categorical variable in data analyses [17, 28]. One consequence of treating type A as a typology might be the findings that typically type Bs tend to act differently from type As [45], not more or less intense as one would expect from conceptualizing type A as a continuum. More importantly, treating type A as a typology may have contributed to the absence of a dose-response relationship between type A and coronary disease [33, 56; cf. 28]. If one takes seriously either the original definition of type A as a continuum of behaviors or the suggestion in this paper that the SI is measuring a continuum of hyperreactivity elicited by challenging events, it would be wise to develop further and to use continuous measures of type A in future studies. At least, the hypothesis that type A might be best considered as a continuum merits testing.

Another assessment issue only alluded to earlier, but of major theoretical import to the definition of type A, is the failure to take seriously that type A is considered to be a set of overt behaviors resulting from a set of predispositions in a person and the appropriately challenging environment. Rather, type A has been treated (at least implicitly) as a trait variable without consideration of environmental elicitors. For example, the Western Collaborative Group Study, the first prospective study of the type A risk factor, did not include measures of the participants' life situation. Only their type A behavior was assessed. Furthermore, the measures of type A were expected to be somewhat reliable across the duration of the study, regardless of the changing life situation of the participants.

Treating type A as a trait variable has had two consequences. First, there has been a failure to specify in a systematic way the 'appropriately challenging' situations that produce type A behavior. A recent review [42] has revealed that behavioral differences between As and Bs are elicited by circumstances that (a) are moderately competitive; (b) are uncontrollable; (c) require endurance; (d) require slow, careful work, and (e) employ a broad focus of attention. However, these are a posteriori descriptions of elicitors of type A behavior. A priori descriptions of elicitors are needed.

Second, there has been a neglect of the frequency with which 'appropriately challenging' situations occur for any particular individual. The result of this oversight might be to underestimate the true coronary risk associated with type A. For example, two individuals might exhibit a similar frequency of type A behaviors during the SI, but a dissimilar frequency of type A behaviors during daily activities because the frequency of 'appropriately challenging' circumstances differ for the two people. Presumably the person with a higher frequency of challenging situations would be at higher risk. Thus, while assessment of type A based on a simple preponderance of type A behaviors during the SI is sufficient for predicting coronary heart disease, assessment of type A behavior based on a preponderance of type A behavior during daily activities may further improve type A's predictive power. In any case, knowledge of type A behaviors during daily activities will certainly improve understanding of the nature of the type A construct.

A final assessment issue concerns measures of disease endpoint. Just as different aspects of pattern A appear to be measured by different operational definitions of pattern A, so too might different aspects of pattern A relate to different clinical manifestations of coronary disease. While it is recognized that atherosclerosis is a basic substrate for all coronary heart disease, it is also thought that one or more of a variety of other pathopsychological processes precipitate the complications of atherosclerosis and give coronary heart disease its several clinical syndromes [30]. Consistent with this reasoning are data reported [24, 25, 30] which indicate that different facets of the behavior pattern are associated with future angina and myocardial infarction patients. Future angina patients report that they are reactive to environmental stimulation and frustration and openly competitive in many areas of their lives, but do not feel rushed for time. On the other hand, future myocardial infarction victims report they do *not* consider themselves harddriving and competitive and, in fact, they try to avoid interpersonal competition. They do, however, have a sense of involvement with work.

Additional support for this point comes from the 10,000 man prospective Israeli Heart Study. Future angina patients tended to report more life problems, had higher anxiety scores, and generally showed greater reactivity to environmental stress than did persons remaining healthy. No such trends were observed for future myocardial infarction victims [51]. Similarly, the Framingham Type A Scale, which is related to reporting adverse affect, including anxiety, appears to predict angina, but not infarction unless it is accompanied by angina [21].

New Assessment Directions

We have described what the operational definitions appear to measure and discussed some problems in refining the type A concept caused by the ways type A has been assessed. We now are ready to discuss three promising directions that take an assessment approach to understanding pattern A behavior and its associated coronary proneness.

The first direction to be discussed arose out of a concern that a large proportion of the population is classified as type A, but there is a relatively low incidence of coronary heart disease in type As [56]. The low specificity and sensitivity of the type A variable has led some investigators to suspect that the pathogenic mechanisms contributing to coronary heart disease are not distributed evenly throughout the type A group [18, 62]. Thus, it is possible that the physiological changes which lead to coronary disease appear only for some type A people. It is also possible that other psychosocial factors beside type A are related to these changes. These possibilities have led some investigators to begin to develop standardized ways to measure cardiovascular and neuroendocrine reactivity in response to laboratory tasks and to ascertain the behavioral characteristics, including type A, of reactors [18, 39, 40; *Dembroski and MacDougall,* this volume]. By such efforts, the field of coronary-prone behavior is broadened and increased specificity of the type A variable is likely.

A note of caution, however, is relevant here. It is important to remember in these efforts that the physiological and neuroendocrine mechanisms implicated in coronary heart disease are not well understood and their role in coronary heart disease is currently under debate in the biomedical community [57, 58]. Furthermore, sympathetic reactivity, which is thought to account for type A's coronary proneness, has not been firmly established as a predictor of clinical coronary heart disease, whereas type A has [42]. Thus, it is important to continue to make connections with type A until advances can be made in understanding pathogenic mechanisms.

A second promising direction for refining the type A construct comes from attempting to measure type A-like behaviors in samples that differ in cultural background and in incidence rates of coronary heart disease from the original validation sample. If type A-like behaviors have predictive significance for coronary heart disease and for the mechanisms by which type A is thought to exert its pathogenic influence in other populations, then the overlap between type A measured in the original validation sample and type A-like behaviors measured in other populations can increase understanding of the coronary-prone core of type A behavior.

An illustration of this approach comes from the analyses by *Cohen* et al. [8] of data from a prospective study of Japanese Americans in Hawaii. In that study, type A measured by the JAS was related to the prevalence of coronary heart disease. However, the dimensions of type A were organized differently in this sample than in the validation sample of Caucasian Americans. That is, instead of factors S (speed and impatience), H (hard-driving competitiveness), and J (job involvement) emerging from the factor analyses of JAS items, portions of the original factors H and S including having a temper, hurrying a speaker, and an orientation toward hard-driving, competitive behavior emerged on one factor. The two other factors that emerged from the analyses were a hardworking factor and a strong job orientation factor. Analyses of the association of these factors with heart disease showed that men who reported being hard-driving and Westernized had the highest prevalence of disease. Strong job orientation and hardworking factors were unrelated to disease. Distinctions such as these probably could not be discerned as easily in American populations since in these populations hard-driving and hardworking behaviors are often closely related to one another. In the Japanese culture, it is relatively easy to find a hardworking person and relatively difficult to find a hard-driving person. In this group with low coronary heart disease rates, it was possible to distinguish these two concepts from one another with a resulting increased understanding of type A behavior.

Another illustration of this approach comes from work on the origins of type A. Several groups of investigators are assessing overt type A-like behaviors in children and adolescence and relating them to the pathogenic mechanisms suspected of accounting for type As' coronary risk [34, 43, 49, 50]. If specific type A-like behaviors do have the same predictive significance in children for cardiovascular reactivity, for example, as they do in adults, the overlap between type A measured in adults and type A-like behaviors measured in children can aid in identifying the critical core of pattern A behavior. Furthermore, it would suggest when in the life span type A behaviors might become associated with coronary risk. After all, the development of atherosclerosis is a life-long process, which can begin in the first or second decade of life. In any event, understanding the etiology of pattern A can lead to increased understanding of the type A construct itself.

The third and final promising direction (to be discussed here) that can promote understanding of type A is comprehensive measurement of coronary-prone behavior. There has been a tendency to study type A and its effects in isolation and without consideration of how other behavioral risk factors might interact with the type A variable in producing its effects. Thus, it has not been possible to benefit from research on other behavioral risk factors in an effort to understand what type A is and why it is coronary-prone. In light of the low specificity and sensitivity of the type A variable, it is particularly worthwhile to make connection with literature on coronary-prone behaviors defined more broadly. Take the following illustration as an example. One of the reasons suggested by *Scherwitz* et al. [62] for the low specificity and sensitivity of type A is that those type As who remain healthy have some sort of protective mechanism against coronary risk. Stated differently, those type A cardiac patients may lack some important protective mechanism. One important protective mechanism against disease appears to be social support, i.e. reporting that one has friends and family to rely on [1, 31; *Henry*, this volume]. It is reasonable to suggest that the hostility component of type A interferes with developing an adequate social network and disturbs ongoing social and work relationships. Thus, hostile type As may increase their susceptibility to coronary disease because they lack social support. However, measuring type A in isolation would not permit uncovering this aspect of the coronary-prone core of type A.

Another possible reason for the low sensitivity and specificity of type A is that the pathogenic aspects of type A may be elicited only by a specific inhospitable environment. For example, some evidence indicates that an incongruity between the status of one's background and the present is related to incidence of coronary heart disease [16, 64]. Type As may be more likely to experience this incongruity in status than are Bs because they expect and do advance rapidly in their career [47, 52]. More importantly for the present argument, it also seems likely that an environment that makes salient the discrepancy between one's original and present status would elicit, in particular from the type A, continued striving to maintain one's status. Presumably the continual struggle to earn one's position is accompanied by pathophysiological processes inimical to cardiovascular health. If this notion is correct, then the risk associated with type A is exacerbated by a specific inhospitable environment. Indeed, similar reasoning is advanced by *Glass* [17] when he suggested that the interaction of type A and uncontrollable life events is particularly detrimental to cardiovascular health.

Other behavioral risk factors deserve attention in the effort to place type A in the context of coronary-prone behaviors. Life events, particularly those concerning work, anxiety, depression, bereavement, life problems, work overload, and anger are among the behavioral variables associated with coronary disease that are candidates for further study in relation to type A [9, 22, 24, 25, 51, 65]. It should be noted that while comprehensive measurement of these and other coronary-prone behaviors can increase understanding of type A, it also can broaden the focus of investigations and permit the development of more sophisticated, albeit complex etiologic models of person-environment interactions in the pathogenesis of coronary disease.

Conclusions

This paper has considered assessment issues in coronary-prone behavior. Evidence concerning what each of the three operational definitions of type A measure was reviewed. This review made apparent that the three operational definitions measure different aspects of type A and that some problems have resulted from the way type A is assessed. In order to correct these oversights, it is recommended that type A be assessed in a comprehensive manner and on a continuum, that environmental elicitors of type A be measured, and that specific classifications of coronary heart disease be utilized. By doing such, refinements in the definition of the type A coronary-prone behavior pattern are possible. The paper concludes with a discussion of three promising directions in the area of assessment: development of stable measures of physiological responsivity to standardized environmental events; measurement of type A-like behaviors in samples that vary in cultural background and in incidence rates of coronary heart disease from the original sample in which type A was validated; and comprehensive assessment of type A along with other behavioral risk factors for coronary heart disease. While the paper has focused on understanding type A and its associated coronary-risk from an assessment perspective, it also suggests that future research should broaden its focus beyond type A. In this way, more sophisticated, albeit complex, etiologic models of person-environment interactions in the pathogenesis of coronary disease can be developed.

Acknowledgement

This paper was written during the tenure of an Established Investigatorship from the American Heart Association with funds contributed in part by the American Heart Association Pennsylvania Affiliate and was facilitated by Grant No. NIH-RO1 HL 25767-02. The author thanks *David Krantz* for his critical evaluation of an earlier version of this paper.

References

1   Berkman, L.F.; Syme, L.: Social networks, host resistance, and mortality. A nine year fol-low-up study of Alameda County residents. Am. J. Epidem. *109:* 186–204 (1979).

2   Bortner, R.W.: A short rating scale as a potential measure of pattern A behavior. J. chron. Dis. *22:* 87 (1969).

3   Bortner, R.W.; Rosenman, R.H.: The measurement of pattern A behavior. J. chron. Dis. *20:* 525–533 (1967).

4   Caffrey, B.: Reliability and validity of personality and behavioral measures in a study of coronary heart disease. J. chron. Dis. *21:* 191–204 (1968).

5   Carver, C.S.; Coleman, A.E.; Glass, D.C.: The coronary-prone behavior pattern and the suppression of fatigue on a treadmill test. J. Personal. soc. Psychol. *33:* 460–466 (1976).

6   Carver, C.S.; Glass, D.C.: Coronary-prone behavior pattern and interpersonal aggression. J. Personal. soc. Psychol. *36:* 361–366 (1978).

7   Chesney, M.A.; Black, G.W.; Chadwick, J.H.; Rosenman, R.H.: Psychological correlates of the type A behavior pattern. J. behav. Med. *4:* 217–229 (1981).

8   Cohen, J.B.; Syme, S.L.; Jenkins, C.D.; Kagan, A.; Zyzanski, S.J.: Cultural context of type A behavior and risk for CHD. A study of Japanese American males. J. behav. Med. *2:* 375–384 (1979).

9   Cottington, E.M.; Matthews, K.A.; Talbott, E.; Kuller, L.H.: Environmental events pre-ceding sudden death in women. Psychosom. Med. *42:* 567–574 (1980).

10 Dembroski, T.M.: Reliability and validity of methods used to assess coronary-prone behavior; in Dembroski et al., Coronary-prone behavior (Springer, New York 1978).

11 Dembroski, T.M.; MacDougall, J.M.; Herd, J.A.; Shields, J.L.: Effects of level of challenge on pressor and heart responses in type A and B subjects. J. appl. soc. Psychol. *9:* 209–228 (1979).

12 Dembroski, T.M.; MacDougall, J.M.; Lushene, R.: Interpersonal interaction and car-diovascular response in type A subjects and coronary patients. J. hum. Stress *5:* 28–36 (1979).

13 Dembroski, T.M.; Weiss, S.M.; Shields, J.; Haynes, S.; Feinleib, M. (eds): Coronary-prone behavior (Springer, New York 1978).

14 Friedman, M.; Brown, M.A.; Rosenman, R.H.: Voice analysis test for detection of behavior pattern. J. Am. med. Ass. *208:* 828–836 (1969).

15 Friedman, M.; Rosenman, R.: Type A behavior and your heart (Knopf, New York 1974).

16 Gillum, R.F.; Paffenbarger, R.S.: Chronic disease in former college students. Am. J. Epidem. *108:* 289–298 (1978).

17 Glass, D.C.: Behavior patterns, stress, and coronary disease (Erlbaum, Hillsdale 1977).

18   Glass, D.C.: Type A behavior: mechanisms linking behavioral and pathophysiologic pro-
      cesses; in Siegrist, Halhuber (eds), Myocardial infarction and psychosocial risks (Springer,
      New York 1981).
19   Glass, D.C.; Krakoff, L.R.; Contrada, R.; Hilton, W.F.; Kehoe, K.; Mannucci, E.G.; Col-
      lins, C.; Snow, S.; Elting, E.: Effect of harassment and competition upon cardiovascular
      and catecholaminic response in type A and type B individuals. Psychophysiology *17:* 453–
      463 (1980).
20   Glass, D.C.; Snyder, M.L.; Hollis, J.: Time urgency and the type A coronary-prone
      behavior pattern. J. appl. soc. Psychol. *4:* 125–140 (1974).
21   Haynes, S.G.; Feinleib, M.: Type A behavior and incidence of coronary heart disease in
      the Framingham Heart Study; in Denolin, Psychological problems before and after myo-
      cardial infarction. Adv. Cardiol., vol. 29, pp. 85–95 (Karger, Basel 1982).
22   Haynes, S.G.; Feinleib, M.; Kannel, W.B.: The relationship of psychosocial factors to
      coronary heart disease in the Framingham Study. III. Eight-year incidence of coronary
      heart disease. Am. J. Epidem. *111:* 37–58 (1980).
23   Haynes, S.G.; Levine, S.; Scotch, N.; Feinleib, M.; Kannel, W.B.: The relationship of
      psychosocial factors to coronary heart disease in the Framingham Study. I. Methods and
      risk factors. Am. J. Epidem. *107:* 362–383 (1978).
24   Jenkins, C.D.: Psychologic and social precursors of coronary disease. New Engl. J. Med.
      284: 244–255, 307–317 (1971).
25   Jenkins, C.D.: Recent evidence supporting psychologic and social risk factors for coronary
      disease. New Engl. J. Med. *294:* 987–994, 1033–1038 (1976).
26   Jenkins, C.D.: A comparative review of the interview and questionnaire methods in the
      assessment of the coronary-prone behavior pattern; in Dembroski et al., Coronary-prone
      behavior (Springer, New York 1978).
27   Jenkins, C.D.; Rosenman, R.H.; Friedman, M.: Replicability of rating the coronary-prone
      behavior pattern. Br. J. prev. soc. Med. *22:* 16–22 (1968).
28   Jenkins, C.D.; Rosenman, R.H.; Zyzanski, S.J.: Prediction of clinical coronary heart dis-
      ease by a test of the coronary-prone behavior pattern. New Engl. J. Med. *23:* 1271–1275
      (1974).
29   Jenkins, C.D.; Zyzanski, S.J.; Rosenman, R.H.: Progress toward validation of a com-
      puter-scored test for the type A coronary-prone behavior pattern. Psychosom. Med. *33:*
      193–202 (1971).
30   Jenkins, C.D.; Zyzanski, S.J.; Rosenman, R.H.: Coronary-prone behavior: one pattern or
      several? Psychosom. Med. *40:* 25–43 (1978).
31   Joseph, J.G.; Syme, S.L.: Social affiliation, risk factors, and CHD. Proc. Annu. Meet. Am.
      Heart Association Council on Epidemiology, Washington 1981.
32   Krantz, D.S.; Glass, D.C.; Schaeffer, M.A.; Davia, J.E.: Behavior patterns and coronary
      disease: a critical evaluation; in Cacioppo, Petty, Perspectives in cardiovascular psycho-
      physiology (Guilford, New York 1982).
33   Krantz, D.S.; Sanmarco, M.E.; Selvester, R.H.; Matthews, K.A.: Psychological correlates
      of progression of atherosclerosis in men. Psychosom. Med. *41:* 467–475 (1979).
34   Lawler, K.A.; Allen, M.T.; Critcher, E.C.; Standard, B.A.: The relationship of psycholog-
      ical responses to the coronary-prone behavior pattern in children. J. behav. Med. *4:* 203–
      216 (1981).
35   Lovallo, W.R.; Pishkin, V.: Type A behavior, self-involvement, autonomic activity, and
      the traits of neuroticism and extraversion. Psychosom. Med. *42:* 329–334 (1980).

36 MacDougall, J.M.; Dembroski, T.M.; Krantz, D.S.: Effects of types of challenge on pressor and heart rate responses in type A and B women. Psychophysiology *18:* 1–9 (1981).

37 MacDougall, J.M.; Dembroski, T.M.; Musante, L.: The structured interview and questionnaire methods of assessing coronary-prone behavior in male and female college students. J. behav. Med. *2:* 71–83 (1979).

38 Manuck, S.B.; Corse, C.D.; Winkleman, P.A.: Behavioral correlates of individual differences in blood pressure reactivity. J. psychosom. Res. *23:* 281–288 (1979).

39 Manuck, S.B.; Craft, S.A.; Gold, K.J.: Coronary-prone behavior pattern and cardiovascular response. Psychophysiology *15:* 403–411 (1978).

40 Manuck, S.B.; Garland, F.N.: Coronary-prone behavior pattern, task incentive, and cardiovascular response. Psychophysiology *16:* 139–142 (1979).

41 Matarazzo, J.D.; Wiens, A.N.: The interview: research on its anatomy and structure (Aldine-Atherton, New York 1972).

42 Matthews, K.A.: What is the type A (coronary-prone) behavior pattern from a psychological perspective? Psychol. Bull. *91:* 293–323 (1982).

43 Matthews, K.A.; Angulo, J.: Measurement of the type A behavior pattern in children: assessment of children's competitiveness, impatience anger, and aggression. Child Dev. *51:* 466–475 (1980).

44 Matthews, K.A.; Brunson, B.I.: Allocation of attention and the type A coronary-prone behavior pattern. J. Personal. soc. Psychol. *37:* 2081–2090 (1979).

45 Matthews, K.A.; Glass, D.C.: Type A behavior, stressful life events, and coronary heart disease; in Dohrenwend, Dohrenwend, Stressful life events and their contexts (Prodist, New York 1981).

46 Matthews, K.A.; Glass, D.C.; Rosenman, R.H.; Bortner, R.W.: Competitive drive, pattern A, and coronary heart disease: a further analysis of some data from the Western Collaborative Group Study. J. chron. Dis. *30:* 489–498 (1977).

47 Matthews, K.A.; Helmreich, R.L.; Beane, W.E.; Lucker, G.W.: Pattern A, achievement-striving and scientific merit: Does pattern A help or hinder? J. Personal. soc. Psychol. *39:* 962–967 (1980).

48 Matthews, K.A.; Krantz, D.S.; Dembroski, T.M.; MacDougall, J.M.: The unique and common variance in the Structured Interview and the Jenkins Activity Survey measures of the type A behavior pattern. J. Personal. soc. Psychol. *42:* 303–313 (1982).

49 Matthews, K.A.; Siegel, J.M.: The type A behavior pattern in children and adolescents: assessment, development, and associated coronary-risk; in Baum, Singer, Handbook of health and medical psychology, vol. 2 (Erlbaum, Hillsdale 1982).

50 Matthews, K.A.; Volkin, J.I.: Efforts to excel and the type A behavior pattern in children. Child Dev. *52:* 1283–1289 (1981).

51 Medalie, J.H.; Goldbourt, U.: Angina pectoris among 10,000 men. Am. J. Med. *60:* 910–921 (1976).

52 Mettlin, C.: Occupational careers and the prevention of coronary-prone behavior. Soc. Sci. Med. *10:* 367–372 (1976).

53 Nielson, W.R.; Dobson, K.S.: The coronary-prone behavior pattern and trait anxiety: evidence for discriminant validity. J. consult. clin. Psychol. *48:* 546–547 (1980).

54 Rahe, R.H.; Hervig, L.; Rosenman, R.H.: The heritability of type A behavior. Psychosom. Med. *40:* 478–486 (1978).

55 Rosenman, R.H.: The interview method of assessment of the coronary-prone behavior pattern; in Dembroski et al., Coronary-prone behavior (Springer, New York 1978).

56   Rosenman, R.H.; Brand, R.J.; Jenkins, C.D.; Friedman, M.; Straus, R.; Wurm, M.: Coro-
      nary heart disease in the Western Collaborative Group Study: final follow-up experience
      of 8½ years. J. Am. med. Ass. *233:* 872–877 (1975).
57   Ross, R.; Glomset, J.A.: The pathogenesis of atherosclerosis. 1. New Engl. J. Med. *295:*
      369–377 (1976).
58   Ross, R.; Glomset, J.A.: The pathogenesis of atherosclerosis. 2. New Engl. J. Med. *295:*
      420–425 (1976).
59   Sales, S.M.: Differences among individuals in affective, behavioral, biochemical and
      physiological responses to variations in work load; doct. diss., Ann Arbor (1969). Disserta-
      tion Abstracts International, 1969 (University Microfilms No. 60-18098).
60   Scherwitz, L.; Berton, K.; Leventhal, H.: Type A assessment and interaction in the
      behavior pattern interview. Psychosom. Med. *39:* 229–240 (1977).
61   Scherwitz, L.; Berton, K.; Leventhal, H.: Type A behavior, self-involvement, and car-
      diovascular response. Psychosom. Med. *40:* 593–609 (1978).
62   Scherwitz, L.; Leventhal, H.; Cleary, P.; Laman, C.: Type A behavior: consideration for
      risk modification. Health Values: Achieving High Levels of Wellness *2:* 291–296 (1978).
63   Schucker, B.; Jacobs, D.R.: Assessment of behavioral risk of coronary disease by voice
      characteristics. Psychosom. Med. *39:* 219–228 (1977).
64   Shekelle, R.B.; Ostfeld, A.M.; Oglesby, P.: Social status and incidence of coronary heart
      disease. J. chron. Dis. *22:* 381–394 (1969).
65   Theorell, T.; Lind, E.; Floderus, G.: The relationship of disturbing life changes and emo-
      tions to the early development of myocardial infarction and other serious illnesses. Int. J.
      Epidemiol. *4:* 281 (1975).
66   Van Egeren, L.F.: Social interactions, communications, and the coronary-prone behavior
      pattern: a psychophysiological study. Psychosom. Med. *41:* 2–18 (1979).
67   Van Egeren, L.F.: Cardiovascular changes during social competition in a mixed motive
      game. J. Personal. soc. Psychol. *37:* 858–864 (1979).
68   Vickers, R.: A short measure of the type A personality; unpublished manuscript, Ann
      Arbor (1973).
69   Waldron, I.: The coronary-prone behavior pattern, blood pressure, employment and
      socio-economic status in women. J. psychosom. Res. *22:* 79–87 (1978).
70   Williams, R.B.; Haney, T.L.; Lee, K.L.; Kong, Y.; Blumenthal, J.A.; Whalen, R.E.: Type
      A behavior, hostility, and coronary atherosclerosis. Psychosom. Med. *41:* 539–550 (1980).
71   Zyzanski, S.J.; Jenkins, C.D.: Basic dimensions within the coronary-prone behavior pat-
      tern. J. chron. Dis. *22:* 781–795 (1970).

6 Occupational Setting and Coronary-Prone Behavior in Men and Women

Margaret A. Chesney

Work is an integral part of the type A (coronary-prone) behavior pattern definition, that emphasizes aggression, ambitiousness, competitiveness, and work orientation [28]. The importance of work to type A behavior is also reflected in the tools used in its assessment that emphasize questions about the worksetting [34]. Moreover, there are strong indications that work environments elicit and reward the type A behavior pattern [9]. In this paper, the relationship between the world of work and the type A behavior pattern in women and in men will be reviewed. First, the prevalence of type A behavior in men and women will be presented. Type A behavior and coronary heart disease (CHD) risk in working and non-working women will be compared to provide insight into the relative contribution of work to the behavior pattern. The possibility that the importance of work in type A behavior may be an artifact of the measurement evices' reliance on work, rather than to the work itself, will be discussed. Second, the relationship between occupational achievement and type A behavior will be reviewed. Achievement in terms of traditional sex roles as well as the relationship of sex roles to type A behavior will be included in this review. Third, the interaction between the behavior pattern and specific working conditions will be discussed as a mechanism by which type A behavior leads to CHD risk. Finally, future directions for research on coronary-prone behavior in the occupational setting will be proposed.

Type A Behavior Prevalence and the World of Work

The coronary-prone behavior pattern is associated with increased prevalence and incidence of CHD, and with coronary atherosclerosis in both men and women [*Rosenman*, this volume]. Men show a higher prevalence of the type A behavior pattern than women [17, 38]. This sex difference may reflect some inherited sex differences in aggressiveness but is more likely to be due to sex differences in socialization [24, 34].

A higher prevalence of type A behavior has been found among working women as compared to non-working women [17, 35, 38], indicating the importance of work in the behavior pattern. Using the Jenkins Activity Survey (JAS) to measure type A behavior, *Waldron* [35] found a higher prevalence of type A among women employed full-time (i.e. more than 30 h per week) than among homemakers (i.e. not employed outside the home) and women employed part-time. Similarly, *Haynes* et al. [17, 18] found a strong relationship between type A behavior in women and working using a 6-item scale drawn from the Framingham Study interview questionnaire. Women who had been employed over half their adult lives had type A scores almost identical to those of men, and higher than women who worked less than half their adult lives.

Type A and the Working Woman

Individual as well as environmental factors have been discussed in an attempt to account for the higher prevalence of type A behavior among working women [34]. Women who are achievement-oriented and hard-driving, i.e. type A, may be more likely to pursue careers and less likely to leave the work force once a member. Studies showing a higher need for achievement among employed women [1, 22] support this hypothesis as does the finding that the relationship between type A behavior and working is stronger among women who work because they prefer to than among women working in response to financial pressure [38]. This preference for work may account for the higher JAS type A scores observed among employed women in their mid-thirties than employed women in their mid-twenties [38]. Also consistent with the concept of type A women expressing a need for achievement, non-working type A women were found to be more involved in volunteer work activities than non-working type B women [35].

Work pressure is another factor that may play a role in the higher levels of type A behavior among working women. The stresses and strains associated with working may elicit type A behavior in women. Compared to homemakers, gainfully employed women have considerably less free time [31] yet they often carry many of the same child-rearing and housekeeping responsibilities as their non-working counterparts. Such time and work pressure would likely be stronger for working women in their mid-thirties than those in their mid-twenties since more women in the former group have children [38]. *Waldron* [34] found that type A women are more likely than type B women to work in jobs they preferred and to keep a job even when they feel burdened by the dual demands of their job and home. This finding is consistent with research which show type A men and women persist in tiring treadmill testing and report less fatigue than type Bs [6, 39].

Type A and Work: A Measurement Artifact?

It is important to note that *Waldron's* studies showing a link between type A and non-traditional work roles for women relied on the JAS, a type A measure initially developed and refined in research with male subjects. It is possible that her findings concerning type A behavior and work among women may be an artifact of using measures that were developed for men and emphasized work.

From this perspective it is interesting to look more closely at the Framingham Study [16–18], which used a type A scale that is less related to work than the JAS, and which has been related to CHD outcome data.

Controlling for the standard CHD risk factors, type A behavior as assessed by the Framingham 6-item scale was found to predict CHD incidence among working women and housewives [16]. (Women who had worked over half of their lives outside the home were classified 'working women'; otherwise, women were classified as 'housewives' [17].) Working women had higher type A scores and higher CHD incidence rates than housewives (7.8 and 5.4%, respectively) but this difference was not significant. Among the working women, clerical workers had the highest CHD rate (10.6%), nearly twice that of housewives [15]. The observed incidence of CHD in the housewives group is undoubtedly influenced by the 'healthy worker effect' [25]. That is, certain women are selected into the workforce because they are relatively healthy, while less healthy women, who are less able to seek, obtain, or hold jobs, become housewives [32]. In summary, the results of the Framingham Study indicate that the relationship between work and type A behavior is not an artifact of measurement and that both work and the behavior pattern are related to CHD incidence.

Occupational Achievement and Type A Behavior

Initial studies of type A behavior in the occupational setting focused on correlates of the behavior pattern. A relationship between type A behavior and occupational status was found in a study of 2,010 males from 23 occupational groups from 67 different worksites [5]. Among the occupational groups studied were physicians, air traffic controllers, train dispatchers and scientists. A 49-item type A scale developed by *Sales* [29] was administered along with other self-report measures to assess job stress and psychological strain, among other variables. Although relationships between type A behavior and stress variables were examined, the only significant correlate of type A behavior was occupational status. Similar relationships between type A behavior (assessed by the JAS) and work status were found in a study of 943 white-collar, middle-class males from five organizations in Buffalo, New York [26], and in the Western Collaborative Group Study [41].

The relationship between occupational status and type A behavior was observed for both women and men in the Framingham Study [18] and in the Chicago Heart Association Detection Project in Industry [30, 34]. In the Chicago Detection Project, socioeconomic status as defined by education and occupation was positively related to type A on the JAS among 5,347 employed men and women. With regard to women, when the effects of age and occupational status were controlled, women were found to have type A scores that are equivalent to those for men [34].

The type A behavior pattern is associated with achievement among men and women. *Mettlin* [26] found the type A behavior pattern to be related to rapid career development among males, as indicated by rank and income relative to age. Men with high type A scores in the JAS reported their employers as having high expectations for the quality and quantity of work performed, and for the competitiveness of their work. From his research, *Mettlin* [26, p. 367] concluded, 'type A behavior is integral to the modern occupational career and that attempts to alter the occurrence of type A behavior in the general population might conflict with valued aspects of the individual's career and may therefore meet with significant resistance.'

Although type A behavior is associated with occupational status, no studies have yet documented a relationship between the behavior pattern, and advancement or achievement in employed women. However, the behavior pattern has been shown to be related to achievement orientation as reflected by upward educational mobility among women [34] and in achievement among college students [36].

The type A behavior pattern may contribute more to achievement success in traditional male roles than in female roles [35]. As discussed previously, succes in the vocational sphere as reflected by occupational status is related to the behavior pattern in women. However, type A behavior is not related to factors that might be considered measures of success from the perspective of the traditional female role, i.e. marital status and husband's occupational status [35].

The research on the prevalence and occupational correlates of type A behavior suggests that type A behavior is more consistent with the traditional male sex-role. *Mix and Lohr* [27] studied the relationship between sex-role orientation as defined by the Bem Sex-Role Inventory [2] and scores on a student form of the JAS [14] and found a significant positive correlation between type A behavior and self-rated masculine sex-role characteristics for both male and female college students. Being of the male sex accounted for only a small proportion of the variance in type A scores. These findings are consistent with the hypothesis that higher prevalence of type A behavior in males results from social modeling and reinforcement of male sex-role stereotypes. As women acquire these stereotyped characteristics that are consistent with career orientation and achievement in the workplace, their rates of type A behavior and, perhaps, CHD will increase.

Behavior Pattern and Work Environment Interaction

The original conceptualization of the type A behavior pattern, described type A behavior as a characteristic response pattern that is evoked by challenges in the social and physical environment. More recently attention has been turned to this interaction as the arena where the behavior pattern's response to challenge triggers a pathophysiologic process which leads eventually to clinical manifestations of CHD. Laboratory research focusing on this interaction is providing evidence that, under certain challenging situations, type As more than type Bs show the neuroendocrine and cardiovascular responses to stress that are thought to be aspects of this pathophysiologic process. As challenging environments, occupational settings are of interest because they may trigger the neuroendocrine and cardiovascular responses that are part of the pathophysiologic process in type As [*Dembroski and MacDougall, Schmidt, Williams*, this volume].

Much of the early research on the interface between type A behavior and work environments focused on differences between descriptions type As and type Bs gave to their work settings. One such study [20] compared managers classified as type A or type B by the Structured Interview (SI). Type As reported longer work weeks, working more discretionary hours, higher work loads and work competition, difficulty in satisfying conflicting demands and heavier supervisory responsibilities than type Bs. Another related study [21] examined the techniques type As used to cope with the pressures at work. Type As relied on changing to a different *work* activity for coping, a technique found to be the least effective of those studied. Thus, rather than 'cope' with challenging stress by diversion or relaxation, type As 'dig in' and continue work activity.

In a study of 127 senior administrators of Canadian correctional institutions, *Burke and Weir* [3] found significant relationships between type A scores on the 44-item type A scale developed by *Sales* [29] and work demands, stressful work-related life events, interference of work with home life, and marital dissatisfaction. On the other hand, higher scores on this type A scale were significantly related to self-esteem and life satisfaction. These findings indicate that type As describe their work as challenging and experience some negative consequences of this challenge in terms of non-work-related life factors (e.g. marital dissatisfaction), but, rather than being a source of distress, the challenge of their jobs is a source of self-satisfaction.

The research examining the relationship between type A behavior and CHD risk factors assessed in the work settings is less consistent than that looking at the relationship of type A behavior and challenge at work. In one study *Howard* et al. [19] observed type A managers to have significantly higher blood pressures than did type B managers. The relationships between type A behavior and serum cholesterol and triglycerides were found to be U-shaped with extreme type As and type Bs having higher levels than moderate type As and type Bs. In the Framingham Study [18], type A behavior was significantly related to blood pressure among male white-collar workers, and inversely related to serum cholesterol among male white- and blue-collar workers. In their study of correctional institution administrations, *Burke and Weir* [3] also examined the relationship between type A and CHD risk factors, finding few significant associations. Although type A scores were directly related to pounds overweight, they were inversely related to systolic blood pressure and serum cholesterol. *Burke and Weir* [3] suggest that their method of type A assessment may account for the lack of relationships between type A behavior and CHD risk. However, in another study [8] the type A SI was used to assess the behavior pattern in 384 middle managers in an aerospace industry and no direct relationships between the behavior pattern and CHD risk factors were found.

Type A Behavior and Person-Environment Fit

Research that has focused on the interaction between the person and his or her work environment, i.e. the person-environment fit, may be providing some insight into the link between CHD risk and type A behavior in the work setting. The person-environment fit concept suggests that a lack of fit constitutes a challenge or stressor. As with the research showing type A response to challenge in the laboratory, type As show enhanced cardiovascular arousal in response to the challenge of a poor person-environment fit. Type A individuals are described previously as deriving self-satisfaction from work pressure. Thus, type As experience a lack of 'fit' in work settings characterized by little work pressure. In an examination of such a situation, type As reported more distress and showed more arousal in terms of catecholamine and cortisol excretion and heart rate during inactivity than during strenuous mental work [13]. The opposite pattern was found for type Bs. That is, type B persons reported more distress and showed higher levels of arousal during strenuous mental work than inactivity. Thus, both type As and type Bs showed cardiovascular response levels that were higher when there was a lack of fit.

In the study of 384 middle managers in an aerospace industry [8] referred to previously, similar significant person-environment interactions were observed. The type A behavior pattern has been found to be correlated with measures of autonomy and extroversion [7]. Type A managers in work environments that do not encourage autonomy, or where peer cohesion (allowing expression of extroversion) is low, were found to have higher blood pressures. Conversely, type B managers had higher blood pressures in work environments that encourage autonomy and peer involvement. Type B managers also had higher systolic blood pressures in work environments low in physical comfort (i.e. poor lighting, too cold, etc.) than type B managers in comfortable work environments. There was no relationship between work environment, physical comfort and blood pressure of type As. Perhaps type As are so job-involved, they are insensitive to their physical surroundings just as they were found to focus on task performance in treadmill testing and not report fatigue [6, 39].

It is difficult to generalize the person-environment concept to women because the appropriate work environment 'fit' for type A and type B women is not known, given the dual role expectations and rapid social changes. One study of women managers [12] found that women classified as type A based on the Bortner Self-Rating Scale reported higher levels of frustration, irritation and anxiety than their type B associates. Although irritation or hostility has long been considered an aspect of the type A behavior pattern [28], the type A behavior pattern is not related directly to anxiety [7]. However, in certain situations, interactions between type A behavior and environmental factors have shown a relationship to anxiety. For example, type A computer users reported more anxiety than type B users when confronted with a major stressor in their work environment – a computer shutdown [4]; type A managers reported significantly more anxiety when in a work environment in which they were under the control of others than when they were in an environment that allowed them to be in control [10]. Perhaps women managers, as well as many other working and non-working women, may be uncertain about their roles and, thus, experience a chronic lack of fit with their work and home environments.

Work-Related Coronary-Prone Behaviors

The Framingham Study identified work-related behaviors that predict clinical coronary events during an 8-year follow-up [16]. The research reviewed thus far was limited to the relationship between type A behavior and CHD risk factors. The Framingham Study [16], on the other hand, identified work-related coronary-prone behaviors that are independent of the standard CHD risk factors. Among white-collar working males, type A behavior and suppressed hostility were significantly related among men between 45 and 64 years of age. Type A behavior was not significantly related to CHD incidence among blue-collar males. This lack of predictive power with blue-collar workers may relate to the fact that the behavior pattern was formulated primarily within white-collar settings and may not generalize well to blue-collar workers. However, while the number of promotions received was not associated with incidence of CHD among white-collar workers, it was significantly associated with CHD among blue-collar workers. In summary, the Framingham Study indicates that the challenge of promotions at work is coronary-prone for male blue-collar workers, whereas, type A behavior and hostility are coronary-prone for male white-collar workers.

Among women, type A behavior and suppressed hostility were found to be independently associated with CHD incidence [16]. When housewives and working women were examined separately, different coronary-prone behaviors emerged. For the 350 housewives studied, a self-description as easygoing, type A behavior, and tension predicted CHD incidence. Type A behavior and tension were so highly correlated that when they both were in a multivariate analysis, tension accounted for the predictive contribution of type A behavior. When the tension scale was excluded from the analysis, type A emerged as a significant predictor. Thus, for housewives, coronary-prone behaviors include specific descriptions of tension (e.g. difficulties piling up, trouble sleeping) or type A behaviors, as well as a self-report of being easygoing. This inconsistency between behaving in a tense, type A manner, and reporting oneself as 'easygoing' is similar to the type As who do not report fatigue on treadmill testing, or who obtain self-satisfaction through work pressure.

Type A behavior and suppressed hostility were significant predictors of CHD incidence among the 387 working women studied [15]. As noted previously, within the group of working women, the 125 clerical workers were found to be at greater risk of CHD. After controlling for standard risk factors, suppressed hostility, non-support from boss and family responsibility emerged as significant predictors of CHD incidence among clerical workers. Interestingly, none of the standard risk factors including age, systolic blood pressure, serum cholesterol and cigarette smoking were associated with CHD risk. These findings indicate that it is the interaction between the clerical worker, her roles, and her work environment that is coronary-prone. Specifically, the clerical worker who has the challenge of family and work responsibility, who is in a job without autonomy and control, who receives little support from her boss – the person in control, and who suppresses the anger and frustration she feels is at elevated risk for CHD. The coronary-prone situation of the clerical worker is consistent with research suggesting that both a lack of control over challenging situations [14] and hostility may be coronary-prone components of the type A behavior pattern [23, 40].

Future Directions and Conclusions

Type A behavior is more prevalent among men than women and, within women, more prevalent among working than non-working women. This latter comparison suggests that women, responding to the western emphasis on achievement, are moving into the competitive working world despite traditional roles of homemaking and child-rearing. Research is needed to examine the relative contributions of personality or individual achievement orientation and the work environment in fostering type A behavior and increasing risk of CHD among men and women.

The relationship between type A behavior and achievement in terms of traditional sex roles reveals a sex difference. Achievement in terms of type A behavior is more consistent with the masculine sex role, suggesting that aspects of the male role in western societies contribute to men's higher rates of CHD [33, 37]. This conclusion leads directly to the question of whether it is possible to maintain or even strengthen the positive work-related correlates of the type A behavior pattern, such as occupational status and achievement, while reducing those correlates that contribute to disease.

The final section of this chapter identified situations in which features of the work environment have been found to interact with the type A behavior pattern resulting in changes in cardiovascular and neuroendocrine arousal. Interestingly, none of these interactions indicates negative effects as yet for such job features as productivity, heavy work loads or long hours. Instead, these interactions highlight the need for a better understanding of how to match individuals with work environments. Further, more process-oriented research in naturalistic settings is needed to identify the coronary-prone aspects of the interaction between the work environment and the type A behavior. As these features are identified, interventions can be tailored to specific situations that are shown to be associated with risk rather than advocating broad life-style changes. As this research progresses it will be important to study women as well as men because there is evidence from laboratory research that differences may exist between the sexes in the types of situations that evoke coronary-prone behavior and the accompanying neuroendocrine and cardiovascular arousal that is thought to lead over time to clinical manifestations of CHD [23].

Cross-cultural studies have shown that as men were exposed to and endorsed western work ethics, originally low CHD rates rose to levels equal to that for white American males [11]. A similar phenomenon may be underway with regard to American females. Research is needed to examine the process of integration of American females into the occupational setting. This research may help elucidate the development and full expression of the coronary-prone aspects of the interaction between type A behavior and work, which in turn would provide a basis for interventions that would not endanger the productivity, rewarding and self-satisfying aspects of the type A behavior pattern.

References

1   Baruch, R.: The achievement motive in women: implications for career development. J. Personal. soc. Psychol. 5: 260–267 (1967).
2   Bem, S.L.: The measurement of psychological angrogyny. J. consul. clin. Psychol. 42: 155–162 (1974).
3   Burke, R.J.; Weir, T.: The type A experience: occupational and life demands, satisfaction and well-being. J. hum. Stress 6: 28–38 (1980).
4   Caplan, R.D.; Jones, K.W.: Effects of work load, role ambiguity, and type A personality on anxiety, depression, and heart rate. J. appl. Psychol. 60: 713–719 (1975).
5   Caplan, R.D.; Cobb, S.; French, J.R.P.; Harrison, R.V.; Pinneau, S.R.: Job demands and

worker health. Publ. No. (NIOSH) 75–160 (US Department of Health, Education, and Welfare, Washington 1975).

6   Carver, C.S.; Coleman, A.E.; Glass, D.C.: The coronary-prone behavior pattern and the suppression of fatigue on a treadmill test. J. Personal. soc. Psychol. *33:* 460–466 (1976).

7   Chesney, M.A.; Black, G.W.; Chadwick, J.H.; Rosenman, R.H.: Psychological correlates of the coronary-prone behavior pattern. J. behav. Med. (in press).

8   Chesney, M.A.; Sevelius, G.; Black, G.W.; Ward, M.M.; Swan, G.E.; Rosenman, R.H.: Work environment, type A behavior and coronary heart disease risk factors. J. occup. Med. (in press).

9   Chesney, M.A.; Rosenman, R.H.: Type A behavior in the work setting; in Cooper, Payne, Current concerns in occupational stress (Wiley, London 1980).

10   Chesney, M.A.; Ward, M.M.; Black, G.W.; Swan, G.E.; Rosenman, R.H.: Type A/B and environmental control: too much or too little (Am. Psychological Ass., New York 1979).

11   Cohen, J.B.: The influence of culture on coronary-prone behavior; in Dembroski, Weiss, Shields, Haynes, Feinleib, Coronary-prone behavior, pp. 243–252 (Springer, New York 1978).

12   Davidson, M.H.; Cooper, C.L.; Chamberlain, D.: Type A coronary-prone behavior and stress in senior female managers and administrators. J. occup. Med. *22:* 801–805 (1980).

13   Frankerhaeuser, M.; Lundberg, U.; Forsman, L.: Note on arousing type A persons by depriving them of work. J. psychosom. Res. *24:* 45–47 (1980).

14   Glass, D.C.: Behavior patterns, stress and coronary disease (Erlbaum, Hillsdale 1977).

15   Haynes, S.G.; Feinleib, M.: Women, work and coronary heart disease: prospective findings from the Framingham Heart Study. Am. J. Publ. Hlth *70:* 133–141 (1980).

16   Haynes, S.G.; Feinleib, M.; Kannel, W.B.: The relationship of psychosocial factors to coronary heart disease in the Framingham Study. III. Eight-year incidence of coronary heart disease. Am. J. Epidem. *111:* 37–58 (1980).

17   Haynes, S.G.; Feinleib, M.; Levine, S.; Scotch, N.; Kannel, W.B.: The relationship of psychosocial factors to coronary heart disease in the Framingham Study. II. Prevalence, of coronary heart disease. Am. J. Epidem. *107:* 384–492 (1978).

18   Haynes, S.G.; Levine, S.; Scotch, N.; Feinleib, M.; Kannel, W.B.: The relationship of psychosocial factors to coronary heart disease in the Framingham Study. I. Methods and risk factors. Am. J. Epidem. *107:* 362–383 (1978).

19   Howard, J.H.; Cunningham, D.A.; Rechnitzer, P.A.: Health patterns associated with type A behavior: a managerial population. J. hum. Stress *2:* 24–31 (1976).

20   Howard, J.H.; Cunningham, D.A.; Rechnitzer, P.A.: Work patterns associated with type A behavior: a managerial population. Hum. Relat. *30:* 825–836 (1977).

21   Howard, J.H.; Rechnitzer, P.A.; Cunningham, D.A.: Effective and ineffective methods for coping with job tension. Publ. personnel Mgmnt *Sept./Oct.:* 317–326 (1975).

22   Kriger, S.F.: nAch and perceived parental child-rearing attitudes of career women and homemakers. J. vocat. Behav. *2:* 419–432 (1972).

23   MacDougall, J.M.; Dembroski, T.M.; Krantz, D.S.: Effects of types of challenge on pressor and heart rate responses in type A and B women. Psychophysiology *18:* 1–9 (1981).

24   Matthews, K.A.: Assessment and developmental antecedents of the coronary-prone behavior pattern in children; in Dembroski, Weiss, Shields, Haynes, Feinleib, Coronary-prone behavior, pp. 207–217 (Springer, New York 1978).

25   McMichael, A.J.; Haynes, S.G.; Tyroler, H.A.: Observations on the evaluation of occupational health. J. occup. Med. *17:* 128–131 (1975).

26   Mettlin, C.: Occupational careers and the prevention of coronary-prone behavior. Soc. Sci. Med. *10:* 367–372 (1976).

27   Mix, J.; Lohr, J.M.: The relationship between sex, sex-role orientation and coronary-prone behavior in college students. Proc. Society for Behavioral Medicine, San Francisco 1979.

28   Rosenman, R.H.: The interview method of assessment of the coronary-prone behavior pattern; in Dembroski, Weiss, Shields, Haynes, Feinleib, Coronary-prone behavior (Springer, New York 1978).

29   Sales, S.M.: Differences among individuals in affective, behavioral, biochemical and psychological responses to variations in work load; doct. diss. No. 72-14, p. 822 (University Microfilms, Ann Arbor 1971).

30   Shekelle, R.B.; Schoenberger, J.A.; Stamler, J.: Correlates of the JAS type A behavior pattern score. J. chron. Dis. *29:* 381–394 (1976).

31   Szalai, A. (ed.): The use of time (Mouton, The Hague 1972).

32   US Department of Health Education, and Welfare, Public Health Service. The prevalence of disabling illness among male and female workers and housewives. Publ. Hlth. Bull., No. 260 (US Government Printing Office, Washington 1941).

33   Waldron, I.: Why do women live longer than men? J. hum. Stress *2:* 2–13 (1976).

34   Waldron, I.: Sex differences in the coronary-prone behavior pattern; in Dembroski, Weiss, Shields, Haynes, Feinleib, Coronary-prone behavior, pp. 199–206 (Springer, New York 1978).

35   Waldron, I.: The coronary-prone behavior pattern, blood pressure, employment and socioeconomic status in women. J. psychosom. Res. *22:* 79–87 (1978).

36   Waldron, I.; Hickey, A.; McPherson, C.; Butensky, A.; Gruss, L.; Overall, K.; Schmader, A.; Wohlmuth, D.: Relationships of the coronary-prone behavior pattern to blood pressure variation, psychological characteristics, and academic and social activities of students. J. hum. Stress *6:* 16–27 (1980).

37   Waldron, I.; Johnston, S.: Why do women live longer than men? II. J. hum. Stress *2:* 19–30 (1976).

38   Waldron, I.; Zyzanski, S.; Shekelle, R.B.; Jenkins, C.D.; Tannebaum, S.: The coronary-prone behavior pattern in employed men and women. J. hum. Stress *3:* 2–18 (1977).

39   Weidner, G.; Matthews, K.A.: Reported physical symptoms elicited by unpredictable events and the type A coronary-prone behavior pattern. J. Personal. soc. Psychol *36:* 1213–1220 (1978).

40   Williams, R.B.; Haney, T.L.; Lee, K.L.; Kong, Y.; Blumenthal, J.A.; Wahlen, R.E.: Type A behavior, hostility, and coronary atherosclerosis. Psychosom. Med. *42:* 539–549 (1980).

41   Zyzanski, S.J.: Associations of the coronary-prone behavior pattern; in Dembroski, Weiss, Shields et al., Coronary-prone behavior (Springer, New York 1978).

7 The Sympathetic-Adrenal and Pituitary-Adrenal Response to Challenge: Comparison between the Sexes[1]

Marianne Frankenhaeuser

This paper is concerned with the experimental study of how healthy males and females cope with the psychosocial challenges of their everyday existence. Interest is focussed on psychological mediators of the activity of the sympathetic-adrenal medullary system with the secretion of the catecholamines adrenaline and noradrenaline, and the pituitary-adrenal cortical system with the secretion of cortisol. Our recent approaches to problems in this area of research are reviewed against the background of earlier studies from our laboratory [9, 11, 12] as well as relevant work from other laboratories.

Catecholamines and cortisol both have key functions in human stress and coping processes: as sensitive indicators of the stressfulness of person-environment transactions, as regulators of vital bodily functions and, under some circumstances, as mediators of bodily reactions leading to disease. Since most psychoneuroendocrinologists engaged in stress and coping research have restricted their efforts to one of the adrenal systems, knowledge about their relative sensitivity to different psychosocial stressors has until recently been meager.

Our approach to these problems has been guided by the notion that the effectiveness of psychosocial factors in arousing the adrenal-cortical and the adrenal-medullary systems is determined by the person's cognitive appraisal of the balance between the severity of the situational demands, on the one hand, and his or her personal coping resources, on the orther.

Another basic concept is that neuroendocrine responses to the psychosocial environment reflect its emotional impact on the individual, and that objectively different environmental conditions may evoke the same neuroendocrine responses because they have a common psychological denominator. These formulations are linked conceptually to *Mason's* [32] theory, empha-

[1] The research reported in this paper has been supported by grants from the Swedish Medical Research Council (Project No. 997), the Swedish Council for Research in the Humanities and Social Sciences, and the Swedish Work Environment Fund (Project No. 80/162).

zising the susceptibility of different neuroendocrine systems to the specific emotional component of different environmental settings.

The ability to exert control over one's own activities is generally recognized as a major determinant of the stressfulness of person-environment transactions. It is agreed that, over the long run, controllability facilitates adjustment and enhances coping effectiveness, although the effort involved in exerting control may be associated with a temporary increase in arousal [2]. Conversely, lack of control may have widespread negative consequences, among which is a state of 'learned helplessness' [40] which, in turn, may lead to depression. The animal models of *Seligman* [40], *Henry* [19] and *Weiss* [42] form the basis of much current research on the helplessness-hopelessness dimension in human behavior.

In our studies of healthy persons, to be outlined in this paper, the emphasis is on sympathetic-adrenal and pituitary-adrenal responses to controllable and non-controllable situations. Catecholamines in urine are determined fluorimetrically [1, 6] and cortisol in urine by radioimmunoassay [7, 38]. A key finding is that, in general, catecholamine and cortisol secretion rates are reduced as personal control increases. Insofar as high levels of circulating catecholamines and cortisol are pathogenic, reducing their release by increasing control may have far-reaching implications for health and well-being.

Recent support for this line of reasoning comes from several sources. Of particular interest are Swedish national survey data showing that the correlation between cardiovascular disease and work overload is high only when overload is combined with low decision latitude, i.e. low control over one's own work situation [24].

These findings pose several questions concerning the mechanisms underlying the relationships between health and behavior. By exposing healthy males and females to well-defined laboratory and real-life situations differung with regard to controllability, and measuring their responses on the psychological and physiological level, we hope to throw light on the mechanisms involved.

The Effort-Distress Model

Results from a large number of studies, in which we have obtained self-reports from subjects under laboratory and real-life conditions, have lead us to focus on two components of psychological arousal: effort and distress [13, 31]. Effort and distress may be experienced either singly or in combination, and these two aspects of psychological arousal seem to be differentially associated with catecholamine and cortisol secretion. These psychoneuroendocrine relationships may be conceptualized as follows:

Effort without distress is a joyous, happy state, which is accompanied by catecholamine secretion, whereas cortisol secretion may be actively suppressed.

Effort with distress is probably the state most typical of our daily hassles. It is accompanied by an increase of both catecholamine and cortisol secretion. Most of our studies concern this category. For instance, mental work carried out under conditions of either stimulus underload or overload will typically evoke feelings of effort as well as distress and, consequently, both the catecholamine and the cortisol level will rise.

Distress without effort means giving up, feeling helpless. Such a state, as we know from animal experiments [20] and clinical-psychiatric studies [39], is accompanied by an outflow of cortisol.

The key question is how to achieve the state of effort without distress. Our data point to personal control as an important modulating factor in this regard. A lack of control is almost invariably associated with feelings of distress, whereas being in control may prevent a person from experiencing distress. Hence, personal control tends to act as a buffer, reducing the negative arousal affects, and thereby changing the balance between sympathetic-adrenal and pituitary-adrenal activity.

These principles will be illustrated by data from two laboratory situations: a low-control situation, characterized by 'effort with distress', and a high-control situation, characterized by 'effort without distress'. In the low-control situation, the subjects were given a 1 h vigilance task, which consisted in pressing a key in response to each randomly occurring intensity change in a weak light signal. In the high-control situation the subjects performed a choice-reaction task, designed so as to induce a high degree of personal control and feelings of competence and mastery [15]. To this end, each session started with a preparatory period, in which the subject was encouraged to try out different stimulus rates in order to arrive at his or her 'preferred work pace', i.e. the pace perceived as optimal in terms of well-being as well as efficiency. The task proper did not begin until the subjects felt confident about their choice of pace for the subsequent period of sustained work. Every 5 min the subject was given the opportunity to modify his/her stimulus rate so as to maintain an optimal pace throughout the 1 h session. Hence, the situation was both predictable and controllable to a very high degree. According to self-reports, these experimental arrangements were successful in creating a work situation where each person felt confident of his/her ability to predict and control the pace of work and, at the same time, felt pleasantly challenged and motivated to perform well.

The results are shown in figure 1. Diagram 1a shows self-reports of distress and effort, expressed as percentages of self-reports obtained in a neutral non-work (baseline) situation. It is seen that the low-control task induced both effort and distress. The high-control task induced effort, but distress fell below baseline, i.e. the work situation was experienced as more pleasant and stimulating than the non-work (baseline) condition.

The neuroendocrine pattern is shown in figure 1b. During the low-control task, which induced both distress and effort, adrenaline as well as cortisol increased. In other words, the effort made in performing the high-control task was accompanied by adrenaline increase, whereas the lack of distress was reflected in the decrease of cortisol. Thus, in this highly controllable situation the pituitary-adrenal systems was 'put to rest'.

These results contribute to our understanding of the selective response of the pituitary-adrenal and the sympathetic-adrenal system to psychologically different conditions. In short, pituitary-adrenal activation was associated with the negative feelings of distress in the low-control situation, and sympathetic-adrenal activation was associated with the positive feeling of effort in the high-control situation. Our results are consistent with those of *Ursin* et al. [41], who identified a 'cortisol factor' and a 'catecholamine factor' by factor analysis of data from a study of parachute trainees. In a general way, the results from these studies of human beings fit the animal model proposed by *Henry and Stephens* [20] according to which the sympathetic-adrenal system is activated when the organism is challenged in its control of the environment, whereas the pituitary-adrenal system is associated with the conservation, withdrawal response.

A point of special interest, illustrated rather strikingly by the data in figure 1, is the bidirectional nature of the pituitary-adrenal response. This implies that environmental changes can either elevate or suppress the secretion of cortisol. In our study, adrenal-cortical suppression occurred under conditions characterized by high controllability/predictability. This finding is consistent with data from animal experiments [26], indicating that reinforcement is an important cognitive factor mediating suppression of the adrenal-cortical system. Relevant human data are available from a study by *Rodin* [36] of elderly persons, and a study by *Vernikos-Danellis* et al. [43] of U-2 pilots. In both these studies a high level of personal control was found to be associated with low cortisol secretion.

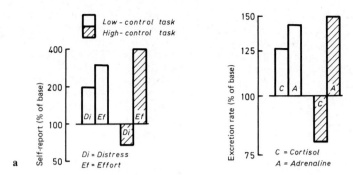

Fig. 1. Mean values for self-reports of distress and effort **(a)** and cortisol and adrenaline excretion **(b)** in male and female students. Values obtained during a low-control task and a high-control task are expressed as percentages of values obtained during a baseline condition [data from ref. 15].

Type A Behavior and Controllability

There is an interesting link between the concept of control and rushed competitive, aggressive type A behavior, which constitutes an independent risk factor in coronary heart disease [37]. This has been emphasized by *Glass* [18] who points to fear of loosing control as a major threat in the lives of type A persons.

Insofar as controllability is a significant psychological concept in coronary-prone behavior, interesting information should be gained by comparing stress and coping responses in type A persons and type Bs (i.e. persons lacking type A characteristics) in our high-controllability situation (described above). We wanted to know whether the rush and time urgency characteristic of type As would manifest itself in their choosing a faster work pace than type Bs and, if so, whether the faster tempo of the type A persons would be reflected on the subjective and neuroendocrine level.

Figure 2 shows choice of work pace, reaction time and number of correct responses over a 1-hour session for university students classified as type A or type B on the basis of their answers to a Swedish 33-item questionnaire [27], modelled on the 'speed and impatience' and 'hard-driving' components of the Jenkins Activity Survey (JAS) [21]. The As and Bs selected for our experiments represented the highest and lowest quartiles for each sex of the total distribution of 460 university students. Since there were no significant sex differences in achievement variables, the males and females were grouped together. As shown in figure 2, achievement behavior differed distinctly

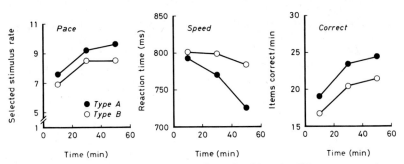

Fig. 2. Successive mean scores for type A and type B subjects for different aspects of performance on a 'high-control' choice-reaction task, i.e. self-selected work pace (max. pace = 11), reaction time, and number of correct responses [data from ref. 15].

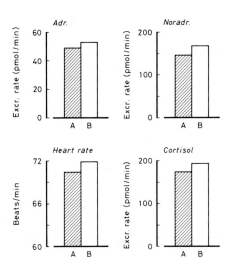

Fig. 3. Mean values for adrenaline and noradrenaline excretion, heart rate, and cortisol excretion for type A and type B subjects in a 'high-control' choice-reaction task [data from ref. 15].

between the type A and B groups. Not only did type A persons select a faster pace, thus subjecting themselves to a greater total work load, they also coped more effectively with this load than did type B persons with their lesser load. Thus, type As responded faster to individual stimuli, yet maintained a higher level of accuracy and, hence, achieved a larger number of correct responses in the time allowed.

Our next question was whether the superior performance of type A persons was associated with greater costs on the subjective level. According to self-reports this was not the case. For example, the increase in effort from the baseline to the experimental conditions was of the same magnitude in As as in Bs. (Here we have a sex difference which will be considered in the next section.) Nor was there any appreciable difference between As and Bs with regard to sympathetic-adrenal and pituitary-adrenal activation (fig. 3). Thus, when allowed to work at their own pace, type As did not show the hyperresponsiveness manifested under other kinds of challenge [4, 5]. It is worth noting that our data do not cover possible aftereffects and, hence, do not tell us whether type As took longer to 'unwind' and return to baseline.

We interpret our results as showing that the type A person, when in control of the situation, sets his or her standards high, copes effectively with the self-selected heavy load, and does so without mobilizing excessive physiological resources. There is an interesting parallel between this experimental illustration of how type As cope with an acute work load and epidemiological data [21, 25], showing that persons high in 'job involvement' (i.e. one of the major components of type-A behavior) had a relatively lower incidence of coronary heart disease than those high in the 'hard-driving' and 'speed and impatience' factors [28].

One could speculate that conditions which call for effort and activate the sympathetic-adrenal system are potentially harmful, primarily when they also induce feelings of distress and pituitary-adrenal activation. Conditions which evoke effort but no distress would, according to this line of reasoning, be less threatening to health.

Insofar as type As are not worn out by their heavy work load as such, we must look elsewhere for factors contributing to their vulnerability. Some of our data point to lack of strategies for coping with non-work conditions as a major weakness of the type A person. We found that type B subjects were consistently less aroused (according to self-reports and sympathetic-adrenal indices) when asked to remain unoccupied in the laboratory than when asked to do arithmetic under noise exposure. In contrast, type As tended to be equally aroused or more aroused when deprived of work than when given work to do [16]. In line with this general tendency to rebel against passivity, type As secreted significantly more cortisol than type Bs during a prolonged vigilance task, but not during rapid information processing [30].

Comparison between the Sexes

The effort-distress model presented above applies to both sexes. However, although the general pattern of subjective and adrenal-hormonal activation is the same for males and females, there is a distinct sex difference

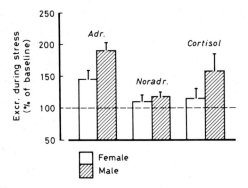

Fig. 4. Means and standard errors for adrenaline excretion (expressed as percentages of baselines) in female and male groups during stress induced by an IQ test, a color-word conflict test, and venipuncture. The first diagram is based on data from *Johansson and Post* [23], the other two on data from *Frankenhaeuser* et al. [14].

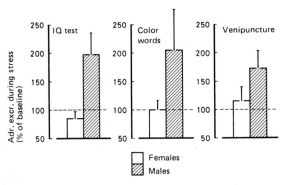

Fig. 5. Means and standard errors for adrenaline, noradrenaline, and cortisol excretion in female and male high-school students. Values obtained during a matriculation examination are expressed as percentages of values obtained during a day of ordinary school work [data from ref. 17].

in the magnitude of the response: women report less intense effort and, accordingly, secrete less catecholamines.

A series of studies from my laboratory [10, 11] shows that, in general, women are less prone than men to respond to achievement demands by increased catecholamine secretion. During rest and relaxation, sex differences in catecholamine excretion are generally slight (provided one allows for body weight), but in challenging performance situations consistent differences appear. This is true for adrenaline in particular, but the tendency is the same for noradrenaline.

Figure 4 summarizes data from various studies [14, 23]. Each diagram shows the adrenaline excretion in a stress situation, expressed as a percentage of a baseline value obtained at the same time of day under relative inactivity, during which the sexes did not differ markedly. Stress in the different experiments shown in figure 4 was induced by intelligence testing, a color-word conflict task, and venipuncture. The common characteristic of all diagrams is the lack of adrenaline increase during stress in the females and, in contrast, the significant rise in the males. The picture was similar for noradrenaline. (Cortisol data are not available from these early studies.) The mean age range in the different experiments was 18–35 years. Other data from our laboratory show a similar sex difference for 12-year-olds [22] and 4-year-olds [29].

Next, we compared males and females in a real-life stress situation, which was more severe than the relatively mild situations depicted in figure 4. This was a 6-hour examination which formed part of matriculating from high-school in Finland [17]. In figure 5 examination-stress values have been expressed as percentages of values obtained during ordinary school work. (Since the latter is also somewhat stressful, the increase in neuroendocrine activity is smaller than it would have been, if true baseline values had been available.) In this rather intense stress situation, the females did increase their adrenaline secretion to a significant degree, but the rise was significantly greater for the males. The pattern was similar for cortisol. Thus, these results tell us that during severe stress women do respond in a manner similar to men, but to a lesser degree.

An important point is that the females did not perform less efficiently than the males in any of the situations described. Insofar as there were any sex differences in performance, they favored the women.

It is worth noting that the picture with regard to male-female differences was the same for plasma catecholamines determined by a radioenzymatic technique [33] as for fluorimetrically determined urinary catecholamines. Figure 6 shows data from a recent experiment in our laboratory [8], where blood samples were drawn from healthy males and females performing a color-word conflict task during carotid-baroreceptor stimulation by neck-suction. Plasma adrenaline was significantly higher in the male than in the female group. As in earlier studies, the sex difference in noradrenaline pointed in the same direction but did not reach significance.

The fact that women respond less than men in terms of catecholamine excretion, when faced with the pressure to achieve, may mean that they have a more 'economic' way of coping. Thus, their costs of adapting to achievement demands may be lower. This could have a bearing on the sex differences

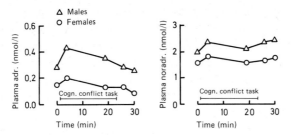

Fig. 6. Successive mean values for plasma adrenaline and noradrenaline for groups of healthy males and females before, during, and after a cognitive-conflict task performed during carotid-baroreceptor stimulation by neck-suction [data from ref. 8].

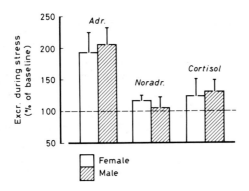

Fig. 7. Means and standard errors for adrenaline, noradrenaline, and cortisol excretion in female and male engineering students. Values obtained during a cognitive-conflict task are expressed as percentages of values obtained during an inactivity period [data from ref. 3].

in health. In short, we are led to speculate that the greater vulnerability of males to, for example, coronary heart disease, could be related to their more intense, and more frequent, neuroendocrine stress responses. And this, in turn, leads to the question of genetically versus culturally determined sex differences in behavior.

To the extent that stress and coping responses are learned, differences between the sexes in this respect are likely to be reduced as the social roles of males and females become more equal. One way of approaching this problem is to study differences between women who have adopted different social roles, the hypothesis being that those who have taken on a male role in, for example, their professional life, would tend to exhibit the neuroendocrine stress responses typical of men. Our results show that, on the whole, such 'non-traditional' females do tend to respond to achievement demands by the increase in adrenaline secretion which we have found to be typical of males.

This is true of female engineering students, selected from the most male-dominated branches in a Swedish school of engineering [3]. Figure 7 shows that the female students increased their adrenaline excretion almost as much as their male fellow students when performing a cognitive-conflict task.

Studies in progress show that the same is true for female bus drivers whose work schedule is identical with that of their male colleagues, as well as for female lawyers doing the same intellectual work as male lawyers.

There is no unequivocal interpretation of these results. The similarities between the sexes might arise from these women being constitutionally like men in terms of responding to achievement demands, and this may be the reason why they have chosen a male work role. The second possibility is that these women have, so to speak, been shaped by their vocational role. We know from retrospective reports of the female engineering students that as children they played conventional girls' games and showed no sign of tomboyism. As adults, however, they had adopted a typical 'male interest profile', perhaps as a result of the social pressure to be 'real engineers'.

Let us turn now from person-characteristics to situation-characteristics. A hypothesis that we are examining at present is that females tend to be more vulnerable when challenged in areas in which, by tradition, they are expected to show more competence than males. So far, we have considered only situations which challenge the so-called male area of competence: asserting oneself in relation to others, performing, producing and the like. In the so-called female area of competence, emphasis is on helping other people to maintain harmonious relationships. We are led to wonder how men and women respond to situations which pose demands in the female area of competence. In this area it is much harder to do controlled experiments. However, we have had the opportunity of carrying out a study which deals with the traditional female area: home, family, children [29].

We compared mothers and fathers when they both took their 3-year-old child to hospital for a check-up. In this demanding but non-competitive situation the women secreted at least as much adrenaline, noradrenaline and cortisol as the men. This underscores our point that psychological factors are powerful determinants of neuroendocrine stress responses.

Let us look, finally, at the pattern of correlations between catecholamine excretion during stress and achievement-related variables in the two sexes [35]. Figure 8, based on data from the subjects who (at the age of 18) partici-

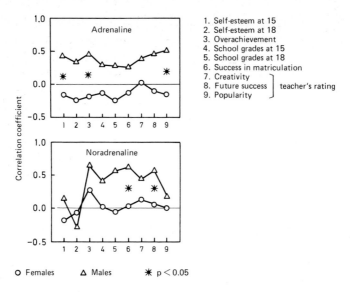

1. Self-esteem at 15
2. Self-esteem at 18
3. Overachievement
4. School grades at 15
5. School grades at 18
6. Success in matriculation
7. Creativity
8. Future success ⎤ teacher's rating
9. Popularity ⎦

O Females   △ Males   ✳ p < 0.05

Fig. 8. Product-moment coefficients of correlation between values for adrenaline and noradrenaline excretion of male and female high-school students during an examination (at age 18) and values for psychological functions (obtained at age 15 and/or 18) [data from ref. 35].

pated in the matriculation-examination study described above (fig. 5), shows that, for the males, adrenaline and noradrenaline excretion correlated positively with a number of achievement-related variables: self-esteem, overachievement, success in school work, success in the matriculation examination, and teachers' ratings of creativity, future success and popularity. In the female group, the corresponding correlations were close to zero or negative.

The male data seem to offer a fairly straightforward interpretation: they paint the picture of an 'achieving boy' whose catecholamine secretion during stress appears to be part and parcel of a constructive effort to cope with a challenging, competitive situation.

The correlations on which this picture is based are persistently fairly low, but strikingly consistent. Moreover, strong support for the validity of these correlations comes from the fact that correlations were highly similar between catecholamine excretion during stress and psychological data obtained when the subjects were 15 and 18 years old.

For the females, the correlational pattern is much less informative, a majority of the correlations being very low. Those coefficients which are high enough to merit attention have, in most cases, the opposite sign to those in the male group.

One could speculate that achievement for females has a more complex and mixed meaning than for males. Following this line of reasoning we are looking to the socialization process for possible interpretations. Available data [34] tell us that girls are trained to be more flexible in responding to situational changes and to discriminate more closely between different social cues than boys. This might be why females tend to respond more selectively to challenge and more economically in the sense that they master many stressful situations without calling upon their bodily reserves to the same extent as their male counterparts.

Boys tend to be more consistently achievement-oriented in a variety of situations and, as we have seen, almost invariably respond with catecholamine increase. This could have a bearing on the wider issue of the health differential between the sexes. One could speculate that, as sex roles are changing, males, freed of some traditional expectations, might develop new and more healthful ways of coping with stress.

References

1   Andersson, B.; Hovmöller, S.; Karlsson, C.-G.; Svensson, S.: Analysis of urinary catecholamines. An improved auto-analyzer fluorescence method. Clinica chim. Acta *51:* 13–28 (1974).

2   Averill, J.R: Personal control over aversive stimuli and its relationship to stress. Psychol. Bull. *80:* 286–303 (1973).

3   Collins, A.; Frankenhaeuser, M.: Stress responses in male and female engineering students. J. hum. Stress *4:* 43–48 (1978).

4   Dembroski, T.M.: MacDougall, J.M.; Lushene, R.: Interpersonal interaction and cardiovascular response in type A subjects and coronary patients. J. hum. Stress *5:* 28–36 (1979).

5   Dembroski, T.M.; MacDougall, J.M.; Shields, J.L.: Physiological reactions to social challenge in persons evidencing the type A coronary-prone behavior pattern. J. hum. stress *3:* 2–10 (1977).

6   Euler, U.S.v.; Lishajko, F.: Improved technique for the fluorimetric estimation of catecholamines. Acta physiol. scand. *51:* 348–355 (1961).

7   Ficher, M.; Curtis, G.C.; Ganjam, V.K.; Jeshlin, L.; Perry, S.: Improved measurement of corticosteroids in plasma and urine by competitive protein-binding radioassay. Clin. Chem. *19:* 511–515 (1973).

8   Forsman, L.; Lindblad, L.-E.: Effect of mental stress on baroreceptor mediated changes in blood pressure, heart rate, plasma catecholamines and subjective responses in healthy human beings. Psychosom. Med. (in press).

9   Frankenhaeuser, M.: Behavior and circulating catecholamines. Brain Res. *31:* 241–262 (1971).

10 Frankenhaeuser, M.: Psychoneuroendocrine sex differences in adaptation to the psycho-social environment; in Carenza, Pancheri, Zichella, Clinical psychoneuroendocrinology in reproduction (Academic Press, New York 1978).

11 Frankenhaeuser, M.: Psychoneuroendocrine approaches to the study of emotion as related to stress and coping; in Howe, Dienstbier, Nebraska Symp. on Motivation 1978 (University of Nebraska Press, Lincoln 1979).

12 Frankenhaeuser, M.: Psychoneuroendocrine approaches to the study of stressful person-environment transactions; in Selye, Selye's guide to stress research, vol. I (Van Nostrand Reinhold, New York 1980).

13 Frankenhaeuser, M.: Psychobiological aspects of life stress; in Levine, Ursin, Coping and health (Plenum Press, New York 1980).

14 Frankenhaeuser, M.; Dunne, E.; Lundberg, U.: Sex differences in sympathetic-adrenal medullary reactions induced by different stressors. Psychopharmacology *47:* 1–5.

15 Frankenhaeuser, M.; Lundberg, U.; Forsman, L.: Dissociation between sympathetic-adrenal and pituitary-adrenal responses to an achievement situation characterized by high controllability. Comparison between type A and type B males and females. Biol. Psychol. *10:* 79–91 (1980).

16 Frankenhaeuser, M.; Lundberg, U.; Forsman, L.: Note on arousing type A persons by depriving them of work. J. psychosom. Res. *24:* 45–47 (1980).

17 Frankenhaeuser, M.; Rauste-von Wright, M.; Collins, A.; Wright, J. von; Sedvall, G.; Swahn, C.-G.: Sex differences in psychoneuroendocrine reactions to examination stress. Psychosom. Med. *40:* 334–343 (1978).

18 Glass, D.C.: Behavior patterns, stress, and coronary disease (Erlbaum, Hillsdale 1977).

19 Henry, J.P.: Understanding the early pathophysiology of essential hypertension. Geriatrics *31:* 59–72 (1976).

20 Henry, J.P.; Stephens, P.M.: Stress, health, and the social environment. A sociobiological approach to medicine (Springer, New York 1977).

21 Jenkins, C.D.; Zyzanski, S.J.; Rosenman, R.H.: Progress toward validation of a computer-scored test for the type-A coronary-prone behavior pattern. Psychosom. Med. *33:* 193–202 (1971).

22 Johansson, G.; Frankenhaeuser, M.; Magnusson, D.: Catecholamine output in school children as related to performance and adjustment. Scand. J. Psychol. *14:* 20–28 (1973).

23 Johansson, G.; Post, B.: Catecholamine output of males and females over a one-year period. Acta physiol. scand. *92:* 557–565 (1974).

24 Karasek, R.A.: Job socialization and job strain: the implications of two related psycho-social mechanisms for job design; in Gardell, Johansson, Working life. A social science contribution to work reform (Wiley & Son, New York 1981).

25 Kenigsberg, D.; Zyzanski, S.J.; Jenkins, C.D.; Wardwell, W.I.; Licciardello, A.T.: The coronary-prone behavior pattern in hospitalized patients with and without coronary heart disease. Psychosom. Med. *36:* 344–351 (1974).

26 Levine, S.; Weinberg, J.; Brett, L.P.: Inhibition of pituitary-adrenal activity as a consequence of consummatory behavior. Psychoneuroendocrinology *4:* 275–286 (1979).

27 Lundberg, U.: Type A behavior and its relation to personality variables in Swedish male and female university students. Scand. J. Psychol. *21:* 133–138 (1980).

28   Lundberg, U.: Psychophysiological aspects of performance and adjustment to stress; in Krohne, Laux, Achievement, stress and anxiety (Hemisphere, Washington 1980).

29   Lundberg, U.; Chateau, P. de; Winberg, J.; Frankenhaeuser, M.: Catecholamine and cortisol excretion patterns in three-year-old children and their parents. J. hum. Stress. *7:* 3–11 (1981).

30   Lundberg, U.; Forsman, L.: Adrenal-medullary and adrenal-cortical responses to understimulation and overstimulation. Comparison between type A and type B persons. Biol. Psychol. *9:* 79–89 (1979).

31   Lundberg, U.; Frankenhaeuser, M.: Pituitary-adrenal and sympathetic-adrenal correlates of distress and effort. J. psychosom. Res. *24:* 125–130 (1980).

32   Mason, J.W.: Emotion as reflected in patterns of endocrine integration; in Levi, Emotions: their parameters and measurement (Raven Press, New York 1975).

33   Peuler, J.D.; Johnson, G.A.: Simultaneous single isotope radioenzymatic assay of plasma norepinephrine, epinephrine and dopamine. Life Sci. *21:* 625–636 (1977).

34   Rauste, M.: The image of man among Finnish boys and girls. Rep. Dep. Psychol., University of Turku, Turku 1975, No. 41.

35   Rauste-von Wright, M.; Wright, J. von; Frankenhaeuser, M.: Relations between sex-related psychological characteristics during adolescence and catecholamine excretion during achievement stress. Psychophysiology *18:* 362–370 (1981).

36   Rodin, J.: Managing the stress of aging: the role of control and coping; in Levine, Ursin, Coping and health (Plenum Press, New York 1980).

37   Rosenman, R.H.; Brand, R.J.; Sholtz, R.I.; Friedman, M.: Multivariate prediction of coronary heart disease during 8.5-year follow-up in the Western Collaborative Group Study. Am. J. Cardiol. *37:* 903–910 (1976).

38   Ruder, H.J.: Guy, R.L.: Lipsett, M.B.: A radioimmunoassay for cortisol in plasma and urine. J. clin. Endocrin. Metabol. *35:* 219–224 (1972).

39   Sachar, E.J.: Psychological factors related to activation and inhibition of the adrenocortical stress response in man. A review; in Wied, Weijnen, Prog. Brain Res., vol. 32 (Elsevier, Amsterdam 1970).

40   Seligman, M.: Helplessness (Freeman, San Francisco 1975).

41   Ursin, H.; Baade, E.; Levine, S.: Psychobiology of stress (Academic Press, New York 1978).

42   Weiss, J.M.: Psychological factors in stress and disease. Sci. Am. *226:* 104–113 (1972).

43   Vernikos-Danellis, J.; Goldenrath, W.L.; Dolkas, C.B.: The physiological cost of flight stress and flight fatigue. US Navy Med. M. *66:* 12–16 (1975).

8 Behavioral and Psychophysiological Perspectives on Coronary-Prone Behavior[1]

Theodore M. Dembroski, James M. MacDougall

This chapter describes a series of studies underway in our laboratory designed to clarify and refine the concept of coronary-prone behavior. This research is directed specifically toward (a) determining which specific aspects of the multidimensional type A pattern are consistently linked to coronary heart disease (CHD), morbidity, and mortality; (b) establishing the degree to which these components and other psychological dimensions are related to potentially pathologic patterns of cardiovascular reactivity in everyday life; (c) exploring the degree to which cardiovascular reactions in the laboratory are predictive of similar cardiovascular responses in daily life, and (d) identifying factors important in promoting type A behavior and concomitant patterns of cardiovascular reactivity.

Components of the Type A Pattern and CHD Morbidity and Mortality

During the past decade an extensive literature has developed which documents the association of the type A behavior pattern with at least some manifestations of CHD [15, 23]. In spite of this progress, it must be recognized that the specificity value of the type A pattern for predicting coronary-related diseases is quite low, since the majority of adult males in a variety of subpopulations in the United States have been found to show the behavior pattern to a substantial degree and, yet, only a small subset of these persons will develop clinically manifest heart disease at an early age. Clearly, many behavioral, environmental, and constitutional factors modultating this relationship remain unidentified. If the concept of coronary-prone behavior in general, and the type A pattern in particular, is to have further utility, it is important to identify those features of the pattern, plus as yet unrecognized additional components, which are essential to the behavior-disease linkage.

[1] Preparation of this chapter in which research from our laboratory is reported was supported by research Grant HL-22809 awarded to the authors by the National Heart, Lung, and Blood Institute, National Institutes of Health.

Our basic research objective is to go beyond the global A/B behavior pattern designation by scoring separately various components of the multidimensional type A pattern [39; and appendix for details on component scoring system]. This reanalysis involves rescoring tape recordings of the standard Rosenman and Friedman structured interview (SI) from extant studies which have related global type A designations to various manifestations of CHD. The data base relevant to this objective has been obtained from SI tapes generated by (a) the prospective Western Collaborative Group Study (WCGS), (b) SI tapes on patients who have undergone coronary angiographic testing at several different medical centers, and (c) an extant heritability study of twins. Each of these ongoing projects is described below.

Prospective Relationship between Components of the Type A Pattern and Incidence of CHD

In spite of its limitations, the type A behavior pattern (TABP) as classically measured by the SI and Jenkins Activity Survey (JAS) is likely to remain with us for some time to come because of the data base established in the WCGS. In the meantime, data available from the WCGS can continue to contribute to further refinement of the concept of coronary-prone behavior. For example, a promising first step in this regard is illustrated by a study by *Matthews* et al. [32], who showed that some components of the Friedman-Rosenman TABP appear to have greater strength of association with CHD than others. For example, speed of activity, achievements, and job involvement were not related to *overt* manifestations of CHD. The attributes that were related primarily reflected potential for hostility, competitiveness, impatience, irritability and vigorous voice stylistics. Further reanalyses of the WCGS data are important for several reasons. First, there was no linear relationship reported between SI-derived categories of type A (i.e. different levels of type A behaviors) and CHD in the WCGS. It is possible that the lack of a dose-response relationship between levels of type A and CHD was due to inappropriate weighting of certain components of the TABP in designating subjects as more or less extreme type A. For this reason, component scoring of the SI to provide continuous rather than dichotomous variables for the total pattern and its components can be used to reexamine this issue with extant WCGS data. Second, and along the same line, certain attributes of the TABP can be examined to determine their relationship to *different* manifestations of CHD, e.g. silent myocardial infarction (MI) vs angina vs symptomatic MI. For example, *Jenkins* [22] in a small scale study (25 cases vs 50 controls) reported that sense of time urgency, job promotions, and past achievements were most characteristic of those manifesting *silent* MI. As mentioned earlier, such analyses make it clear that the conceptual and operational definitions of coronary-prone behavior are presently in a evolving state and eventually will only partially overlap with the original Friedman and Rosenman conceptualization of the TABP [8]. In other words, reanalyses of the WCGS data will suggest which elements of the pattern may be related to pathophysiological processes and which may be benign correlates. Third, some evidence suggests that type A may be related to violent death, mild forms of illness, and alcoholism [14, 19, 24, 38]. Work is needed to determine the nature of such relationships and the possible mechanisms involved. Component analyses of type A make possible examination of the relationship of various aspects of the pattern to a variety of endpoints other than CHD in the WCGS. In this regard, several specific hypotheses are being tested. For example, *Rose* et al. [38] somewhat surprisingly found a tendency for JAS defined type Bs to develop hypertension during the course of a 3-year prospective study of air traffic controllers. Since the JAS and SI do not correlate very well [28, 34], it is possible that JAS-defined type Bs who score as SI-defined type As may be prone to develop hypertension. This issue, too, can be examined along with test of the anger-in vs anger-out hypothesis concerning the development of essential hypertension [1], using rated stylistics derived from the SI. Fourth, reanalyses also permit examination of some assessment issues. *Rosenman* [39] has been the only investigator to rate all subjects in the WCGS. *Jenkins* [22] and *Matthews* et al. [32] each rated small samples of the WCGS in their respective studies, but each did so as a single rater using procedures that did not provide reliability and validity data. It is essential to determine whether *independent research teams*, each using two or more independent raters can produce similar results. The component scoring system which we have developed [34; see Appendix] is suitable for this purpose because it has been shown to be reliable and valid among a variety of different researchers [*Chesney, Krantz, Glass, Matthews, Rosenman*, personal communication]. Other issues in the assessment area are also being examined. There is a strong current tendency for researchers to find about 70% of their sample to be SI-defined type As. In the WCGS the frequency was approximately 50%. Have the scoring procedures changes since 1960? Have the interviews become more challenging? Has the percentage of type As increased in the population during the past two decades? Use of two separate research teams for reinspection of the WCGS data will help to address some of these issues.

The Relationship between Components of the Type A Pattern and Arteriographically Determined Severity of Atherosclerosis

We believe that it is also important to explore the relationship of components of type A to arteriographically documented severity of atherosclerosis. To our knowledge this issue has not been systematically explored by any research group. There is ample rationale for doing so. For example, *Williams* et al. [43] showed that MMPI-defined hostility and the SI-defined TABP each made independent contributions in predicting angiographically documented severity of atherosclerosis. Research of this kind can be extended in a number of ways. For example, use of the MMPI in their study offers the opportunity for exploring the relationship between MMPI defined hostility and ratings of hostility in the Rosenman interview. Other components can be explored in the same manner. Similarly, component analyses of the interviews in the *Williams* et al. [43] sample will allow us to determine whether the same factors that predicted CHD in the component analyses of the WCGS interviews also predict severity of atherosclerosis. In addition, examination of similar data from other institutions will allow cross-validation of any relationship uncovered in the *Williams* et al. [43] data. The same procedure will be applied to data collected at additional medical centers that include samples that *have and have not* shown a relationship between globally defined type A and extent of coronary disease. Study of such samples will provide the additional opportunity for examining quality of interviews *and* the degree of agreement with different researchers in assessing global type A. In other words, assessment issues similar to those described above will be examined, and, in this regard, comparisons will be made between different samples and procedures used to obtain them.

Heritability of Components of the Type A Pattern in Adult Male Twins

The finding of a relationship between type A in fathers and offspring raises the issue of whether type A behavior has a genetic determinant [4]. However, study of 190 pairs of twins, identical vs fraternal, revealed no significant heritability estimate for the type A pattern as assessed by the SI scored by *Rosenman* alone [37, 40]. The same study did disclose a significant heritability estimate for type A (JAS-defined), activity level, and impulsiveness as measured by self-reports. These findings are consistent with those of a subsequent twin study (n = 56 pairs) in which only a modest genetic component was reported for the 'hard-driving' subscale of the JAS [33]. A more accurate picture of the influence of genetic factors on pattern A, however, must await further research. Type A assessment in adulthood is based on the exhibition of a simple preponderance of type A behaviors. Thus, individuals can be classified as type A for several reasons. One type A individual, for example, could be very impatient, but not at all concerned about excelling at work. Another type A might be very patient and careful, but at the same time persistent and aggressive in his approach. As mentioned above, the global type A classification is an imprecise measure of specific behaviors, and studies of the concordance of global type A between twin pairs may mask genetic contributions to a subset of type A behaviors. In order to illucidate the heritability of type A, heritability of individual type A behaviors must be ascertained, since some components of the type A pattern may have an heritable base. As *Matthews* [31] has observed, there is evidence that activity level has an heritable base and that related characteristics such as achievement striving, competitiveness, aggressiveness (at least in males) emerge in childhood and are relatively stable over time [3, 25]. Data are thus needed on the heritability of components of the TABP with special attention devoted to those attributes most closely associated with CHD. A component reanalysis of the taped interviews (n = 380) employed in the *Rahe* et al. [37] twin study is presently underway to accomplish this goal. The results will have obvious implications for research on the etiology of components of the TABP pattern and as noted above, may be useful to future intervention research.

Autonomic Reactivity as a Stable Individual Difference Variable

Just as many type As will remain free of clinically manifest CHD, research from our laboratory and others' reveals that only a relatively small subset of type A persons are prone to exaggerated autonomic reactivity in response to standardized laboratory challenge. The observed frequency of such persons is approximately twice as great among type As as Bs. Thus, although showing a statistical association with the type dimension, the tendency toward patterns of excessive cardiovascular reactivity may well be considered a stable individual difference variable of itself, and direct study of it may allow us to explore more efficiently a possible coronary-prone tendency. Therefore, since a predisposition toward excessive cardiovascular reactivity only partially overlaps with type A as presently defined, a second objective of our research is to investigate the relationship of both these individual difference variables, i.e. various type A attributes and laboratory-identified extreme patterns of cardiovascular reactivity, to the frequency and patterning of cardiovascular responses in daily life in adult, male managers while engaged in normal workday activities. The identification of individuals who evidence transsituational tendencies toward exaggerated physiological arousal provides a potentially efficient method for refining the concept of coronary-prone behavior. By identifying those aspects of the current definition of type A which are common to such persons – in conjunction with relevant aspects of the social and physical environment – it may be possible to greatly strengthen the specificity value of the construct.

In addition to its potential utility for sharpening the definition of coronary-prone behavior, investigation of how cardiovascular response in one circumstance (e.g. during the SI) is predictive of cardiovascular response in other circumstances in the laboratory and in everyday life is important for several additional reasons. First, measures of physiological reactivity may offer a means of transcending the error inherent in purely behavioral assessment procedures by providing a more direct determination of those individuals who are coronary-prone by virtue of their patterns of physiological response regardless of its constitutional or behavioral origins. Second, investigation of various maneuvers for inducing physiological response and the ability of such maneuvers to predict stable physiological responses in everyday life may yield valuable information on potential procedures to be used should a prospective study of physiological reactivity and CHD prove warranted. Third, if such research does establish a link between challenge-induced physiological response and incidence of CHD, the information on such maneuvers would be important for any development of diagnostic tools for clinical use. Fourth, paradigms used in the proposed research may prove valuable in testing the effectiveness of various intervention programs designed to reduce excessive physiological reactivity should such responses be firmly linked to CHD endpoints.

To date, our assessments of individual differences in ANS reactivity have utilized a variety of laboratory paradigms in which specific situational variables have been experimentally manipulated in order to assess their effects on persons typed as pattern A or B. This work and parallel research in other laboratories has demonstrated that globally defined type A college students and working adults show greater cardiovascular reactivity changes indicative of ANS arousal to a variety of performance challenges than do their type B counterparts [12, 20, 21]. Additional data suggest that those components of the SI which were reported to be most predictive of CHD incidence in the WCGS are also most predictive of challenge-induced reactivity [9–11, 27]. A next logical step in the analysis is to discover whether (a) type A and the components as assessed by the current SI are also predictive of cardiovascular reactivity in day-to-day life and (b) whether reactivity measures obtained in our laboratory paradigms are themselves predictive of reactivity patterns in daily life. Published data bearing on the first question are inconsistent. An early study by *Friedman* et al. [18] reported catecholamine production differences in extreme SI-defined As and Bs during the work day, but not at night. Studies by *Manuck* et al. [29] and *Waldron* et al. [42] provide some evidence that JAS-defined type A working adults and college students show higher blood pressure (BP) levels during their daily activities. By contrast, *Rose* et al. [38] found no difference in BP levels of JAS-defined As and Bs in the high-stress daily activities of air traffic controllers; and *DeBaker* et al. [7] found no difference between SI-defined As and Bs in catecholamine excretion, heart rate (HR), or ECG abnormalities in Belgium factory workers. Finally, *Stokols* et al. [41] reported mixed results, with JAS-defined type Bs showing relatively higher systolic blood pressure (SBP) under high commuting stress and type As higher levels under moderate stress levels. These findings strongly suggest that the TABP, however assessed, is not invariably associated with differentially higher levels of ANS responsivity in daily life and that situational factors and other person variables may be critical in modulating this behavior pattern/physiology linkage.

Concerning the second issue, to our knowledge there are no published data concerning the degree to which laboratory measures of ANS cardiovascular reactivity are predictive of similar measures obtained in daily life. Our own work and a paper by *Manuck and Garland* [30] demonstrate moderate test-retest correlations for BP and heart rate reactivity during similar laboratory tasks. A small-scale pilot study conducted in our laboratory found that SBP and HR changes in students in response to the stress of taking an in-class quiz (but not listening to a lecture) were nearly identical to the values obtained during a moderately stressful reaction time task in the laboratory. In all, however, the existing data do not permit us to evaluate the degree to which laboratory measures of type A and related constructs and/or direct assessment of ANS reactivity are predictive of physiological responses in daily life.

Resolution of this issue is the goal of an ongoing project being conducted at the Western Electric Plant in Omaha, Nebraska, in collaboration with Drs. *Eliot and Buell.* The project is designed to answer the following specific questions: (a) What is the extent of individual differences in physiologic responding to various laboratory situations including the type A interview? (b) Can consistent transsituational patterns of cardiovascular reactivity be distinguished among individuals? (c) What is the nature of the relationship between physiologic reactivity observed in the above maneuvers and static measures of physiologic risk factors, contemporary medical status, psychological or behavioral attributes, and job performance, stress, satisfaction, etc.? (d) What is the extent of individual differences in physiologic reactivity during the working day? (e) Are these physiologic reaction differences in the job environment stable over a 6-month period? (f) What initial assessment procedures, including physiologic ractivity in the psychophysiologic maneuvers, predict physiologic reactivity on the job? (g) How does physiologic reactivity during the working day relate to job performance, stress, satisfaction, etc.? (h) How does physiologic reactivity both in psychophysiologic testing and on the job relate to risk factors, illnesses, accidents, absenteeism, etc.? (i) What assessment procedures either singly or in combination predict such job-related events? (j) How do the data collected from Western Electric personnel compare with those studied in other industries?

The use of impedance cardiography [26, 36] during the laboratory assessment phase of this study is an essential feature of this research, since much of our work to date suggests considerable individual variation not only in the magnitude but also in the patterns of cardiovascular reactions to laboratory challenges. A major dimension of this variation appears to be the relative degree to which BP elevations are produced by β-adrenergic effects on the myocardium as opposed to elevations engendered by net increases in total peripheral resistance. Although intercorrelations among change values of SBP, diastolic blood pressure (DBP), and HR provide some clues concerning the relative contribution of these two factors, the moderate range of changes seen in many of the laboratory paradigms precludes precise identification of the ANS mechanisms involved. Simultaneous measurement of stroke volume and BP/HR changes will help us to identify qualitatively distinct *patterns* of cardiovascular reactivity which may have important implications for different disease states. For example, subjects who are most likely to develop sustained hypertension may have peripheral vascular resistance that is inappropriately high for the levels of BP measured [5, 17]. By contrast, subjects who are most likely to develop CHD may have exaggerated sympathetic nervous system activity with high levels of cardiac output and peripheral resistance which is normal or decreased below normal during behavioral procedures. Information of this type may also, for example, help resolve the apparently contradictory finding that cardiovascular reactivity in various laboratory paradigms is positively associated with frequency of minor illnesses [14, 35], but level of BP reactivity in the day-to-day activities of air traffic controllers was negatively correlated with illness frequency [38].

The basic plan of the Western Electric study involves several stages: (a) recruitment of volunteers and initial screening for CHD/hypertension; (b) administration of a physical examination and collection of basic demographic and health information; (c) psychophysiological testing and collection of psychological data, and (d) ambulatory monitoring during daily activity. The psychophysiological protocol involves collection of baseline measures of BP, HR, ECG, and stroke volume, followed by successive exposure to the SI, a difficult history quiz, mental arithmetic, and a challenging video game. This is followed by a monitoring period, during which participants receive 2 days of on-the-job monitoring for physiological reactivity using portable Avionics blood pressure/ECG units. Both the week and days in which a given person is monitored are randomized across the participants.

Data are now available for 30 participants. Of these, 28 completed the entire laboratory test sequence, while 2 persons were terminated early due to the repeated occurrence of previously unsuspected ectopic beats and excessive BP elevations. The analysis of the data is still in progress, but several interesting features have already emerged. First, of the 30 participants, only 5 could be typed as pattern B, while the remainder fell into the type A (n = 23) and type X (n = 2) categories. Although this extremely uneven split was not unexpected, it again clearly points out the need for more refined component analyses if the specificity value of the type A concept is to be improved.

Second, meaningful analyses of type A/B differences could not be performed due to the small number of type B subjects. More refined component analyses are presently underway, and it is possible that some of the components associated with type A (e.g. quickness of responding) will evidence a more robust association with reactivity levels.

Third and of greater immediate import for this discussion and for the study of cardiovascular reactivity as a distinct individual difference variable are the data obtained using the impedance cardiograph instrumentation. As we had anticipated, we observed extremely large individual differences in the magnitude of all cardiovascular parameters monitored. Table I provides an

Table I. Cardiovascular changes for entire sample (n = 28) observed during interview, TV pong, and mental arithmetic phases of psychophysiological testing

	Interview				TV pong game				Mental arithmetic			
	$\bar{X}$	SD	range		$\bar{X}$	SD	range		$\bar{X}$	SD	range	
			min	max			min	max			min	max
△ SBP, mm Hg	+17.8	7.7	0	+35	+22.3	9.7	+ 6	+51	+21.2	13.0	−13	+62
△ DBP, mm Hg	+ 9.5	4.7	0	+19	+ 7.6	6.5	− 3	+20	+ 8.0	6.2	− 4	+20
△ HR, bpm	+ 6.1	4.8	− 3	+16	+ 9.5	11.0	− 4	+49	+10.6	8.6	− 6	+25
△ SVI ml/m²	+ 0.9	5.2	−10.4	+13.5	+ 1.3	6.9	−13.7	+18.7	+ 2.6	7.6	−17.8	+17.1
△ COI liters/min/m²	+ 0.31	0.41	− 0.59	+ 1.27	+ 0.46	0.77	− 1.25	+ 1.76	+ 0.64	0.77	− 1.62	+ 2.39
△% TPR	+ 2.5	15.3	−25	+32	− 0.3	23.5	−35	+71	− 5.1	25.3	−35	+92

SVI = Stroke volume index; COI = cardiac output index; TPR = total peripheral resistance.

overview of the changes seen for the entire sample. As noted above, the cardiac output measures obtained through impedance cardiography are best expressed in terms of changes from baseline since these measures have shown the greatest agreement with other more widely used techniques and since the primary interest of the project lay in individual differences in *reactivity* to situational stress. Inspection of these data reveals that the average cardiovascular response to the laboratory challenges was substantial, and a smaller number of persons showed extremely large reactions inconsistent with the minimal physical demands of the situation.

More detailed analyses of the individual data suggested that the 28 participants could be grouped into three subcategories based upon the *patterning* of their cardiovascular response to the challenge of the various tasks. The first group consisted of 9 individuals who responded to all tasks with increased stroke volume (SV) and cardiac output and diminished computed total systemic resistance. These data are presented in the top of figure 1 (group A), where SV and cardiac output changes are expressed as indices adjusted for total body surface area – SV index (SVI) in ml/m² = SV in ml/total body surface area in meters; cardiac output index (COI) in liters/min/m² = cardiac output (CO) in liters/min/total body surface area in meters – and computed total peripheral resistance expressed as a percentage change relative to baseline. A second subgroup of these subjects (group B) responded to all tasks with diminished SV and cardiac output and heightened peripheral resistance. These data are displayed in the center portion of the figure. Finally, a large subgroup of 16 individuals (group C) tended to show BP elevations

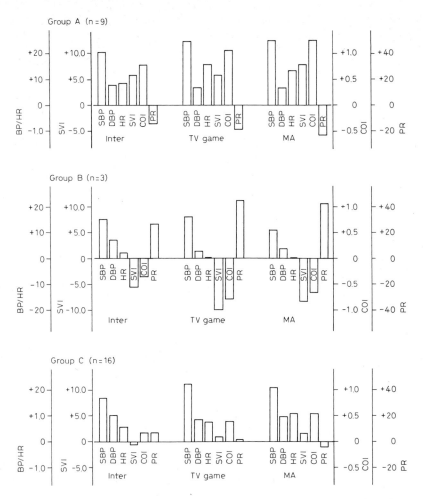

Fig. 1. Patterns of cardiovascular response to laboratory maneuvers: Type A interview, TV 'Pong' game, and mental arithmetic. See text for abbreviations.

resulting from enhanced output, coupled with relatively small and variable changes in peripheral resistance. This latter group showed the least stereotyping in the patterning of response across the three tasks and, interestingly, was comprised of individuals who showed either very small changes in BP or very large changes. The data from this subgroup are displayed in the lower portion of figure 1. In all, these data provide good support for the hypothesis that stable individual differences exist not only in the magnitude of cardiovascu-

Table II. Blood pressure and heart rate data for subject 02 during psychophysiological testing and ambulatory monitoring

I. Psychophysiological testing

Test period	mm Hg	bpm
Baseline	143/76	73
Interview	175/94	82
TV pong	170/96	88
Mental arithmetic	175/93	94

II. Ambulatory monitoring – morning

Time	mm Hg	bpm	Subject's description of activity
9:00	135/76	75	baseline – sitting quietly
9:15	157/100	80	in office, preparing argument to justify promotions to boss
9:30	161/97	n.a.	as above
9:45	167/104	85	discussing promotion issue with colleague
10:00	144/94	n.a.	putting on coat, distracted by snagged sleeve
10:15	165/105	85	discussing promotion issue with another colleague
10:30	160/97	85	as above
10:45	186/129	95	presenting arguments to boss
11:00	160/100	n.a.	discussing results with staff
11:15	160/100	80	as above

lar response to challenge, but also the patterning of cardiovascular dynamics operating to produce BP elevations, which tend to remain stable regardless of type of task or challenge. Moreover, the findings also demonstrate that impedance cardiography can be efficiently employed in the psychophysiological paradigms discussed in this chapter.

The ambulatory monitoring phase of the pilot study was only recently completed and, as yet, summarized data are available for only a few of the participants. For illustration, we have included the findings from the first of the subjects (02) tested using this procedure. These are presented in table II, along with his data from the various psychophysiological test paradigms. In general, the levels of BP reactivity noted in the various test paradigms are consistent with those observed during the working day itself, although it is noteworthy that 02s confrontation with the plant manager succeeded in producing elevations considerably in excess of those seen for him during the psychophysiological tests. We have encountered few problems in obtaining

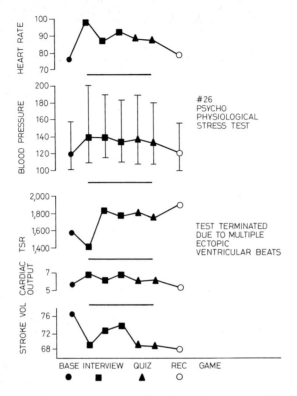

Fig. 2. Levels and patterns of cardiovascular response to laboratory maneuvers of subject number 26.

accurate readings from the ambulatory unit and the participants tested to date report no particular difficulty in adjusting to wearing the unit or in keeping the necessary activity sheets. Overall, the presence of the monitoring unit seems to have little impact on the normal activity of the participants, and in fact there appears to be good-natured involvement in the study from most of the participants.

In general, the findings to date from the pilot study indicate that the procedures and instrumentation discussed here can be successfully employed in a large-scale study of this type, and that the psychophysiological maneuvers developed with college students yield stable individual differences in cardiovascular reactivity among working adults.

We also have some anecdotal evidence that supports the feasibility of psychophysiological testing as a potential diagnostic tool. Figures 2 and 3 contain data derived from one of the subjects (26) whose testing was termi-

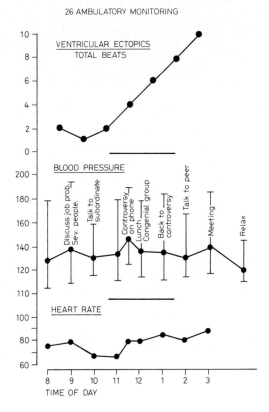

Fig. 3. Cardiovascular response of subject number 26 during ambulatory monitoring in the work place.

nated because he showed multiple ectopic ventricular beats while playing the TV pong game (fig. 2). In fact, at times these irritable beats were so severe that they approached ventricular tachycardia. Inspection of the health records of this 53-year-old subject revealed a recent ECG to be within normal limits, a resting BP of 140/90, and no prescribed medication either by the plant physician or his personal physician. Moreover, the subject was completely unaware of the ectopic beats and in fact pleaded with T.M.D. that he be allowed to finish the TV pong game because it was such fun! Although we insisted that psychophysiological testing be stopped, we did proceed with ambulatory monitoring of this subject.

Figure 3 presents his cardiovascular reactions during the working day. Inspection of these data shows a highly labile BP with levels linked to the vari-

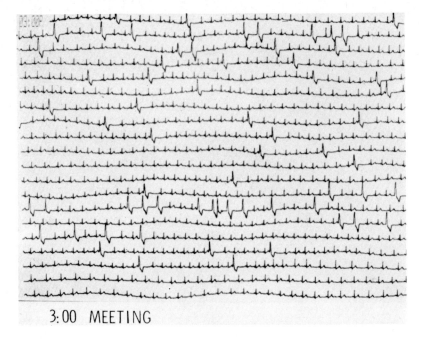

3:00 MEETING

Fig. 4. ECG tracing of subject number 26 during a 3:00 p.m. business meeting.

ous challenges encountered in the job place at different times of day. Note-worthy is the linear increase in premature ventricular contractions as the day progressed. Figure 4 shows his ECG at 3:00 p.m. while engaged in a business meeting. One need not be trained in cardiology to recognize the abnormality of the ECG tracings. We made his records available to both the plant and his personal physician. No medication was prescribed by either physician. Approximately 6 months after we tested this subject, he was admitted to the coronary care unit with an acute MI. Again, it is emphasized that this case history is anecdotal. However, the pilot data reported here and the experiences observed in our program of research clearly show, from a physio-logical perspective, that type A is not synonymous with hyperreactivity, nor is type B invariably associated with hyporeactivity. Moreover, the findings suggest that psychophysiological procedures have potential merit as diagnos-tic tools that can provide information beyond that available from purely behavioral assessment techniques alone.

```
ID:              #:    TIME:        POSITION: Stand, sit, lie
PEOPLE PRESENT: alone, one, several, crowd. INTERACTING:
WHERE:                                       YES   NO
ACTIVITY:
      NONE          physical activity (last 5 min)   CONTINOUS
  VERY LOW          estimated pressure (now)         VERY HIGH
   .DROWSY                                           ALERT
 LEISURELY                                           HURRIED
   RELAXED                                           TENSE
 LETHARGIC                                           ENERGETIC
      IDLE                                           BUSY
      CALM                                           EXCITED
       SAD                                           HAPPY
     ANGRY                                           AMUSED
  VERY LOW          estimated HR                     VERY HIGH
EVEN TEMPERED                                        IRRITATED
   PATIENT                                           IMPATIENT
COOPERATIVE                                          COMPETITIVE

      0                                              100
```

Fig. 5. Self-report form used in conjunction with ambulatory monitoring.

Psychophysiological laboratory maneuvers and ambulatory monitoring taken together also have potentially great usefulness in uncovering relationships between the emotions and physiological processes. The central question is: Do emotional states accurately mirror the physiology? The data from our program of research and those derived from the Omaha study suggest that the answer to this question is both yes and no. Work in our laboratory has consistently revealed little or no difference in reported mood states of type A and B subjects when they significantly differ in challenge-induced BP and/or HR elevations [13]. Figure 5 presents the self-report form used in conjunction with ambulatory monitoring in the Omaha study. Subjects responded to this form each time the monitoring device was triggered throughout the day, i.e. 15 min. Considering only *group* data from the study, the correlation between reported emotion and BP and HR elevations was not significant. However, when *within subject* correlations are considered, mood changes are correlated with changes in physiology. Said differently, suppose subject 1 reports high levels of tension, irritation, excitement, and the like, and subject 2 reports the same levels of emotional arousal. What does that tell us? It tells us that (a) both subjects are psychologically aroused and (b) we can be fairly confident that both are elevated in BP and/or HR over their respective baseline or resting levels. However, the self-report of emotional data tells us very little or nothing about how high each subject's BP or HR is at the time. Although both are elevated above resting levels, subject 1 could be 5 mmHg above baseline, while subject 2 might be 50 mmHg above resting level. And it is conceivable that both subjects might be near their respective maximum levels of both emotional arousal *and* physiological arousal. Thus, if one knows through psychophysiological testing at one point in time that a subject is a 'hot' reactor in a particular situation, and if later the subject reports high emotional arousal in the same situation, one can bet that such a person's BP is highly elevated.

Psychological Concomitants of Individual Differences in Cardiovascular Reactivity

In addition to the behavioral/psychological dimensions tapped by the two major type A assessment procedures (SI and JAS), we are administering a large number of standardized psychological tests to participants undergoing psychophysiological testing. Discriminant analysis will permit the specification of heretofore unidentified characteristics of individuals who evidence inappropriately high levels of cardiovascular reactivity. Behavioral attributes derived from these analyses will then be compared with those which have been related to CHD endpoints described in the first objective and to other endpoints as well, such as frequency of mild illnesses and family history of heart disease. Such data may suggest which behaviors may ultimately qualify for research in primary and secondary prevention programs.

A major assumption underlying this research is that the increased risk of CHD associated with the type A pattern is mediated via a behaviorally based predisposition toward exaggerated ANS/adrenocortical reactivity which is statistically more frequent in type A persons. As noted above, however, our work has shown that this statistical association is only modest for the SI and is quite weak for a variety of paper-and-pencil instruments which purport to assess type A behaviors. Indeed, we were the first to show through analyses of composite data from our laboratory studies that vocal mannerisms and levels of irritability and hostility manifest during the SI seem to carry most of the association burden with physiological reactivity, while self reports of speed, drive, ambition, work load, and so forth are less strongly related to physiological changes [8]. These findings from analysis of SI data suggest that many of the trait characteristics which form the conceptual definition of type A probably are not related to physiological reactivity and, in view of the *Matthews* et al. [32] data may not be related to CHD incidence either.

We are proposing that a constellation of *psychological and behavioral traits* which partially overlap the current definition of type A, lead individuals to respond to various environmental challenges with quantitatively exaggerated although qualitatively normal cardiovascular responses. Using type A and its various stylistic and attitudinal components as a starting point, we are attempting to empirically isolate the psychological factors and the specific elements in the physical/social environment which discriminate subgroups of subjects who evidence consistently high vs low magnitudes of cardiovascular reactivity.

The choice of psychological/behavioral measures to be included in the study was heavily influenced by the fact that the Stanford Research Institute Group has completed an extensive analysis of the relationship of a number of standardized scales to SI-defined type A and to static measures of coronary risk factors and psychological distress in a sample of 400 male aerospace workers in California [6]. In particular, this group has found that (a) SI determinations of type A behavior are poorly related to all other so-called type A scales; (b) variability in these other paper-and-pencil measures of coronary-proneness largely reflects the factors of impatience, anxiety, neuroticism, depression, extraversion, and achievement orientation; (c) two standardized instruments (subscales of Gough Adjective Checklist (ACL) and Thurstone Temperament Schedule) correlate better with SI determinations than does the JAS AB scale; (d) some non-SI measures of coronary-prone behavior correlate with static risk factors (e.g. lipid levels), while the SI is unrelated to such static factors, and (e) measures of involvement in job and social support are negatively correlated with distress and static CHD risk.

Based upon the foregoing and other findings from our own and *Chesney's* work, we have incorporated the following psychological instruments into the Western Electric and our ongoing college student studies, and these will serve as the bases for the psychometric analysis of persons evidencing different types and levels of cardiovascular reaction to the laboratory and day-to-day challenges.

(1) Type A measuring instruments: SI, JAS, Framingham Type A Scale. The SI and JAS have already been factor-analyzed [34], and the data analysis will utilize these derived factor scores.

(2) Gough ACL: 18 scale measure of personality trait characteristics, resolved by *Chadwick* et al. [6] into three factor components: 'impulsive aggressiveness', 'achievement orientation', 'lively extroversion', with the latter dimension moderately correlated with SI determinations.

(3) Eysenck Personality Questionnaire: A highly standardized instrument yielding primary divisions of extroversion and neuroticism which have

been related to physiological reactivity in a variety of studies [16], plus additional subscales for neuroticism and psychoticism.

(4) Sympton Distress Checklist: This instrument yields six subscales related primarily to psychological distress, with heavy loadings on neuroticism and depression.

(5) California Personality Inventory: This is a broadly used and highly standardized measure of non-psychiatric personality dimensions, and was previously employed by *Rahe* et al. [37] in a major twin study of type A described above.

(6) Work Environment Scale: This instrument was developed at Stanford Social Ecology Laboratory for assessing involvement, pressure, support, etc., in the work environment.

(7) Family Environment Scales: This instrument has 10 subscales designed to assess various aspects of the home environment [6].

(8) Brief Hypertension Instrument: This 16-item instrument developed by *Baer* et al. [2] successfully discriminated hypertensives from normotensives in five different samples of subjects. Examples of items include anger arousal, resentment, anxiety, and attention-seeking.

These instruments, along with an extensive health profile questionnaire, have been administered to the 30 participants in the Western Electric study and to 150 male and female college students who have undergone extensive psychophysiological evaluation in the laboratory. A subset of the latter will also undergo ambulatory BP and HR monitoring during normal college activities. The next step in the analysis will involve the identification of those personal and health status variables (e.g. sex, parental hypertension), situational factors (e.g. stress, type of challenge), and psychological-behavioral characteristics (e.g. type A, trait characteristics) which are correlated with distinguishable patterns of cardiovascular hypo- and hyperreactivity. Ultimately, our objective in this regard is to construct an explanatory model of the development and maintenance of pathological cardiovascular reactions to situational stress.

References

1   Alexander, F.: Psychosomatic medicine (Norton, New York 1950).
2   Baer, P.E.; Collins, F.H.; Bourianoff, G.G.; Ketchel, M.F.: Assessing personality factors in essential hypertension with a brief self-report scale. Psychosom. Med. *41:* 321–330 (1979).

3 Block, J.: Lives through time (Bancroft, Berkeley 1971).

4 Bortner, R.W.; Rosenman, R.H.; Friedman, M.: Familial similarity in pattern A behavior: fathers and sons. J. chron. Dis. *23:* 39–43 (1970).

5 Brod, J.; Fencl, V.; Hejl, Z.; Jirka, J.: Circulatory changes underlying blood pressure elevation during acute emotional stress (mental arithmetic) in normotensive and hypertensive subjects. Clin. Sci. *18:* 269–279 (1959).

6 Chadwick, J.H.; Chesney, M.A.; Black, G.W.; Rosenman, R.H.; Sevelius, G.G.: Psychological job stress and coronary heart disease. Technical report to National Institute for Occupational Safety and Health, 1979.

7 DeBaker, G.; Kornitzer, M.; Kittel, F.; Bogaert, M.; VonDurme, J.P.; Vincke, J.; Rustin, R.M.; Degre, C.; DeSchaepdrijven, A.: Relation between coronary-prone behavior pattern, excretion of urinary catecholamines, heart rate, and heart rhythm. Prev. Med. *8:* 14–22 (1979).

8 Dembroski, T.; Caffrey, B.; Jenkins, C.D.; Rosenman, R.H.; Spielberger, C.D.; Tasto, D.L.: Section summary: assesssment of coronary-prone behavior; in Dembroski, Weiss, Shields, Haynes, Feinleib, Coronary-prone behavior (Springer, New York 1978).

9 Dembroski, T.M.; MacDougall, J.M.: Stress effects on affiliation preferences among subjects possessing the type A coronary-prone behavior pattern. J. Personal. soc. Psychol. *36:* 23–33 (1978).

10 Dembroski, T.M.; MacDougall, J.M.; Herd, J.A.; Shields, J.L.: Effects of level of challenge on pressor and heart rate responses in type A and B subjects. J. appl. soc. Psychol. *9:* 209–228 (1979).

11 Dembroski, T.M.; MacDougall, J.M.; Lushene, R.: Interpersonal interaction and cardiovascular response in type A subjects and coronary patients. J. hum. Stress *5:* 28–36 (1979).

12 Dembroski, T.M.; MacDougall, J.M.; Shields, J.L.: Physiologic reactions to social challenge in persons evidencing the type A coronary-prone behavior pattern. J. hum. Stress *3:* 2–10 (1977).

13 Dembroski, T.M.; MacDougall, J.M.; Shields, J.L.; Petitto, J.; Lushene, R.: Components of the type A coronary-prone behavior pattern and cardiovascular responses to psychomotor performance challenge. J. behav. Med. *1:* 159–176 (1978).

14 Dembroski, T.M.; MacDougall, J.M.; Slaats, S.; Eliot, R.S.; Buell, J.C.: Relationship of challenge-induced cardiovascular response to illness, 1981. J. hum. Stress *7:* 2–5 (1981).

15 Dembroski, T.M.; Weiss, S.M.; Shields, J.L.; Haynes, S.G.; Feinleib, M. (eds): Coronary-prone behavior (Springer, New York 1978).

16 Eysenck, H.J.; Eysenck, S.B.G.: Manual for the Eysenck Personality Questionnaire (Educational & Industrial Testing, Service, San Diego 1975).

17 Falkner, B.; Onesti, G.; Angelakos, E.T.; Fernandes, M.; Langman, C.: Cardiovascular response to mental stress in normal adolescents with hypertensive patients. Hypertension *1:* 23–30 (1979).

18 Friedman, M.; St. George, S.; Byers, S.O.; Rosenman, R.H.: Excretion of catecholamines, 17-ketosteroids, 17-hydroxycorticoids, and 5-hydroxyindole in men exhibiting a particular behavior pattern (A) associated with high incidence of clinical coronary artery disease. J. clin. Invest. *39:* 758–764 (1960).

19 Glass, D.C.: Behavior patterns, stress and coronary disease. (Erlbaum, Hillsdale 1977).

20 Glass, D.C.; Krakoff, L.R.; Contrada, R.; Hilton, W.F.; Kehoe, K.; Mannucci, E.G.; Collins, C.; Snow, S.; Eltius, E.: Effect of harassment and competition upon cardiovascular

and catecholaminic responses in type A and B individuals. Psychophysiology *17:* 453–463 (1980).

21 Glass, D.C.; Krakoff, L.R.; Finkelman, J.; Snow, S.; Contrada, R.; Kehoe, K.; Mannucci, E.; Isocke, W.; Collins, C.; Hilton, W.F.: Effect of task overload upon cardiovascular and plasma catecholamine responses in type A and B individuals. Basic appl. soc. Psychol *1:* 199–218 (1980).

22 Jenkins, C.D.: Components of the coronary-prone behavior pattern: their relation to silent myocardial infarction and blood lipids. J. chron. Dis. *19:* 599–609 (1966).

23 Jenkins, C.D.: Behavioral risk factors in coronary artery disease. A. Rev. Med. *29:* 543–562 (1978).

24 Jenkins, C.D.; Rosenman, R.H.; Zyzanski, S.J.: Prediction of clinical coronary heart disease by a test for the coronary-prone behavior pattern. New Engl. J. Med. *290:* 1271–1275 (1974).

25 Kagan, J.; Moss, H.A.: Birth to maturity (Wiley, New York 1962).

26 Karnegis, J.N.; Kubicek, W.G.: Physiological correlates of the cardiac thoracid waveform. Am. Heart J. *79:* 519–523 (1970).

27 MacDougall, J.M.; Dembroski, T.M.; Krantz, D.S.: Effects of types of challenge on pressor and heart rate responses in type A and B women. Psychophysiology *18:* 1–9 (1981).

28 MacDougall, J.M.; Dembroski, T.M.; Musante, L.: The structured interview and questionnaire methods of assessing coronary-prone behavior in male and female college students. J. behav. Med. *2:* 71–83 (1979).

29 Manuck, S.B.; Corse, C.D.; Winkelman, P.A.: Behavioral correlates of individual differences in blood pressure reactivity. J. psychosom. Res. *23:* 281–288 (1979).

30 Manuck, S.B.; Garland, F.N.: Coronary-prone behavior pattern, task incentive and cardiovascular response. Psychophysiology *16:* 136–147 (1979).

31 Matthews, K.A.: Assessment and developmental antecedents of the coronary-prone behavior pattern in children; in Dembroski, Weiss, Shields, et al., Coronary-prone behavior (Springer, New York 1978).

32 Matthews, K.A.; Glass, D.C.; Rosenman, R.H.; Bortner, R.W.: Competitive drive, pattern A, and coronary heart disease: a futher analysis of some data from the Western Collaborative Group Study. J. chron. Dis. *30:* 489–498 (1977).

33 Matthews, K.A.; Krantz, D.S.: Resemblances of twins and their parents in pattern A behavior. Psychosom. Med. *28:* 140–144 (1976).

34 Matthews, K.A.; Krantz, D.S.; Dembroski, T.M.; MacDougall, J.M.: The unique and common variance in the structured interview and Jenkins activity survey measures of the type A behavior pattern. J. Personal. soc. Psychol. *42:* 303–313 (1982).

35 McClelland, D.C.; Floor, E.; Davidson, R.J.; Saron, C.: Stressed power motivation, sympathetic activation, immune function, and illness. J. hum. Stress *6:* 11–19 (1980).

36 Miller, J.C.; Horvath, S.M.: Impedance cardiography. Psychophysiology *15:* 80–91 (1978).

37 Rahe, R.H.; Hervig, L.; Rosenman, R.H.: The heretability of type A behavior. Psychosom. Med. *40:* 478–486 (1978).

38 Rose, R.M.; Jenkins, C.D.; Hurst, M.W.: Air traffic controller health change study. Report to the Federal Aviation Administration, June 1978.

39 Rosenman, R.H.: The interview method of assessment of the coronary-prone behavior pattern; in Dembroski, Weiss, Shields, et al., Coronary-prone behavior (Springer, New York 1978).

40   Rosenman, R.H.; Friedman, M.: Neurogenic factors in pathogenesis of coronary heart disease. Med. Clins N. Am. *58:* 269–279 (1974).

41   Stokols, D.; Novaco, R.W.; Stokols, J.; Campbell, J.: Traffic congestion, type A behavior, and stress. J. appl. Psychol. *63:* 467–480 (1978).

42   Waldron, I.; Hickey, A.; McPherson, C.; Butensky, A.; Gruss, L.; Overall, K.; Schmader, A.; Wohlmuth, D.: Type A behavior pattern: relationship to variation in blood pressure, paternal characteristics, and academic and social activities of students. J. hum. Stress *6:* 16–27 (1980).

43   Williams, R.B.; Haney, T.L.; Lee, Kong, Blumenthal, Whalen: Type A behavior, hostility, and coronary atherosclerosis. Psychosom. Med. *42:* 539–549 (1980).

Appendix

Quantitative Scoring Key for Type A Interviews
    Each of the seven *stylistic* dimensions is scored on a 1–5 point scale, anchored as indicated below.

    1. Loud Voice. Subject's voice is scored for loudness, independently of the other voice stylistics listed below. There is often, but not always, a melodic quality associated with the soft voice.
1   Consistently soft voice.
2   Less than average loudness.
3   Average loudness.
4   Greater than average loudness.
5   Consistently loud voice.

    2. Explovise Speech. Subjects with this attribute usually, but by no means always, have a louder than average voice. The key stylistic here is vigorous emphasis or explosiveness on some words or sentences, particularly simple declarative statements ('Never!' or 'Right! – Right!') or emphatic adjectives ('I'm *always* on time!'). It is the explosiveness of the subject's words with or without other stylistics that is scored. It is often the interviewer's challenges that will trigger maked increases in explosiveness. This is a key point to remember. Look for explosiveness in strings of words *and* during abrupt, single-word answers.
1   Consistently without particular emphasis on key words.
2   Sometimes, but rarely, increases emphasis on words or abrupt declarations.
3   Occasionally shows explosiveness.
4   Frequent explosiveness.
5   Consistently *explosive* declarations, often consisting of single words.

    3. Rapid and Accelerated Speech. The stylistic consists of rapid word production, most often with an acceleration of speech at the end of a long sentence. In the extreme, this may be accompanied by 'word clipping' (failure to pronounce the ending sounds of words or tripping over words, e.g. saying 'immedialy' instead of 'immediately'), word repetition ('yes, yes'), or word ommission ('No!' I 'Never do that!'). Accelerated speech is often observed during attempts at self-justification in response to interview challenges.
1   Consistently slow, measured word production, often accompanied by pauses, 'ahs', or breaks at the end of sentences.

2   Less than average production rate. Generally slow production rate, but with one or two instances of rapid and accelerated speech.
3   About average production rate with instances of both slow, deliberate speech, and rapid and accelerated speech.
4   Faster than average production rate, with few instances of slow, measured speech.
5   Extreme tendency toward high rate of speech, accelerated endings, word clipping, word repetition, and omission.

4. Response Latency. Responses are given with very short latencies and in the extreme occur prior to completion of the question. Also included is 'hurrying' in which the subject attempts to speed up the question by saying 'yes, yes' or 'mm, mm' or some other verbal device.
1   Consistently long latencies (one or more seconds) between the end of the question and the beginning of the answer.
2   Generally long latencies, but a few short latency answers and an absence of 'hurryings'.
3   Occasional short latency responses, but usually an average number with *few* interrupting answers and no more than one or two 'hurryings'.
4   The majority of responses are of a short latency, with a few 'hurryings'.
5   Consistently short latencies with several interruptions and 'hurryings'.

5. Potential for Hostility. This is a difficult dimension to score. Here, it is primarily a clinical judgment. Pay attention to both stylistics and content. Responses are argumentative ('Nobody always does anything'), repeatedly and unnecessarily qualified ('It depends'), pointlessly challenging of the interviewer ('What do you mean by *that*?'). The voice characteristics suggest boredom, condescension, or surliness. Subject's answers to specific questions suggest impatience, anger, or irritability when faced with obstacles ('...Car going too slowly...' '...wait in lines...') and the tendency to make harsh generalizations ('The people here are all narrow-minded'). Extreme levels of hostility may be accompanied by *obscenity* or use of emotion laden words ('I *hate* it here!').
1   No statements with possible hostile content or structure, and no hostile voice stylistics.
2   Some (one or two statements) hostile content, but no hostility in voice stylistics.
3   Two to three potentially hostile statements and perhaps some suggestion of hostility in voice stylistics.
4   Three or more content admissions of hostility or anger and some evidence of hostility in attitude or voice stylistics.
5   Frequent hostility expressed in attitude or voice stylistics.

6. Anger-In. This is a rather straightforward dimension to score. Throughout the interview there are several questions regarding the subject's willingness to express anger, to say something to someone in a frustrating circumstance, to sound the horn at a slow driver, etc. Note that one key question simply asks the respondent whether he/she outwardly expresses anger. If the subject answers in the negative to this question he/she automatically receives a score of 3. However, if subsequently the subject makes two or more statements indicating a willingness to express anger, the score is reduced to 2 in the absence of additional evidence to the contrary. Note that a higher score indicates a tendency to hold anger in.
1   Frequent examples of expressing irritation or anger openly, often in a vociferous manner.
2   Generally admits to outward expressions of anger.

3   Expresses some reluctance to show irritation or anger openly, although will do so in appro-
     priate circumstances and/or admits that anger is sometimes held in.
4   No more than one admission of expressing anger openly and more than one admission
     of *unwillingness* to show anger openly.
5   No statements of expressing irritation or anger openly and several statements reflecting
     an unwillingness to show anger outwardly.

7. Competition for Control of Interview. Subject attempts to gain control of the interview
by interrupting interviewer with lengthy responses, engaging in verbal duets, asking for unnecessary qualifications, or offering extraneous (and sometimes hostile) comments or questions which
divert the direction of the interview. Distinguish simple hostility (negativism) from hostility
directed toward intimidating the interviewer and thus gaining control. The latter, of course, is
also scored as potential for hostility. Excessive qualification without hostile or competitive intent
occurs occasionally. Frequently, subjects who are anxious or type B will show such behavior.
A very good index of verbal competitiveness is the tactic of raising the voice to subdue the interviewer when he/she interrupts the respondent.
1   No tendency to compete; subject passively responds to questions.
2   Possibility of some competitiveness, but no really clear examples.
3   Occasional attempts to compete.
4   Three or more clear examples of verbal competitiveness.
5   Repeated attempts to gain control. Score a 5 only if you perceive an ongoing struggle for
     control of the interview.

8. Quality of Interview. For a variety of reasons, occasionally an interviewer will not conduct the interview properly or in a standardized manner. For example, interviewers might not
be challenging enough or there might be too much extraneous noise while the interview is being
conducted. Therefore, it is important to rate the quality of the interview according to current
standards. [For more details on the SI, see ref. 39].
1   Extremely poor.
2   Marginally acceptable.
3   Adequate.
4   Above average administration.
5   Excellent.

9. Comments. Occasionally a non-type A attribute particularly stands out in a subject, e.g.
physical impairment, neuroticism, low intelligence, etc. Therefore, space is available to make
such comments on the scoring sheet.

Content of Responses
     Content is scored with *total* disregard to stylistics. Each question is scored on a 1–5 scale,
with 1 indicating the complete absence of the trait ('No, I never get impatient') and 5 indicating
that the trait is always present ('I'm always impatient in lines'; 'I hate lines'). Use the 1 and 5
scores only when there is absolutely no doubt about the *extreme* character of the response. A
score of 3 indicated an 'average' level of the trait. In the strong majority of cases either a score
of 2 or 4 is assigned. A mean rating value is computed for all questions making up each dimension. This score is then multiplied by 10 to eliminate the decimal point [see ref. 34 for details
on factor structures].

9 Cardiovascular Reactions and Cardiovascular Risk[1]

Thomas H. Schmidt

Behavioral medicine is a new branch in modern medical science, but its roots may range to the beginning of medical practice. An old story dates back to the 3rd century BC and testifies how the link between social bond, emotion, behavior, physiology and disease was understood by ancient Greek medicine, and how psychophysiology was already used as a diagnostic tool. *Plutarch* [27] tells us that Erasistratos, a physician of the Alexandrian school, was called upon by Seleukos, king of Syria, to heal his sick son Antiochus. After an accurate examination, the physician ordered all women living at the court of the king to pass Antiochus' bed. Feeling the patient's pulse, Erasistratos noticed an acceleration and irregularity when Stratonike, the prince's young stepmother, passed by. The physician told the 70-year-old king his diagnosis. Seleukos was a wise man, and so the cure was easy. The king separated from his wife and Stratonike was married to Antiochus who recovered quite soon.

Nowadays medicine has been confronted with an enormous rise in cardiovascular disease. During the last few decades cardiovascular morbidity and mortality have grown to a vast epidemiological extent. Although we have recognized some early indicators, only about half of the new cases of coronary heart disease (CHD) can be predicted by the standard risk factors, such as elevated levels of serum cholesterol, blood pressure (BP), and cigarette smoking. To improve prediction, which may create better possibilities for prevention, two major strategies can be pursued. One is to look for new, unknown factors; in this regard behavioral and psychosocial predictors have been discovered, and the importance of the type A coronary-prone behavior pattern or the role of social support have, for instance, been explored. A second strategy is to improve and refine the assessment of some of the known factors. This altogether may bring further understanding of and give more insight into the mechanisms leading to the disease.

---

[1] Dedicated to Prof. Dr. *Thure von Uexküll* on the occasion of his 75th birthday.

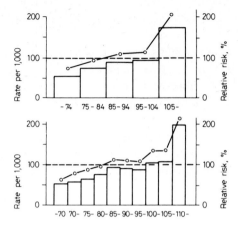

Fig. 1. 12-year rates of myocardial infarction and cardiovascular deaths per 1,000 as a function of DBP calculated from the Pooling Project, which includes data from Albany, Chicago, Framingham, and Tecumseh. The rise in cardiovascular risk with rising DBP derived from first measurement taken is apparent whether BP values are broken down by 10 units (upper) or 5 units (lower) mm Hg. Above average risk occurs at about DBP of 85 mm Hg [26].

No doubt, up to now, the risk factor with the most practical value is height of BP, which appears to be in a dose-response relationship to cardiovascular morbidity and mortality. What many epidemiological studies reveal clearly is that the lower the systolic/diastolic BP, measured on one or more occasions, the lower the risk (fig. 1) [26, 28].

Moreover, reduction of BP clearly has reduced cardiovascular risk over a broad range, and from such intervention studies we cannot even determine at present the lowest value at which further reduction of BP would not reduce the risk. For example, in the Hypertension Detection and Follow-up Program the group with the lowest diastolic BP (90–94 mm Hg), which still received very strict antihypertensive treatment (in a stepped care program), showed a clear reduction in mortality of 22% compared to a traditionally treated group (referred care) whose BP was lowered only by a few mm Hg less [18]. Such investigations indicate that the optimal value appears to be the lowest BP which is compatible with physical and mental efficiency. From a physiological point of view, of course, there should be a BP value below which if not cardiovascular mortality, then at least overall mortality should increase. But epidemiological studies have not to my knowledge been able to detect this, and we might find in the future that

BP could be much lower before it becomes a risk on the other side of the coin.

As BP is not a stable phenomenon, but shows circadian variations and is dependent on situational influences to a great extent, we might have a good chance of improving its power of prediction if we have more detailed and accurate information about how the individual's BP reacts during the course of the day and night. So we have to explore today diagnostic strategies that ancient Erasistratos already practiced; using modern facilities, like ambulatory monitoring, we can monitor our daily activities and hope thus to recognize more precisely causes and possible cures of this 20th century epidemic.

Emotional and Circadian Influences

Through emotional influences, numerous environmental conditions can have a triggering function in BP reactions. With regard to this close connection between emotional behavior and BP rises in Germany, *von Uexküll and Wick* [42] coined the conception of situational hypertension ('Situationshypertonie'). The linkage between environmental stimuli and emotional behavior is to a great extent probably determined by learning processes, and thus neutral stimuli can acquire the ability to trigger physiologic reaction patterns because of the individual learning history.

An experiment that happened to occur by chance may illustrate this connection between environmental stimuli and physiologic reaction patterns as well as the modification of this linkage depending on emotional cues and on what could be called an internal readiness for reaction. For special diagnostic reasons a continuous BP measurement was carried out in a 24-year-old woman over a period of several days. The continuous intraarterial measurement was registered on paper tape every 15 min for 15 s, whereby a recorder standing near the patient's bed automatically switched itself on with a soft humming sound. The BP measurement was commenced in the morning. The patient had to keep to strict bed rest because of the measurements, and during the day nothing out of the ordinary was observed (fig. 2a). Shortly after 9 p.m. the patient wished to sleep, and turned the light off; she was feeling anxious and was wondering whether her BP values were 'good' or not. At 9.15 p.m. the recorder switched itself on again with a soft hum, as it had done every 15 min throughout the day. The BP rose within 7 heart beats systolically more than 40 mm Hg and diastolically 35 mm Hg; the heart rate was also accelerated by 20 bpm, but fell again to the original level as soon as the maxi-

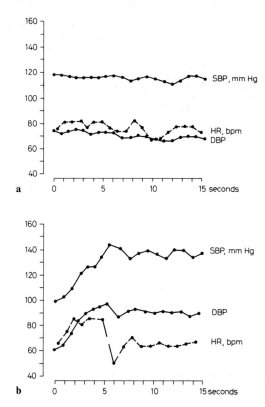

Fig. 2. Beat-to-beat analysis of BP and HR during an interval of 15 s in a 24-year-old patient at bed rest. **a** At daytime there are no major changes of these parameters during automatic registration of intraarterial BP every 15 min. **b** At night, in an anxious state, the soft noise during recording evokes stereotyped reactions of BP and HR every 15 min. SBP = Systolic, DBP = diastolic BP.

mal pressure rise was reached (fig. 2b). These cardiovascular reactions then showed a stereotyped repetition to the same extent every 15 min. Apparently, the patient attached a specific meaning to the sound of the recorder during the night: in her anxiety it became a tormenting waking stimulus with the accompanying physiological changes. Eventually the patient found her futile attempts at going to sleep 'too stupid', and at 12.30 a.m. she began to read. During this period, the rises in BP and heart rate (HR) discontinued. A renewed attempt at sleeping between 3 and 5 a.m. again led every quarter of an hour to stereotyped rises in BP and HR within a few seconds by more than 40 mm Hg systolically. This phenome-

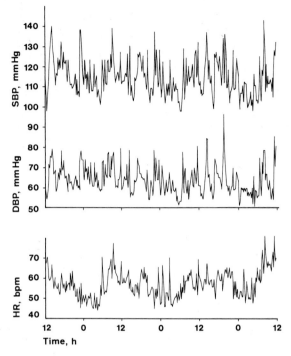

Fig. 3. BP and HR variations in a 40-year-old normotensive patient during the course of 3 days at strict bed rest. Units of observation were derived by averaging every 15 min BP values from 10 heart beats. SBP= Systolic BP; DBP= diastolic BP.

non was repeated during the entire night more than 20 times. The patient then at last decided to give up her futile attempts at sleep and to remain awake: the BP and HR reactions disappeared. During the following nights when the patient slept after she had been reassured, these reactions did not recur.

The above example makes it evident how rapidly, and through very slight external stimuli, considerable cardiovascular reactions can be evoked, even during apparent calmness, when there is a corresponding internal readiness and expectation. The slight humming sound connected with the measuring procedure was capable of producing a distinct cardiovascular reaction, and perhaps this was only because it gained a specific subjective meaning during attempts at sleep during that particular night. In other words, if the stimulus loses its specific anxiety-inducing meaning, i.e. when reading or after the decision 'to be awake', during the day or during other nights, it also loses its specific cardiovascular effects. Many such conditioning processes

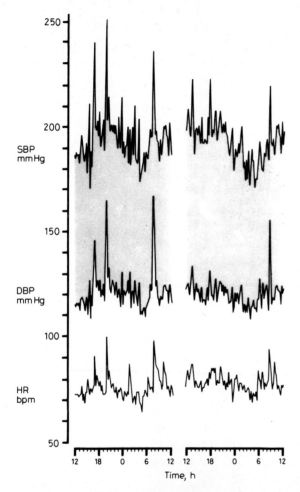

Fig. 4. BP and HR variations in a 31-year-old yet untreated hypertensive patient during the course of 2 days at strict bed rest (see also fig. 3 for units of observation). SBP = Systolic BP; DBP = diastolic BP.

may have an impact on our daily lives. Even at strict bed rest strong cardiovascular reactions can in general be detected in normotensive as well as hypertensive patients (fig. 3, 4).

In 10 untreated hypertensive patients the average maximal BP range during 24 h at strict bed rest was 62 mm Hg for systolic BP (SBP) and 42 mm Hg for diastolic BP (DBP), when intraarterial BP was registered and averaged every quarter of an hour for 10 heart beats; in 10 normotensive

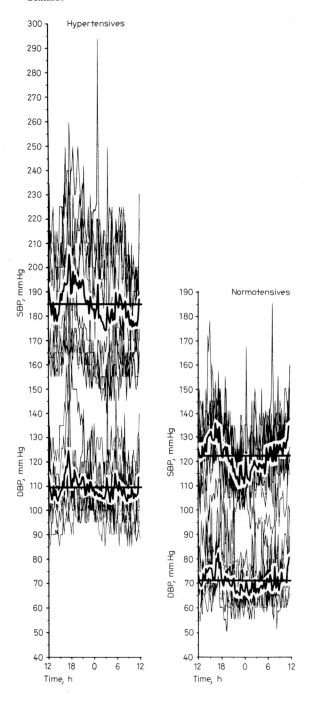

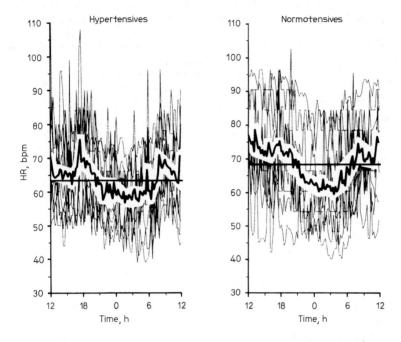

Fig. 6. Mean and individual circadian variation in HR (see fig. 5 for more detail).

patients this BP range was still 52/39 mm Hg. These are enormous changes if compared to the growing risk already appearing in BP steps of 10 or even 5 mm Hg, when measured in epidemiological studies just on one occasion with the Riva-Rocci method, which is, of course, not as accurate as intra-arterial measurements.

Mean value curves of the circadian variation such as in figures 5 and 6, calculated in hypertensive or normotensive patients over the course of 24 h, hide these situational pressure rises as they depend on momentary environmental influences which vary in time and patients. Therefore, the mean circadian fluctuation in these curves is considerably less, and its range of oscillation does not show a difference between the hypertensive and normotensive group with SBP changes of only about 30 mm Hg and DBP changes of about

Fig. 5. 24-hour mean and mean circadian variation (thick lines) as well as individual circadian variation (thin lines) of SBP and DBP in 10 normotensive and 10 untreated hypertensive patients during bed rest. These data were derived from continuous intraarterial BP measurement by averaging the values of 10 heart beats every 15 min [see also ref. 36].

Table I. Variance components (%) of SBP, DBP, PP, and HR in 10 normotensive and 10 hypertensive patients

	Blood pressure			Heart rate
	systolic	diastolic	pulse pressure	
Normotensives				
Between patients	36	26	67	68
Between trials (BT)	14	10	3	10
Error variance (EV)	50	64	31	22
Ratio EV/BT	3.6	6.4	10.3	2.2
Hypertensives				
Between patients	74	51	78	51
Between trials	5	6	2	8
Error variance	21	43	19	41
Ratio EV/BT	4.2	7.2	9.5	5.1

20 mm Hg, although the SBP fall at night takes a longer time to reach its minimum in the hypertensive group and shows a higher rise in the morning at wakening time [33, 35].

An analysis of the different components of the total BP variance can reveal the importance of unsystematic situational BP changes. The total variance of all measured BP values is composed of three components: (1) differences in BP levels, i.e. differences of 24-hour mean values between patients (between patients); (2) BP differences at different times in the mean circadian oscillation (between trials), and (3) error variance, which includes the different situational reactions of the patients.

These variance components are calculated in table I for SBP, DBP, pulse pressure (PP), and HR in the normotensive and hypertensive groups separately, as percentage of the total variance. Normotensives were defined as patients with 24-hour mean values below 140/90 mm Hg and hypertensives with 24-hour mean values above 159/93 mm Hg. The difference of the variance components 'between patients' in BP is partly dependent upon this arbitrary definition, as there is an upper limit for the normotensive group but not for the hypertensive group. In all of the cardiovascular parameters the variance component 'between trials', which constitutes the mean circadian variation, has the smallest percentage. The error variance represents the portion of the total variance which is not explained by differences between the

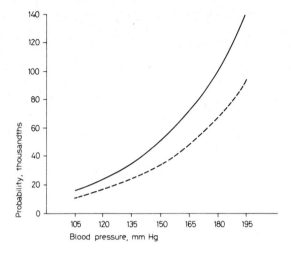

Fig. 7. Risk in cardiovascular morbidity depending on lowest (——; T= 23.62) versus highest (– – –; T= 14.95) SBP (Framingham Study 18-year follow-up) in 30- to 79-year-old men [21].

patients BP, PP, or HR level or by the mean circadian variation, but it includes all unsystematic situational changes during 24 h. This error variance explains quite a considerable amount of BP variance, as can be seen in table I. The ratio error variance/between trials gives an estimate of how much more of the variance can be explained by the different situational reactions of the patients than by the common circadian variation, and this is about 4 times more for SBP, 6–7 times for DBP, around 10 times for PP, and twice as much for HR in normotensives as well as 5 times in the hypertensive patients [36].

These results demonstrate the much greater role situational changes play compared to the circadian fluctuations. The fact that situational BP reactions already occur to such a great extent during physical inactivity at bed rest points to the decisive importance of psychological and emotional factors in daily BP regulation. As these BP changes explain even at bed rest a relatively large proportion of the total variance, they might well be regarded as a potential risk factor.

Epidemiological studies point also to the possibility of a more detailed assessment of BP improving prediction. In the Framingham Study lowest as well as highest SBP from repeated measurements are seen to contribute to cardiovascular morbidity (fig. 7) [21], and SBP lability in normotensive men and women seems to be associated with the development of hypertension during the course of 12 years [20]. Moreover, 3 DBP measurements appear to be a better predictor for the development of hypertension than just one DBP value [30, 39b], and reactions of DBP in the cold pressor test have been related to the incidence of CHD over the course of a 20-year prospective study [22]. All these data suggest that height, duration, and frequency of situational BP rises also influence cardiovascular risk, although the question remains still unanswered whether these BP reactions contribute to the risk just by increasing the mean BP or whether they bear additionally a risk of their own. We may ask why we have inherited the ability to react in this way and why we are exposed to those reactions to such an enormous extent even at rest, although this appears to be not only unnecessary but also harmful.

Evolutionary and Physiological Aspects

As *Konrad Lorenz* [25] has pointed out, every living organism is in each of its structural and functional characteristics determined by the course evolution has followed. This is true for all living creatures, including their morphology and physiology, their perception, behavior and emotions, and generally for all psychic functions, up to and inclusive of human reason [29]. *Charles Darwin* described the interplay of spontaneous genetic changes (the term mutation was introduced later by *De Vries*) and natural selection as the main causes of the extraordinary adaptation of organisms to their environment. Of course, he already understood his theory of evolution in this broad sense. When *Alfred Russel Wallace,* the independent codiscoverer of the theory of evolution, argued in public about his opinion concerning the human mind being free of the consequences of natural selection, *Darwin* [3] wrote to him in 1869: 'I hope you have not murdered too completely your own and my child.'

The organisms achieved the fitness and suitability of their organization through the processes of mutation, new combinations of genes by sexual reproduction, and natural selection. Random changes took place in the genetic code, and those genotypes better adapted to the environmental conditions survived, leaving a greater number of descendants. That is to say, genotypes with ill-fated adaptation left fewer descendants and died out. If the environmental conditions change, natural selection advances some of the existing genetic variations within a certain species and suppresses others. After a corresponding space of time, a new, better genetic adaptation to the changed conditions has been achieved.

In analyzing form and function of living systems, there are two major tasks: one is to describe the system in its momentary state; the second is to find out how it has developed in that way rather than another. It is the same question the English philosopher *David Hume* put at the center of his considerations: 'How does the mind work, and why does it work in such a way and not another?' Living structures and functions are always a compromise formed by different and often opposing selection pressures, and for a deeper understanding science has to ask the evolutionary question: 'Of what use are these structures and functions?' which means that we want to understand their values for survival.

Under such perspectives we have to ask with regard to BP, why has evolution not provided us all with an optimal low BP, which guarantees a maximal span of life? One explanation could be that a higher BP is connected with other advantages in the selection processes, or at least that it has been connected with advantages in the phylogenetic past and therefore a higher cardiovascular risk has been allowed for. Another reason could be found in a rapid change of environmental conditions which have an effect on BP, with time being too short for genetic adaptation. Consider the possibility that nowadays BP is such an impressive predictor of morbidity and mortality because today in many human societies the natural life expectancy predominating the greater part of our evolution has been considerably prolonged through the control of other factors which used to shorten life.

From a theoretical point of view, longevity, by itself, cannot be expected in general to be an evolutionary advantage if there is sexual reproduction. This is the case only under special conditions, as for instance if parental care gives the descendants of that species a better chance for survival of the adaptive gene pool. Preprogrammed short lives could have an advantage in the more rapid succession of generations, as they enable a faster genetic adaptation to environmental change. The average length of a species' life is probably a compromise between different counteracting selection pressures, however, measuring which presents the real problem. Knowledge about the effective selection pressures working on us is the basis for a better understanding also of very important factors in human epidemiology; it is these factors we wish to manipulate, for instance by extending life through early antihypertensive treatment.

A selection pressure is only then directly and clearly measurable in terms of mortality rates if it concerns populations before their age of reproduction. Later on opposing factors may occur, the effects of which can scarcely be isolated in detail. Cardiovascular mortality does not reach its peak until well after the initial age of reproduction. It thus appears possible that the long-term effects of a high BP or of a higher BP reactivity, which may partially depend on the physiological adaptations to high BP, must be allowed for, because it may be associated at a younger age with advantages in the selection process.

The circulatory function certainly serves to adapt the organism to the tissue's changing requirements; this has to be regarded as a regulatory system for the tissue's supply. The basis for this is a blood volume adapted to the requirements, as well as a sufficient pressure gradient between arteries and veins. The tissue's changing requirements demand a complex regulatory system which can change the total blood flow in the cardiovascular system as well as relative blood flows to the various vascular areas, according to their needs. Height of arterial BP, determined by cardiac output and peripheral vascular resistance, as well as BP changes, are mainly responsible for height and variations of the pressure gradient. Situational BP rises increase the pressure gradient for the time of their duration, i.e. with unchanged resistance they enable a higher blood flow at the same time, or the same blood volume can be transported against a higher resistance.

Situational BP rises enable rapid shifts of blood volume from one area in the body to another. As the investigations of *Brod* [2] have shown whether a situational BP rise is produced by a rise in peripheral vascular resistance, or in cardiac output, or both, there is always a shift of blood volume to the musculature. This reaction pattern is integrated in the hypothalamus and commonly has been called the hypothalamic defense reaction [1, 6]. It includes a centrally initiated inhibition of vagal influences to the heart and a sympathetic activation of heart, venous system, and most parts of the arterial vascular system, which leads, with the exception of the vessels in the musculature, to vasoconstriction; in contrast, muscle vessels dilate, enabling a better blood supply to the muscle [9]. The humoral reactions consist of adrenalin being released from the adrenal medulla [14], the ACTH-cortico-steroid system being activated in the pituitary gland and adrenal cortex [8], as well as a neurogenic release of renin [4, 44], and thus the inclusion of the angiotensin-aldosterone mechanism. Many stimuli can elicit this prepro-grammed reaction pattern and with it situational BP rises. As muscular activation is associated with vasodilatation of the appropriate vessel areas, this physiologic reaction pattern guarantees a better blood supply to the working musculature and hinders a sudden pressure fall, which otherwise could result because of the necessary vasodilatation during a motor action. Here we can see why numerous environmental stimuli are able to elicit this defense reaction as a cardiovascular preparation and adjustment to imminent motor action. The environment, so to speak, has to be under continuous observation for the possibility or probability of an acute danger, in which case the organism must be able to react immediately with a powerful motoric action. Obviously, it is quite possible, then, for situational pressure peaks to occur most of the time in the absence of real need; that is when no motoric action is necessary. On the other hand, a powerful motoric response without preceding cardiovascular adjustment would otherwise lead to a quick fatigue of working muscles, which could have fatal consequences in acute danger. Viewed in this way, the usefulness of the defense reaction becomes directly evident, and so we can understand why the organism is programmed to react with even more situational pressure rises than are actually necessary. Said differently, the reaction is usually not needed, but fortunately it is there in times of real need.

The organism's ability to link this reaction pattern together with new environmental stimuli through learning processes is of great importance. It can thus probably be evoked as a conditioned response, enabling a better preparation and adaptation of circulation to a great variety of environmental conditions in which it would be necessary for the organism to have a motoric response. In other words, easier release of the hypothalamic defense reaction could have been an advantage during evolution under certain environmental conditions. But what may have been an important and necessary advantage for survival in the short run can be a risk in the long run. Inappropriate release of the defense reaction places more stress and strain on the heart and the circulatory system, which may heighten the risk for the development of hypertension, CHD and earlier death [*Buell and Eliot*, and *Herd*, this volume]. So this genetically preprogrammed hypothalamic defense reaction appears to be a mechanism for helping to speed up the redistribution of blood flow from the kidneys, splanchnic area, skin etc. to the musculature – an adaptation of the organism's presumable need in emergency situations like fight or flight. The point is, however, how many times do we fully use our muscles to fight or flee in modern 20th century existance? Perhaps in this context the most frequently used muscles are only the vocal cords.

In humans, the defense reaction pattern responds in a very sensitive way already to a great variety of environmental stimuli, as for instance different mental tasks. If these tasks and the measurement procedures are standardized to a high degree, it can be shown that strength and duration of the defense reaction depends on the specific stimulus [*Engel*, this volume]. In relation to the theory of *Lacey and Lacey* [24], of a varying activation pattern

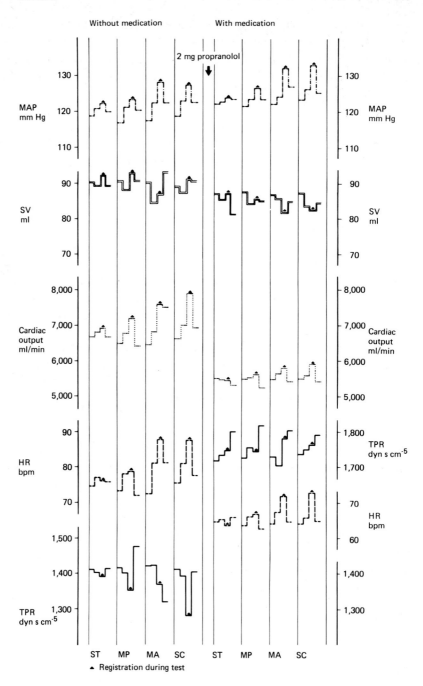

Without medication   With medication

2 mg propranolol

MAP mm Hg

SV ml

Cardiac output ml/min

HR bpm

TPR dyn s cm⁻⁵

MAP mm Hg

SV ml

Cardiac output ml/min

TPR dyn s cm⁻⁵

HR bpm

ST   MP   MA   SC   ST   MP   MA   SC

▲ Registration during test

of the cardiovascular system with experimental conditions involving processes such as sensory intake or sensory rejection, we investigated 30 patients to examine hemodynamic response patterns of different tasks. In this study the role of β-sympathetic mechanisms were investigated by use of propranolol [34, 39].

In four different task situations intraarterial BP (in the brachial artery) as well as the cardiac output (thermodilution method) at 1-min intervals were determined. The total peripheral resistance was calculated from these parameters. The four task situations were set in random sequence and consisted of: observation of stroboscopic light flashes (ST; with a frequency of 10 Hz); detecting the missing part (MP) of a picture shown on a slide, out of an intelligence test (Hawie); solving a mental arithmetic (MA) problem; and forming a sentence out of 5 words all beginning with the same letter of the alphabet (SC). For each task situation four recordings were made at 1-min intervals: (1) at rest before the task; (2) at task announcement (by slide); (3) during the task, shown by a slide, and (4) at rest after the task.

Figure 8 gives an overview of the reactions in the 30 patients of the main variables which were investigated during the four task situations including the four periods of measurement each before and after the intravenous administration of 2 mg propranolol. The reactions of the mean arterial pressure (MAP), stroke volume (SV), cardiac output, HR, and total peripheral resistance (TPR) are displayed in figure 8. During the different task situations variably marked increases of MAP can be seen; they occur through correspondingly variably marked increases of cardiac output, which again arise from correspondingly differentiated increases of HR. The results of an Anova and of linear orthogonal contrasts revealed (independent of propranolol effects) higher reactions for the latter three variables as well as for SBP and DBP in task MA and SC compared to ST and MP (MAP: $T = 7.21$, $p < 0.001$; cardiac output: $T = 30.6$, $p < 0.001$; HR: $T = 98.2$, $p < 0.001$). The reactions of these variables to ST and to MP, which show a stronger increase, can be differentiated statistically in virtually identical fashion. In addition, the reaction after MA continues longer than that observed after SC.

Fig. 8. Mean changes of main hemodynamic parameters of 30 patients during four different task situations (ST = observation of stroboscopic light flashes; MP = mistake in picture task; MA = mental arithmetic; SC = sentence construction) before and after i.v. injection of 2 mg propranolol. In each task situation four measurements were taken in 1-min intervals: (1) at rest; (2) at task announcement; (3) during the task; (4) at rest after the task. MAP = Mean arterial pressure; SV = stroke volume; TPR = total peripheral resistance.

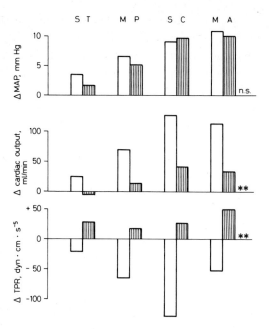

Fig. 9. Mean reactions of Δ mean arterial pressure (MAP), Δ cardiac output, and Δ total peripheral resistance (TPR) during the four task situations without (white columns) and after propranolol injection (shaded columns). There is no significant change in MAP reactions, whereas cardiac output reactions are reduced by propranolol and TPR reactions are changed from a decrease to an increase. ST = Stroboscopic light flashes; MP = missing part of a picture; SC = sentence construction; MA = mental arithmetic. ** $p < 0.001$.

In line with the defense reaction, the different BP rises are induced at simultaneous inhibition of the baroreceptor reflex. Without propranolol, the TPR gives a mirror-like reaction when compared to cardiac output, whereby a rise in cardiac output corresponds to a fall in resistance. Similar to other results [2], the vasodilatory components in the musculature appear to predominate in comparison with the vasoconstriction supposed to take place in the kidney, the splanchnic area, and the skin (fig. 8).

After a subsequent repetition of the experiment using the same kind of tasks but with differing content, as well as after blockade of sympathetic β-receptors with 2 mg propranolol (i.v.), we found essentially the same, variously strong BP reactions corresponding to the different types of tasks. Cardiac output and HR were lowered through propranolol by 20%, or even 16%. Additionally, the strong reactive rises in the tasks MA and SC were lowered more substantially than the only slight reactions observed in the task 'stroboscope flashes' (observation) and 'mistake picture' (cardiac output: T = 4.3, p < 0.001; HR: T = 3.7, p < 0.001), as well as a more prolonged reaction in the MA being shortened. The still existing reactions in cardiac output and HR are certainly mainly determined through changes in the vagal cardiac influence, as propranolol competitively inhibits the effect of catecholamines on the β-receptors. In contrast to the investigation phase without β-blockade, situational rises in TPR (fig. 9) now take place (T = 16.1, p < 0.001). Thus, the α-adrenergic vasoconstriction exceeds β-adrenergic vasodilatation because the receptors are partially blocked. Without propranolol, situational dependent β-adrenergic vasodilatation must here be quantitatively exactly balanced to β-adrenergic cardiac stimulation and the resulting cardiac output rises. Such is the case because the variously strongly marked BP reactions in each task situation remain unchanged, which was also the case in the repetition of the investigation after propranolol administration. In other words, propranolol did not affect BP reactions in these testing situations (fig. 9).

This means, however, that in the investigation phase without propranolol the extent of the β-adrenergically induced rises in cardiac output exactly correspond to the β-adrenergically induced vasodilatation. The thus raised cardiac output then being made available for increased blood flow, probably in the muscular areas, cannot contribute to the rise in BP. The pressure rises must thus be produced by other mechanisms than the blocked β-sympathetic activation of the myocardium. They might partly depend on cardiac output rises mediated by vagal cardiac inhibition (if this is not balanced by cholinergic vasodilatation) as well as on α-adrenergic effects. So this β-adrenergic mechanism does not seem to influence pressure regulation in our investigation, but it does affect redistribution of blood flow in the body. In general, this mechanism can help speed up blood flow to the muscles, but the price is a rise in myocardial oxygen consumption (fig. 10).

Comparing how SBP×HR (PRi) and MAP×cardiac output, which can be regarded as measurements of myocardial oxygen consumption, react during the four task situations before and after propranolol, it can be seen in figure 10 that there is a considerable reduction of the situational reactions produced by β-blockade (p < 0.001). This demonstrates, on the other hand, one of the beneficial therapeutic effects of propranolol, which are important in the treatment of CHD. Propranolol lowers myocardial oxygen consumption especially during cardiovascular stress reactions, and this offers a greater regulatory latitude for the myocardium between the actual oxygen demand

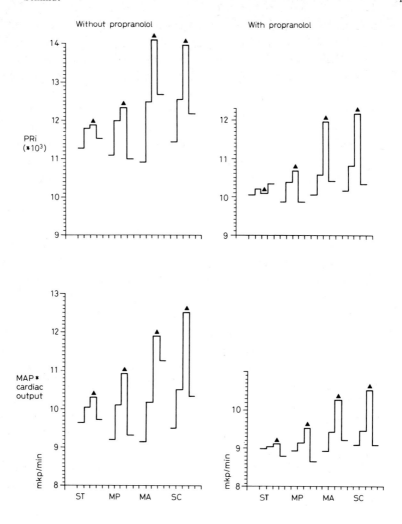

Fig. 10. Changes of pressure-rate index (PRi) and MAP×cardiac output during the four task situations before and after propranolol administration. Propranolol reduces especially the situationally induced rises of these two parameters which can be regarded as indices of myocardial oxygen consumption.

and the highest possible oxygen supply, which of course is reduced by coronary atherosclerosis. It appears that this has to be regarded as a most important cardioprotective mechanism.

Cardiovascular Hyperreactivity in Hypertension

The extent of a BP rise and the amount of the redistribution of blood flow in the body is not only determined by the environmental stimulus, or by psychological, emotional, or behavioral factors and conditioning processes, but it also depends of course on the involved and stimulated physiological systems. The level of response is modified by the reactivity of the entire cardiovascular system, which is affected by the neurohumoral discharge pattern during the hypothalamic defense reaction. Hyperreactivity of the hypothalamic defense area in response to environmental stimuli can be considered in the light of genetic factors. For example, it seems to play an important role in the development of hypertension in spontaneous hypertensive rats [16]. But in established hypertension, cardiovascular hyperreactivity may also only be just a consequence of an adaptation of the vascular system to the elevated pressure.

Folkow's theory of structural autoregulation clarifies the close relationship between functional and structural changes in the vascular system. Prolonged, as well as frequent, situationally induced rises in BP are intercepted in the arterioles, the resistance vessels, and here lead to a gradually increasing hypertrophy of the smooth muscles of the media. The lumen in the arterioles is reduced in relation to the degree of thickness of the vascular wall. The enlarged wall/lumen ratio is thus the structural basis for the raised resistance in fully developed essential hypertension [10, 11]. Morphological investigations have confirmed the close relationship between height of BP and the extent of media hypertrophy in the arteries and the precapillary resistance vessels. Here, the rise in resistance in the proximal portions of the arterioles appears to protect the further distal portions (as well as the capillaries) from a rise in pressure [40].

Structural autoregulation is seen as a normal physiological adaptation of the vascular system to a pressure rise. It plays an important role in every form of hypertension, independent of its origin. Corresponding changes in the vascular system can already be detected in a very early stage of hypertension, as for example in young military service soldiers with borderline hypertension [32]. In its early stages the hypertrophy of the smooth media muscles is still fully reversible, if pressure is reduced; however, an early antihypertensive treatment can obviously still enable an involutional process to take place [17]. If, however, the pressure continues to remain high, as a further reaction connective tissue will be deposited in the vascular wall – a process which appears to be irreversible, even when the pressor stimuli are absent – and the arteriosclerotic process starts [43].

The enlargement of the wall/lumen ratio results in a changed reactivity of the vascular system, through a considerable reactive increase in resistance during vasoconstriction. After this, a similar nervous or humoral pressor stimulus produces a proportionately higher BP rise, corresponding to the size of the wall/lumen ratio in the resistance vessels. Not only vasoconstriction but also vasodilatory effects are increased. In a vascular system adapted to high BP, hypothalamic defense reaction-induced redistribution of blood volume should heavily favor the striated muscles. We can speculate that this could lead to a better performance and less fatigue of the musculature in situations of fight or flight. Thus, a peripheral mechanism, i.e. the morphological changes in the resistance vessels, contributes to hyperreactivity in hypertension. Cardiovascular reactivity is determined through the interaction between central mechanisms such as the extent of changes in the sympathetic and vagal activity, and peripheral mechanisms such as the wall/lumen ratio of the resistance vessels.

Guyton et al. [15] clearly demonstrated that the kidney plays a central role in BP regulation as well as in the development of hypertension. The kidneys compensate elevations of BP by pressure diureses [15], but in hypertension this function is reset at a higher BP level. This can be seen in analogy to the resetting phenomenon of the baroreceptors in hypertension, which function as a short-term barostat. The investigations of *Folkow* et al. [12] point to structural changes of preglomerular arterioles in early hypertension as well as to changes of the wall/lumen ratio in the postglomerular area in the later stages as being a cause of resetting of the long-term barostat kidney. The degree of renal structural autoregulation depends also on height of BP and may therefore be influenced by situational pressure rises, i.e. by strength, duration, and frequency of renal vasoconstriction. Hyperreactivity of pre- and postglomerular vasoconstriction can reduce pressure diuresis and prolong situational pressure rises.

The reactivity of the vascular system depends upon the balance between active contraction and passive distension of the vascular wall as both factors are influenced by the height of BP and the vessel design. As *Folkow* [13] has demonstrated, in order for the same pressure fall to be achieved in the resistance vessels under hypertensive pressure, a vascular system adapted to a normotensive BP has to activate smooth vascular muscle in the arterioles more strongly than in the case of a vascular system already adapted to raised BP. This is the natural result of the thinner vascular wall and the greater wall distensibility. If, on the other hand, the pressure in a hypertensive vascular system is suddenly normalized, e.g. through intense therapy, considerable vascular hyperreactivity ensues from reduced distension at already only slight activation of the smooth vascular muscles. This hyperreactivity at a low pressure can be so marked that often a partial critical vascular occlusion can occur. In addition, this hyperreactivity does not become normal again until the vessel design is readapted to normotensive levels of BP, i.e. when its wall/lumen ratio is reduced. It thus becomes clear that sudden marked fluctuations in pressure can be dangerous for the normotensive as well as for the hypertensive vascular system.

Current dialogue argues about the importance of cardiovascular hyperreactivity being not only a consequence but also a precursor of hypertension. A directly related issue is to what extent hyperreactivity rests on a genetic basis and/or is dependent on environmental factors. Normotensive children of hypertensive parents show stress-induced cardiovascular hyperreactivity [7] and it is known that these children have a higher risk for the development of hypertension. In early or mild hypertension very often a reduced vagal cardiac inhibition and a higher sympathetic influence on the heart and vessels can be demonstrated, which is typical for an activation of the hypothalamic defense area. Moreover, in the early stage of the disease, a higher cardiac output can be normalized by administration of propranolol and atropin [19], whereas in established hypertension cardiac output is normal or subnormal, and total peripheral resistance is elevated due to the structural changes of the resistance vessels.

Investigating the role cardiovascular hyperreactivity may play during the development of essential hypertension, we compared hemodynamic reactions of a normotensive group (N) with a group of hypertensive patients with elevated cardiac output (H1) (mostly with borderline hypertension) and a hypertensive group with elevated TPR (H2). There were 10 patients in each group in the experiment described above. Figures 11 and 12 give a survey of the main hemodynamic variables of group N, H1 and H2 at rest (0), during the propranolol free investigation phase (1), and during the propranolol phase (2).

Anova and linear orthogonal contrast results showed somewhat higher reactions of MAP during all the tasks (without propranolol) in both hyperten-

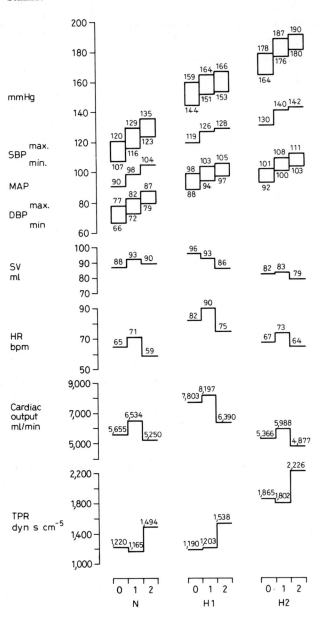

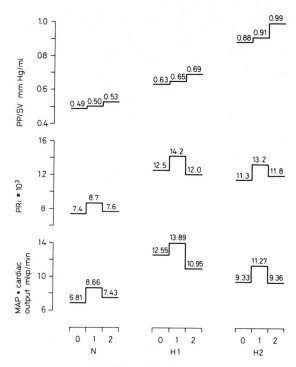

Fig. 12. Mean values of MAP×cardiac output, pressure-rate index (PRi) and pulse pressure/stroke volume (PP/SV) (as an index measurement of aortic rigidity) during investigation phases 0, 1, and 2 (see also legend fig. 11).

sive groups (F = 3.3, p < 0.08), whereas cardiac output reactions seem to be somewhat reduced in group H2, but this reduction is task-dependent and only significant between the groups when the slighter reactions of tasks ST and MP are compared to the more marked ones of MA and SC (T = 2.47, p < 0.007) (fig. 13).

Fig. 11. Mean values of the main hemodynamic variables in three groups of patients (n = 3 × 10): N = normotensives; H1 = hypertensives with elevated cardiac output; H2 = hypertensives with elevated TPR. Investigation phase 0 = mean of two resting values before the experimental procedure begins (initial values). Investigation phase 1 = mean of 16 1-min measurements during the task situation without propranolol. Investigation phase 2 = mean of 16 1-min measurements during the task situations after i.v. administration of 2 mg propranolol. SBP = Systolic BP; MAP = mean arterial pressure; DBP = diastolic BP; SV = stroke volume; TPR = total peripheral resistance.

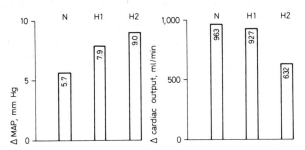

Fig. 13. Mean reactions of MAP and cardiac output in the task situations during the pro-pranolol-free investigation phase of group N, H1, and H2.

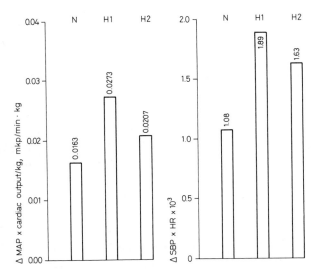

Fig. 14. Mean reactions of MAP× cardiac output/kg and SBP× HR (PRi) during the task situations in group N, H1, and H2.

Higher reactions in both hypertensive groups, which are independent of the effect of propranolol, are found in indicators of myocardial oxygen consumption such as SBP× HR (T= 7.961, p < 0.001) and MAP× cardiac output (T= 2.782, p < 0.007) which was divided by kilograms body weight because of differences between the groups (fig. 14). The latter variable shows also higher situational rises in group H1 than in group H2 (T= 4.455, p < 0.000). Myocardial oxygen consumption is not only raised in hypertension but in comparison to normotension it shows an even higher elevation in response to the tasks. The high cardiac output group H1 shows a stronger sympathetic cardiac drive as cardiac output decreases after propranolol approximately 600 ml more than in group H2 (T = 8.2, p < 0.001) (fig. 11); but this hyperreactivity is not reduced by propranolol. The stronger reactions in group H2 are due to the higher BP level produced through elevated TPR (fig. 11) and therefore to more pronounced structural changes in the arterial vascular system, which is in accordance with a higher index of aortic rigidity calculated from PP and SV (fig. 12). This demonstrates an intricate interplay of functional and structural factors in early as well as established hypertension, and shows clearly the higher impact of environmental stimuli to the heart in both hemodynamic forms of essential hypertension.

Cardiovascular Hyperreactivity and Behavior

Behavior-induced cardiovascular hyperreactivity is by definition not an exaggerated response of the cardiovascular system to all environmental stimuli as it may be in the case of hypertension. It rather depends on the behavior exhibited such as fight-and-flight-related actions, and it may be the case that hyperreactivity plays a more important role as a precursor of CHD than of hypertension. In the USA the type A behavior pattern has been established as an independent risk factor for CHD while showing no substantial relation to hypertension or other traditional risk factors. But there is growing evidence that it is connected, if not with a general cardiovascular hyperreactivity, then with a more specific one, depending mainly on the behavior shown, for instance, in situations of social competition. The type A interview can be regarded as such a situation, and higher SBP or HR rises in type A persons have been demonstrated in several American studies [5, 23]. The important question arises as to what extent the assessment of type A behavior pattern can be transferred to other cultural and language areas, and whether it can also there be proved to be an independent predictor of cardiovascular hyperreactivity as well as of CHD.

The first studies of this kind in Germany are, indeed showing that strong type A characteristics exhibited during the type A interview may be associated with higher cardiovascular reactions, independent of traditional risk factors [31, 37]. In a study with 212 policemen (table II), an age dependency of the type A pattern was found (F = 8.5, p < 0.001).

Table II. Distribution of type A pattern and age in 212 German policemen

Type	n	%	Age	± SD
A1	21	9.9	32.3	± 9.4
A2	101	47.6	27.8	± 9.0
X	28	13.2	24.3	± 6.9
B	62	29.3	23.2	± 6.4
Total	212	100	26.4	± 8.5

Table III. Pearson correlations of type A pattern and component analyses of voice stylistics, clinical ratings of hostility and verbal competitiveness, and age

	Type A	Components				
		1	2	3	4	5
Components						
1 Loud/explosive	0.81					
2 Rapid/accelerated	0.80	0.70				
3 Response latency	0.59	0.45	0.52			
4 Hostility	0.21	0.24	0.16	0.15		
5 Verbal competition	0.42	0.30	0.35	0.38	0.25	
Age, years	0.31	0.33	0.22	0.25	0.05	0.14

This effect might be due to social status, as teachers, administrative employees, and pupils of a police school were interviewed. In ethological terms, type A behavior can be interpreted as a claim to a dominant rank position in the social hierarchy, demonstrated by overt behavior and verbal communication. Therefore, it seems to be comprehensible that older and more senior policemen exhibited more type A characteristics, such as typical speech stylistics (table III). Component analysis reveals that the type A pattern is determined mainly by speech stylistics, such as loud explosive voice, rapid accelerated speech and response latency during the interview.

Many of the investigated parameters, such as the base level BP, HR, PRi, serum cholesterol, LDL-cholesterol etc. were dependent on age, and cardiovascular reactivity is influenced by BP and HR base levels as well as by age. Therefore, in a first step of data analysis, 18 policemen scored as A1

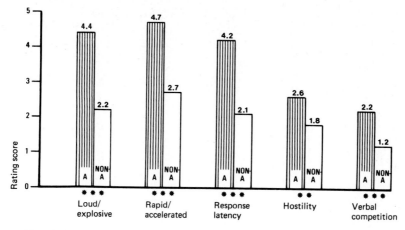

Fig. 15. Component analysis in 18 age-matched policemen exhibiting strong (A1 = A) or no or only rare type A characteristics (B or X = non-A).

(group A) by two independent raters were compared to 18 matched Bs or Xs (group non-A). There were neither differences in SBP, DBP, HR, and PRi at rest between these two groups, nor in total serum cholesterol, LDL-, and HDL-cholesterol, cigarette smoking, or stress experienced during the past week. Component analysis of the interview revealed higher scores in group A for all 5 components, although hostility and verbal competition were scored rather low in these German policemen. Group A also showed higher reactions in HR, SBP, and PRi during the interview (fig. 15, 16).

In the total group of investigated policemen there was a significant relation between type A behavior and higher values of DBP and cholesterol if not controlled for age [37]. But analysis of covariance reveals that these differences must be attributed to age and not to type A behavior (fig. 17, 18).

When age and base values in Ancova are controlled, policemen who exhibit extreme type A characteristics during the interview react more strongly with HR and PRi, indicating a higher adrenergic cardiac activation (fig. 19, 20). These investigations suggest that the type A pattern must be regarded also in Germany as a factor independent of traditional risk factors and that its extreme manifestations are associated with cardiovascular hyper-reactivity.

The main components of type A behavior during the interview, such as loud explosive voice and rapid accelerated speech, etc., can be seen as ritualized forms of social competition in human behavior, and thus as a more

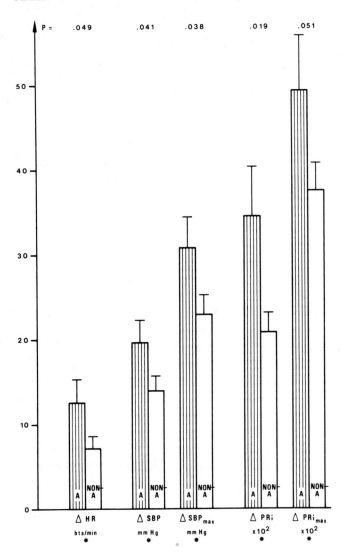

Fig. 16. Mean or maximal cardiovascular reactions during the type A interview in 18 age-matched policemen with strong (A1=A) or no or only rare type A characteristics (B or X=non-A).

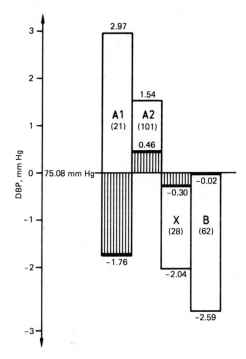

Fig. 17. Group mean DBP at rest for 210 German policemen and above and below group mean values by type A behavior pattern (white columns). When controlled for age the differences between the four groups (F = 2.4, df = 3/209, p = 0.073) disappear (shaded columns).

subtle intraspecific expression of fight-and-flight behavior. This perhaps is a possible explanation of why these characteristics of verbal behavior are associated with cardiovascular hyperreactivity. Additionally, the breathing process may play an important role here, as it is closely related to the cardiovascular system. There are certainly numerous other behavioral influences on cardiovascular reactivity, and one important task is to identify more reliable and potent predictors of cardiovascular hyperreactivity in our daily lives. On the other hand, we have to find out how to influence hyperreactivity in an effective way. We can presume that in contrast to the fight/flight pattern, muscular relaxation is useful; but there are also cognitive and mental attitudes and expectations which can prepare the organism for cardiovascular reactions even in a somewhat relaxed state. Modern as well as ancient relaxation techniques have been investigated and meditation has been found to be one of the best 'behavioral' methods of reducing BP [*Ben-*

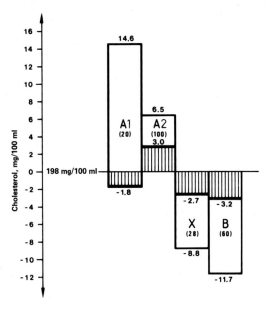

Fig. 18. Mean serum cholesterol levels in 208 German policemen and above and below groups mean values by type A behavior pattern (white columns). When controlled for age the significant differences between the four groups ($F = 3.92$, $df = 3/205$, $p = 0.009$) disappear (shaded columns).

son; Julius and Cottier, this volume], and perhaps even its reactions [*Patel,* this volume]. A general basis of such techniques is to induce a relaxed state, for instance by special breathing exercises or just by breath awareness; then mental strategies are used which calm the mind even further, thus leaving no room for fight/flight-related thoughts. Perhaps here is one reason for the better effect of meditation in BP reduction compared to biofeedback techniques.

Cardiovascular Reactions during Yoga Breathing Exercises

In yoga meditation more complex breathing exercises (pranayama) are often used as a preparation for inducing calmness and relaxation [41]. The roots of these techniques may reach back to prehistoric times and cultures, and these practices are part of a living tradition. In modern medical science, we are just starting to investigate and to understand the deep effects of these

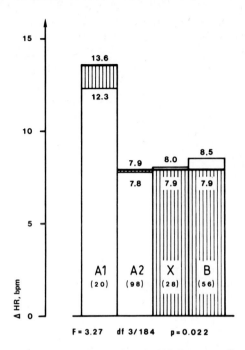

Fig. 19. Mean HR reactions in 202 German policemen during the type A interview in accordance with their behavior pattern. The higher reactions in group A1 can be seen (white columns) which appear to be even higher when controlled for age and initial values (shaded column).

techniques. These breathing exercises can produce extraordinary cardiovascular reactions. The following case report demonstrates such cardiovascular changes during three classical yoga breathing exercises in a 25-year-old Danish man who had been practicing yoga for 5 years [22a, 39a]. These exercises are: (1) sheethali pranayama (cooling whistling breathing); (2) nadi shodan (alternate breathing), and (3) ujjayi pranayama (psychic breathing).

Intraarterial BP was measured in the left brachial artery as well as ECG and the breathing pattern by thoracic expansion using a respiration belt; the recordings were registered on paper and magnetic tape. All exercises are usually practiced in a sitting position with the back as straight as possible, preferable in a meditation pose. Here, the exercises were performed in the lotus pose (legs crossed and each foot resting on the thigh of the opposite leg). All three maneuvers share a basic pattern of slow inhalation (1), holding breath (2), and slow exhalation (3).

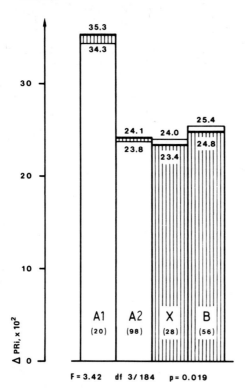

Fig. 20. Mean reactions in PRi during the type A interview. The stronger reactions in group A1 can be seen (white columns) which appear to be even higher when controlled for age and initial values (shaded column).

Sheetali pranayama

(1) In sheetali pranayama teeth are clenched, the corners of the mouth and the lips are stretched as far apart as possible, and the tongue is curled back to the soft palate while a slow and deep inhalation is made through the teeth.

(2) After inhalation the breath is held in a position where the shoulders are raised, both arms are straight, supporting the body with the hands resting on the knees. The perineum is contracted and pulled up (root lock or moola bandha). The head is bent forward with the chin towards the breast (chin lock or jalandhara bandha). Without discomfort, the breath is held as long as possible.

(3) The perineum is relaxed, the head raised, followed by a slow exhalation. Figure 21 shows the results of a beat-per-beat computer analysis of

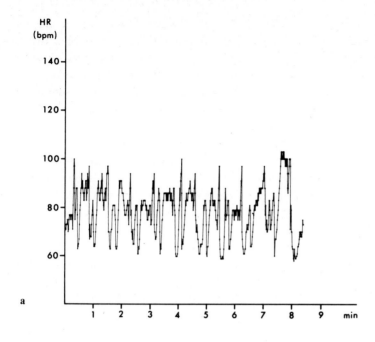

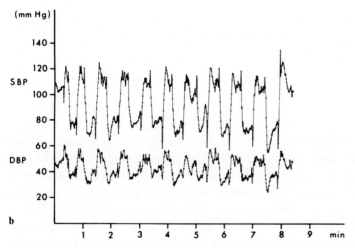

Fig. 21. Beat-to-beat computer analysis of HR **(a)** and BP **(b)** during 10 rounds of sheetali pranayama. BP reduction and HR increases are strictly associated with the phases of holding the breath in.

intraarterial BP (fig. 21b) and of HR (fig. 21a) during ten rounds of sheetali pranayama. From resting BP values of around 105/50 mm Hg and a HR of around 70 bpm, an immediate BP reduction can be seen during phase 2 when breath is held after inspiration and jalandhara bandha (chin lock) and moola bandha (root lock) are performed. During this phase the pressure is lowered to values of about 70/35 mm Hg and the HR rises to 90 bpm. In phase 3 during exhalation BP rises within a few heart beats (about 7) to base levels of 110–120/55–60 mm Hg, and HR is lowered again to 60 bpm. This pattern of cardiovascular reactions is repeated during each cycle of this breathing exercise. During inhalation coolness is felt in the oral area and can be projected to the whole body. After the exercise, calmness and freshness is reported.

Nadi shodan

In nadi shodan inhalation and exhalation are performed alternately through the left and right nostril; the thumb and the ring finger of the right hand are used to close the nostrils, whereby the index and middle finger rest on the forehead. (1) The exercise starts by closing the right nostril with the thumb, and a slow, thorough and soundless inhalation is made through the left nostril. (2) Then the breath is held. (3) After holding the breath, exhalation is made through the right nostril. Then again inhalation is made through the right nostril; breath is held and exhalation is made through the left nostril. This completes one sequence. Five sequences were performed in all. Furthermore, inhalation, holding breath, and exhalation are performed in a fixed ratio of 1:4:2 while counting mentally; here the counting ratio used was 12:48:24.

During this exercise the oscillations of BP and HR described in sheetali pranayama are even more pronounced in height and duration. Figure 22 shows the computer beat-by-beat analysis. Again, during the phase of holding the breath there is an immediate BP reduction down to levels of 40–55/25–30 mm Hg, or even lower, for about 30 s connected with a rise in HR up to 130 bpm. During slow exhalation, there is an immediate BP rise which clearly exceeds base values, reaching peaks just above 150/70 mm Hg; the pressure rise is associated with HR reduction, showing values around 60 bpm. After completion of this exercise base values of 105/50 mm Hg are reached again.

Fig. 22. Beat-to-beat analysis of HR (**a**) and BP (**b**) during nadi shodan. In this yoga breathing exercise most pronounced BP reductions can be seen which last for about 30 s; they are related to a HR rise and correlate strictly with the phase of holding the breath in.

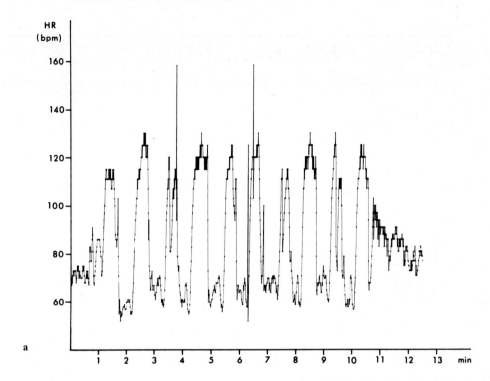

a

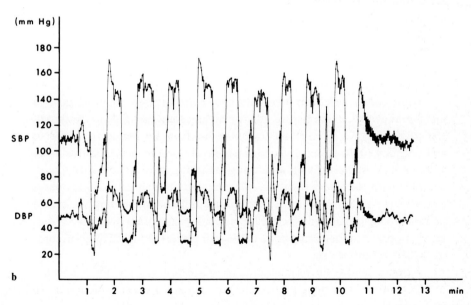

b

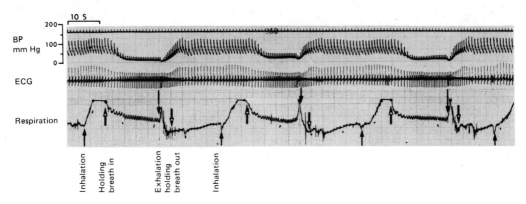

Fig. 23. Original registration of intraarterial BP, ECG, and respiration pattern during ujjayi pranayama. It can be seen how the rhythmical BP fall and rise depends on the breathing phases.

During this exercise the perceived effects are described as immediate relaxation and a more profound 'letting go' of mental and physical tensions while the breath is held, becoming more aware of a feeling of energy and expansion of consciousness. It occurs spontaneously during the time of holding the breath and is reinforced during exhalation. These effects depend on the ability to concentrate on the exercise and not consciously trying to evoke them. The immediate as well as the longer-lasting effects after the exercise are perceived in a very pleasant way, if this exercise is performed correctly, such as an enhanced level of energy, greater sense of physical as well as mental balance, and a clearer and calmer state of mind.

Ujjayi pranayama

During slow and deep inhalation and exhalation through the nose in ujjayi pranayama, a whispering, slightly hissing sound is made in the throat. It is not produced by the soft palate, but comes from further down the throat and is similar to the sound of a child sleeping. It has the same quality during inhalation as well as exhalation. During breathing the tongue is curled back and the tip touches the soft palate. After inhalation the breath is held out for a brief period. There are, then, four phases: inhalation, holding the breath in, exhalation, and holding the breath out. This pranayama is used in various meditation techniques. The timing of the four phases can be changed according to the technique used.

Figure 23 shows the original intraarterial BP curves, and the recordings of ECG and the breathing pattern. In this exercise, a deep reduction in BP again occurs while the breath is being held in, and this is followed by an over-shooting pressure rise during exhalation. In figure 24 the beat-per-beat computer analysis reveals a reaction pattern comparable to the two previous exercises. The BP fall during the time of holding the breath in (values of around 40–55/25–30 mm Hg) is strictly related to a rise in HR (up to 120 bpm) whereas the BP rise during exhalation (130–140/55–65 mm Hg) is associated with HR reduction (to about 60 bpm). In figure 25, the same exercise is performed in a supine position. The cardiovascular reactions are much weaker. From base values for BP of around 105/40 mm Hg, and a HR of 65 bpm, holding the breath produces a BP fall to 80–90/30–35 bpm, and HR rise to 90 bpm. Exhalation is associated with a BP rise to 110/45–50 mm Hg and HR reduction to around 60 bpm.

During this exercise in the sitting position inhalation is associated with a feeling of enhanced energy in body and mind, and exhalation with a relaxing and calming effect as well as a 'letting go' of tension. The phases where breath is held are often connected with a feeling of being more aware and an expansion of consciousness. In the recumbent position, these effects are less pronounced.

Pranayama are important techniques in more advanced yoga, influencing body and mind. The exercises can be performed only in a somewhat relaxed state and they even reinforce relaxation. A better or longer successful performance of nadi shodan for instance, when a higher counting rate is used, is only possible in an even more relaxed state, and already a 'stressful' thought can be a hindrance to holding the breath as long as intended. So this exercise can be regarded as a psychophysiological tool which is designed to improve the intended effects by a correct, better, and prolonged performance. As these exercises can be associated with greatly pronounced cardiovascular reactions, it must be suggested that these changes serve also as a physical basis for the mental effects. There is a similar pattern in all three exercises, but the degree of the hemodynamic changes depends on the technique used. This hemodynamic reaction pattern can be seen in contrast to the hypothalamic defense reaction. As BP reduction and rise in HR are strictly related to the phases of holding the breath where intrathoracic pressure is slightly raised (central venous pressure rises from around 2 up to 15 mm Hg), this reaction might somehow be related to the cardiovascular reflexes seen during the Valsalva maneuver (fig. 26); but it must definitely be regarded as a different pattern, as BP is reduced during all the time of holding the breath. According to Ohm's law, BP is determined by cardiac output and TPR; in this investigation it cannot, however, be seen whether BP reduction

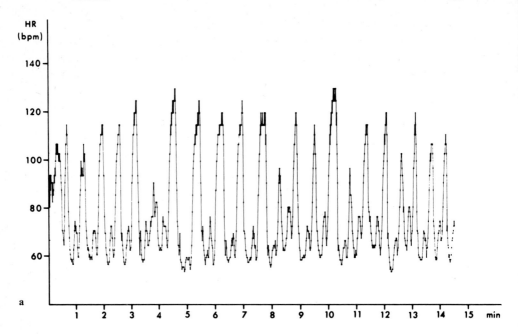

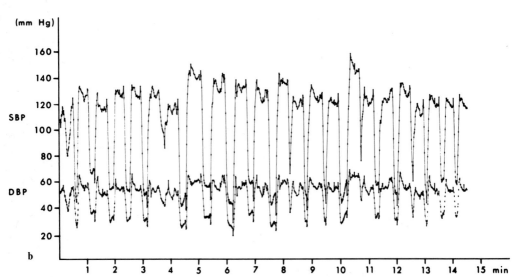

Fig. 24. Beat-to-beat analysis of HR **(a)** and BP **(b)** during ujjayi pranayama performed in the lotus pose.

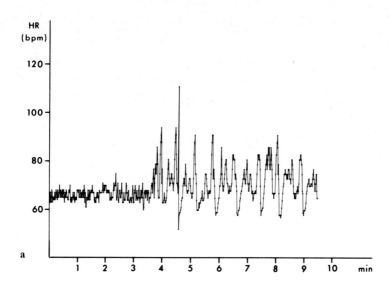

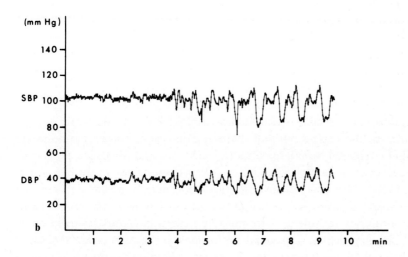

Fig. 25. Beat-to-beat analysis of HR **(a)** and BP **(b)** during ujjayi pranayama performed in the supine position. The exercise starts after 4 min rest.

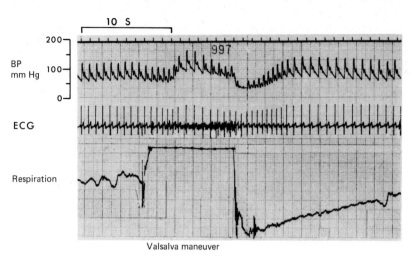

Fig. 26. BP reactions during the Valsalva maneuver in the same subject performing the yoga breathing exercises.

is produced by a fall in cardiac output or TPR by peripheral vasodilatation, or even a reduction in both parameters. The rise in HR points to a reduced SV perhaps by venous pooling, whereby the organism tries to sustain blood flow by a higher HR. In another subject who showed reactions to the same extent, we determined SV by impedance cardiography. During the phase of holding breath, SV was reduced to one third of the values found during exhalation. Only accurate determination of cardiac output can, however, reveal the true hemodynamic nature of this response. It also seems to be related to the orthostatic reaction because the cardiovascular changes are greatly reduced in the supine position. During exhalation, blood volume might slowly be released from large intrathoracic veins and SV might increase as HR decreases. It cannot be said, however, whether a rise in cardiac output or in TPR contributes more to the BP rise. But, it must be assumed that during these breathing exercises, redistribution of blood flow to the inner organs plays an important role as there must be tremendous oscillations in blood flow; they may also be responsible for the mental effects. A phase of reduced blood supply to the brain during the phase of holding the breath in may be followed by a phase of an enhanced flow during slow exhalation. Sheetali pranayama has the mildest effect in lowering BP without overshooting reactions afterwards. Perhaps this is a reason why it has been recommended for people with elevated BP [41]. The other two exercises showed more pronounced physical as well as mental effects. It does not seem to be just the technical procedure of the exercises which produces the effects, for instance by the slightly raised intrathoracic pressure while holding breath. Beginners following the same technique do not show such strong reactions and only after some years of regular practice this subject noticed a strong change in subjective effects and felt to be able to evoke these effects voluntarily during the exercises. The same was true for two further yoga teachers in which we found similar cardiovascular reactions to much the same extent. So the persons have learned through ancient breathing techniques to influence cardiovascular functions in an extraordinary way, thereby influencing the physical and mental condition. It remains open to investigate whether or to what extent these exercises can influence cardiovascular reactions to environmental and emotional stimuli. As the subjective effect of inner calmness is felt for sometime after the exercise or even during the whole day, it might influence the attitude towards environmental stressors and thus the physiological reactions. There is no doubt that the effects are very rewarding for people practicing these exercises when a special level of experience is achieved, and that, of course, might be a reason for good compliance in those people using these techniques.

Final Remarks

Cardiovascular reactions are essential to efficient behavioral adaptation to the physical as well as to the social environment. Evolution has provided us with special preprogrammed reaction patterns such as the hypothalamic defense reaction to serve this purpose. Their protective function in emergency states such as fight or flight may turn into a risk when often evoked without the behavioral consequences such reactions were meant to support. Environmental as well as cognitive-emotional factors influence degree, duration and frequency of such reactions and lead to a behavioral and physiological adaptation that in the past might have been more beneficial than in modern 20th century existence. In this chapter, I have explored a variety of perspectives on cardiovascular reactivity. The purpose was to show the many facets of unexplored environmental, psychological, behavioral, physiological, pathophysiological, and disease linkages. There is a growing need for much more systematic and programmatic research to establish the many parameters possible in this new and exciting area of behavioral medicine.

References

1 Abrahams, V.C.; Hilton, S.M.; Zbrozyna, A.: Active muscle vasodilatation produced by stimulation of the brain stem: its significance in the defence reaction. J. Physiol., Lond. *154:* 491–513 (1960).

2 Brod, J.; Fencl, V.; Hejl, A.; Jorka, J.: Circulatory changes underlying blood pressure elevation during acute emotional stress (mental arithmetic) in normotensive and hypertensive subjects. Clin. Sci. *18:* 269–279 (1959).

3 Darwin, F.: More letters of Charles Darwin (Appleton, New York 1903).

4 Davies, J.O.: The control of renin release. Am. J. Med. *55:* 333–350 (1973).

5 Dembroski, T.M.; MacDougall, J.M.; Shields, J.L.; Petitto, J.; Lushene, R.: Components of the type A coronary-prone behavior pattern and cardiovascular responses to psychomotor performance challenge. J. behav. Med. *1:* 159–176 (1978).

6 Eliasson, S.; Folkow, B.; Lindgren, P.; Uvnaes, B.: Activation of sympathetic vasodilator nerves to the skeletal muscles in the cat by hypothalamic stimulation. Acta physiol. scand. *23:* 333–351 (1951).

7 Falkner, B.; Onesti, G.; Angelakos, E.T.; Fernandes, M.; Langman, C.: Cardiovascular response to mental stress in normal adolescents with hypertensive parents. Hypertension *1:* 23–30 (1979).

8 Folkow, B.; Hedner, P.; Lisander, B.; Rubinstein, E.: Release of cortisol upon stimulation of the hypothalamic defense area in cats. Foersvarsmedicin *3:* suppl. 2, p. 114 (1967).

9 Folkow, B.; Neil, E.: Circulation (Oxford University Press, London 1971).

10 Folkow, B.; Hallbaeck, M.; Lundgren, Y.; Sivertsson, R.; Weiss, L.: Importance of adaptive changes in vascular design for establishment of primary hypertension, studied in man and in spontaneously hypertensive rats. Circulation Res. *32, 33:* suppl. 1, pp. I-2–I-16 (1973).

11 Folkow, B.: Vascular changes in hypertension – review and recent animal studies; in Berglund, Hansson, Werkoe, Pathophysiology and management of arterial hypertension pp. 95–126 (Lindgren & Soener, Moelndal 1975).

12 Folkow, B.; Goethberg, G.; Lundin, S.; Ricksten, S.E.: Structural 'resetting' of the renal vascular bed in spontaneously hypertensive rats (SHR). Acta physiol. scand. *100:* 270–272 (1977).

13 Folkow, B.: Constriction-distension relationships in SHR and NCR resistance vessels. Abstr. 8, 6th Scientific Meet. of the Int. Soc. of Hypertension, Goeteborg 1979, p. 11 (Astra cardiovascular, Goeteborg 1979).

14 Grant, R.; Lindgren, P.; Rosen, A.; Uvnaes, B.: The release of catechols from the adrenal medulla on activation of the sympathetic vasodilator nerves to the skeletal muscles in the cat by hypothalamic stimulation. Acta physiol. scand. *43:* 135–154 (1958).

15 Guyton, A.C.; Young, D.B.; Declue, J.W.; Ferguson, J.D.; McCaa, R.E.; Cevese, A.; Trippodo, N.C.; Hall, J.E.: The role of the kidney in hypertension; in Berglund, Hansson, Werkoe, Pathophysiology and management of arterial hypertension. Proc. Conf. Copenhagen 1975, pp. 78–91 (Lindgren & Soener, Moelndal 1975).

16 Hallbäck, M.: Interaction between central neurogenic mechanisms and changes in cardiovascular design in primary hypertension. Experimental studies in spontaneously hypertensive rats. Acta physiol. scand. suppl. 424 (1975).

17 Hansson, L.; Sivertsson, R.: Rückbildung struktureller Gefässveränderungen nach anti-

hypertensiver Therapie; in Dietz, Ganten, Hofbauer, Lueth, Essentieller Hochdruck und seine Behandlung, pp. 83–87 (Schattauer, Stuttgart 1977).

18 Hypertension Detection and Follow-up Program Co-operative Group: Five-year findings of the hypertension detection and follow-up program. 1. Reduction in mortality of persons with high blood pressure, including mild hypertension. J. Am. med. Ass. *242:* 2562–2571 (1979).

19 Julius, S.; Hansson, L.M.: Hemodynamics of prehypertension and hypertension. Verh. dt. Ges. inn. Med. *80:* 49–58 (1974).

20 Kannel, W.B.; Dawber, T.R.: Hypertension as one ingredient of cardiovascular risk profile. Br. J. Hosp. Med. *11:* 508 (1974).

21 Kannel, W.B.: Importance of hypertension as a major risk factor in cardiovascular disease; in Genest, Koiw, Kuchel, Hypertension physiopathology and treatment, pp. 888–910 (McGraw-Hill, New York 1977).

22 Keys, A.; Taylor, H.L.; Blackburn, H.; Brozek, J.; Anderson, J.T.; Simonson, E.: Mortality and coronary heart disease among men studied for 23 years. Archs intern. Med. *128:* 201–214 (1971).

22a Knudsen, T.; Schmidt, T.H.: Psychophysiological investigations on Yoga breathing exercises. Part 1: Technique. Abstr. 426, 6th World Congr. Int. College Psychosomatic Medicine, Montreal 1981, p. 107 (Montreal 1981).

23 Krantz, D.S.; Schaeffer, M.A.; Davis, J.E.; Dembroski, T.M.; MacDougall, J.M.; Schaffer, R.T.: Extent of coronary atherosclerosis, type A behavior and cardiovascular response to social interaction. Psychophysiology *18:* 654–664 (1981).

24 Lacey, J.J.; Lacey, B.C.: Some autonomic-central nervous system interrelationships; in Black, Physiological correlates of emotion, pp. 206–227 (Academic Press, New York 1970).

25 Lorenz, K.: Vergleichende Verhaltensforschung: Grundlagen der Ethologie (Springer, Wien 1978).

26 Pflanz, M.: Epidemiologie des essentiellen Hochdrucks. Verh. dt. Ges. Kreisl. Forsch. *43:* 20 (1977).

27 Plutarch XLIII (Demetrios); 38.

28 Pooling Projet Research Group : Relation of blood pressure, serum cholesterol, smoking habit, relative weight and ECG abnormalities to incidence of major coronary events: final report of the Pooling Project. J. chron. Dis. *31:* 201–306 (1978).

29 Riedl, R.: Biologie der Erkenntnis: Die stammesgeschichtlichen Grundlagen der Vernunft (Parey, Berlin 1980).

30 Rosner, B.; Polk, B.: The implications of blood pressure variability for clinical and screening purposes. J. chron. Dis. *32:* 451–461 (1979).

31 Rüddel, H.; Langosch, W.; Schiebener, A.; Schmidt, T.H.; Schmieder, R.; Schulte, W.: Kardiovaskuläre Reaktionen während des Typ A Interwiews. Verh. dt. Ges. inn. Med. *87:* 1255–1257 (1981).

32 Sannerstedt, R.; Sivertsson, R.; Lundgren, Y.: Haemodynamic studies in young men with mild blood pressure elevation. Acta med. scand. *200:* suppl. 602, pp. 61–67 (1976).

33 Schmidt, T.H.; Schaefer, N.; Marth, H.: Vergleich tagesperiodischer Schwankungen blutig gemessener Blutdruckwerte bei Normotonikern und Hypertonikern. Verh. dt. Ges. inn. Med. *80:* 298–303 (1974).

34 Schmidt, T.H.; Schonecke, O.W.; Herrmann, J.M.; Krull, F.; Selbmann, H.K.; Schaefer, N.; Uexküll, T. von; Werner, I.: Psychophysiologische Untersuchung zum Verhalten haemodynamischer Kreislaufparameter in verschiedenartigen Aufgabensituationen vor

und nach der intravenösen Gabe von Propranolol. Verh. dt. Ges. inn. Med. *81:* 1747–1751 (1975).

35 Schmidt, T.H.: Tagesperiodische und situative Veränderungen des Kreislaufverhaltens; in Palm, Rudolph, Symp. über den Betablocker Carazolol, pp. 112–135 (Excerpta Medica, Amsterdam 1980).

36 Schmidt, T.H.: Die Situationshypertonie als Risikofaktor; in Vaitl, Essentielle Hypertonie, pp. 77–111 (Springer, Berlin 1982).

37 Schmidt, T.H.: Undeutsch, K.; Dembroski, T.M.; Langosch, W.; Neus, H.; Rüddel, H.: Coronary-prone behavior and cardiovascular reactions during the German version of the type A interview and during a quiz. Activitas nerv. sup., suppl. 3, pp. 241–251 (1982).

38 Schmidt, T.H.; Undeutsch, K.; Dembroski, T.M.; Hahn, R.; Langosch, W.; Neus, H.; Rüddel, H.: Kardiovaskuläre Risikofaktoren and Typ-A-Verhalten. Verh. dt. Ges. inn. Med. *88:* 1203–1210 (1982).

39 Schmidt, T.H.; Schonecke, O.W.; Herrmann, J.M.; Krull, F.; Schaefer, J.; Werner, I.: Stimulusspezifische Reaktionen kardiovaskulärer Grössen bei Normotonikern und Hypertonikern. II. Sylter Symp. über Stress-Forschung, Klappholttal (in press, 1977).

39a Schmidt, T.H.; Knudsen, T.; Rüddel, H.; Schirmer, G.; Thoenes, M.: Psychophysiological investigations on Yoga breathing exercises. Part 2: Physiological effects. Abstr. 516, 6th World Congr. Psychosomatic Medicine, Montreal 1981, p. 129 (Montreal 1981).

39b Souchek, J.; Stamler, J.; Dyer, A.; Paul, O.; Lepper, M.: The value of two or three versus a single reading of blood pressure at a first visit. J. chron. Dis. *32:* 197–210 (1979).

40 Suwa, N.; Takahashi, T.: Morphological and morphometrical analysis of circulation in hypertension and ischemic kidney (Urban & Schwarzenberg, München 1971).

41 Swami Janakananda Saraswati: Yoga, tantra and mediation in everyday life (Rider, London 1978).

42 Uexküll, T. von; Wick, W.: Die Situationshypertonie. Arch. Kreislaufforsch. *39:* 236–271 (1962).

43 Wolinsky, H.: Long-term effects of hypertension on the rat aortic wall and their relation to current aging changes. Circulation Res. *30:* 301–309 (1972).

44 Zanchetti, A.; Stella, A.: Neural control of renin release. Clin. Sci. mol. Med. *48:* suppl. pp. 215–223 (1975).

10 Wet Holter Monitoring: Techniques for Studying Plasma Responses to Stress in Ambulatory Subjects[1]

Joel E. Dimsdale

The careful early research on coronary-prone behavior emphasized meticulous epidemiological studies wherein the association between the type A behavior pattern and various cardiac end points could be demonstrated [3, 21]. This work has established that there is some aspect of the coronary-prone behavior pattern which conveys risk to patients for the development of initial and recurrent coronary events. As a result of this baseline knowledge, research has focused on increasingly finer discriminations relating to coronary-prone behavior. As discussed earlier, considerable work has been devoted to the process of type A assessment per se [5, 14, 17]. Another research direction studies the psychosocial setting wherein type A manifests itself. Until recently, we had little appreciation for the relationship between type A and other aspects of personality functioning. Recent work suggests that type A may be a personality pattern driven to compensate against hopelessness [12] or a pattern related to stress, anger, and anxiety [4].

The other major area of research growth involving type A behavior has focused on the possible pathophysiological mechanisms whereby type A may convey risk. As discussed in earlier papers, some investigators have attempted to relate type A behavior to the extent of coronary artery disease found on angiography. The design of the studies is rather elegant. Patients are evaluated by psychiatrists and psychologists prior to angiography or prior to learning of the results of their angiography; cardiac catheterization is performed by cardiologists. Both psychiatrists and cardiologists are blind to the others' evaluation. Unfortunately, the design of such studies is not so simple. Seven different groups have been using this form of design and have reported inconsistent findings, some groups finding a relationship between type A and vessel disease [1, 10, 28], some groups finding no such relationship [1, 6, 27; *Kornitzer*, pers. Commun.]. Although it is possible that slight variations in the assessment of type A could account for some discrepant findings, the most

[1] This work was supported by a Clinician Scientist Award from the American Heart Association with funds contributed in part by the Massachusetts AHA Affiliate.

likely explanation is that differences in the incoming characteristics of the patients account for the discrepant findings. The factors that help a patient to decide when to come to angiography and where to seek it are very relevant factors which may affect the relationship observed.

Even if there were consistency in the findings relating type A to coronary artery disease, this sort of research endeavor is a discouraging one because it evaluates patients so late in the course of their disease. By the time one comes to angiography, there is little that one can do other than to investigate whether or not coronary artery bypass graft surgery is feasible for the patient. It would be of great interest to examine an earlier pathophysiological site or mechanism whereby behavior appears to convey risk on cardiovascular functioning. It is for these reasons that we have switched our line of research studies from angiographic studies to neuroendocrine studies of emotional expression.

Neuroendocrine Research

An extraordinarily interesting and valuable literature has accumulated from the fields of psychophysiology and neuroendocrinology relating emotional arousal to various biochemical measures. Our own work has concentrated on the development of a new technique for approaching this exciting area. The technique involves the design and utilization of an apparatus that allows one to obtain blood samples in ambulatory subjects as they are exposed to naturalistic stresses that they experience in their everyday lives.

The techniques and machinery are very new. In describing them, it may be well to remember the original model of the Holter ambulatory ECG monitor. That original Holter monitor weighed approximately 20 kg and was carried by backpack. Over the years, medical engineering has successfully miniaturized the Holter ECG monitors so that they can be comfortably worn on the waist. We lack the years of experience in medical engineering for ambulatory blood withdrawal pumps but, nevertheless, the pump apparatus already lends itself easily for use in ambulatory subjects. The limitations of the apparatus will be discussed later in this paper.

The question could be asked: 'Why is it so important to obtain plasma measures as opposed to urinary measures?' For studies that examine catecholamine response, urinary measures are limited because they of necessity integrate over long periods of time. The half-life of plasma catecholamines is on the order of 2 or 3 min, and thus a urinary measure that integrates over an hour or more blurs the short-term responsiveness of the subject [25]. Secondly, the assumption that urinary metabolites and plasma catecholamine metabolites are parallel may not be entirely warranted. Recent work, for instance, has demonstrated that during exercise, urine and plasma catecholamine metabolites follow a very different pattern [24]. Finally, it must be emphasized that the kidney is itself innervated by the sympathetic nervous system and thus the clearance of urinary catecholamine metabolites itself does not remain constant.

Despite all these limitations, considerable valuable work has accumulated regarding urinary catecholamine response to stress [11, 16]. The focus on urinary measures was partially necessitated by the difficulty of measuring plasma catecholamines. Until recently, plasma catecholamine measures have been notoriously difficult and questionable to interpret. However, with the advent of radioenzymatic and high-pressure liquid chromatographic techniques for measuring plasma catecholamines, it is now possible to measure them reliably and on small volumes of blood.

In performing studies of plasma catecholamines, certain methodological precautions must be taken. Because the act of venapuncture itself affects catecholamines notably, some form of indwelling catheter is necessary for obtaining plasma samples. Because plasma catecholamines are so readily oxidized and degraded by other plasma enzymes, the blood must be immediately chilled, centrifuged within a short period of time, and the plasma stored at $-70°C$ [2].

Until recently, the study of plasma catecholamine response to stress had to be performed in the laboratory because of the difficulty of obtaining plasma samples repeatedly through indwelling lines in ambulatory subjects. However, recently, a portable blood withdrawal pump used in conjunction with a heparin-impregnated nonthrombogenic catheter has been developed. Although most work utilizing this pump has focused on pharmacokinetic studies, the pump was used recently in the Air Traffic Controller study to examine cortisol response to job stress [20]. We have worked to modify the pump so that it can obtain appropriate amounts of blood over small periods of time. The pump is small, approximately $9\,cm^2$, and may be worn on the waist (fig. 1). Blood is withdrawn continuously into a vacutainer. Each vacutainer thus represents a memory cell of plasma activity for a given period of time. We have found that integrations of samples over a 3-min interval are appropriate for examining plasma catecholamine response. The only disadvantage to this pump is its fairly primitive method of changing tubes; the tubes must be changed manually by either the subject or a research assistant.

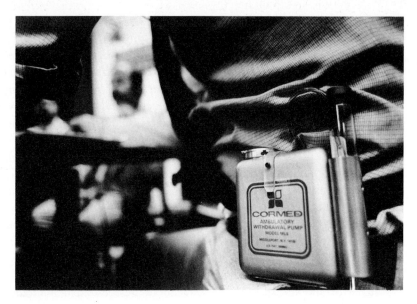

Fig. 1. Ambulatory blood withdrawal pump.

This does not preclude the pump's use in ambulatory subjects, but nevertheless, it would be desirable to improve on this with a portable form of fractional collector. We are currently investigating this possibility.

What are the respective advantages of laboratory-based vs naturalistic studies? The laboratory-based studies are susceptible to careful experimental control, better psychometrics as to self-report measures, and also better psychometrics for behavioral observation. However, given the ethical constraints to laboratory studies, there is a limit to how much deception or how much stress one can impose in the laboratory setting. Thus, naturalistic settings may provide an excellent source of more severe stress. The stress stimulus would be stronger; there would be no ethical restraint in that the subject would have to be immersed in the stress in any event. Furthermore, the examination of the subject's biochemical response to his naturalistic stresses may provide a relevant guide for counseling him regarding possibly desirous life-style modifications.

Because of the different degree of emotional arousal triggered in the laboratory and in vivo, it is possible that the biochemical information may be very different in the two settings, i.e. that the laboratory stress may be fundamentally different from that encountered by individuals out of the labora-

Table I. Experimental and naturalistic observations on plasma epinephrine levels

Experimental	Level pg/ml	Naturalistic	Level pg/ml
Mental arithmetic		Dental procedure [23]	500
Mefford et al. [18]	200	Public speaking [7]	406
Engel et al. [9]	300		
LeBlanc et al. [15]	170		
Williams [26]	120		
Average	197		
Competitive game [13]			
Without harassment	58		
With harassment	105		

tory. Table I compares the plasma epinephrine levels recorded in a number of different studies [7, 9, 13, 15, 18, 23, 26]. The most commonly used laboratory stress studies involve mental arithmetic tasks. As table I indicates, the plasma epinephrine levels obtained under such circumstances are approximately 200 pg/ml. Even when harrassing competitive games are performed in the laboratory, the plasma epinephrine level is still rather low. In contrast, the two studies that have examined naturalistic stresses with simultaneous plasma catecholamine measures have recorded far higher plasma epinephrine levels. During dental procedures, subjects run a level of 500 pg/ml. During public speaking, subjects run a level of 400 pg/ml.

In using the ambulatory blood withdrawal technology, there are five determinants that allow one to select the appropriate blood withdrawal rate. To begin with, one must decide what the acceptable blood loss could be for the subject population. Secondly, one must remember the plasma half-life of the compound. Compounds with a rapid half-life should be sampled frequently whereas compounds with a longer half-life could be sampled over longer intervals of time. Thirdly, the duration of the biological signal is important to consider. Some compounds may be secreted in a very pulsatile fashion whereas others may be secreted more continuously. Once the plasma has been withdrawn and collected in the vacutainer tube, it is important to consider the thermal stability of the compound under study. Compounds such as catecholamines need to be chilled rapidly or else they will be degraded in the vacutainer tube itself. Other compounds such as cholesterol, for instance, could be kept unrefrigerated in the blood collection tube. Finally, one needs to consider the volume requirements for assay. By considering these five parameters, one can readily determine the appropriate rate of blood withdrawal.

Public Speaking as a Natural Model for Stress

I have taken this rather lengthy introduction to emphasize the new aspects of these methodological developments and to explain their rationale. I would now like to discuss their application in a setting that is quite familiar to us. Considerable literature has accumulated regarding the stressful nature of public speaking. Particularly for novice speakers, this is a setting of great anxiety. During formal presentations at case conferences, speakers manifest profound tachycardia and even coupled premature ventricular contractions [19, 22]. For these reasons, we have chosen to examine the response of public speakers and to compare that response to the plasma catecholamine response observed during vigorous exercise and during relaxed conversation. Our baseline measure, relaxed conversation, should not be confused with a 'basal' measure wherein the subject is resting undisturbed. Thus, our baseline value would be expected to be slightly higher than traditional basal measures. Our exercise measure was obtained while subjects were climbing 20 flights of stairs.

Subjects for this study were healthy house officers or junior faculty at Massachusetts General Hospital. Timing of this study was chosen to coincide with the subject's having to present what he regarded as a stressful paper at a public formal medical conference. After giving informed consent, each subject had a nonthrombogenic catheter inserted in an antecubital vein and threaded proximally 3 inches. Distally, the catheter was attached to a portable blood withdrawal pump that was set to withdraw blood at the rate of 1,5 ml/min. Samples were collected over a 3-min period.

Results

Table II demonstrates the profound influence of exercise and public speaking on both norepinephrine and epinephrine [7]. During public speaking, epinephrine roughly triples, whereas during vigorous exercise, norepinephrine roughly triples.

Table II. The effect of exercise and public speaking on plasma catecholamines[1] [from ref. 7]

Subject	Norepinephrine level, pg/ml			Epinephrine level, pg/ml		
	baseline	exercise	speaking	baseline	exercise	speaking
1	470	–	1,767	88	–	333
2	370	1,060	1,003	100	125	333
3	591	1,815	893	106	137	301
4	675	1,772	828	229	230	479
5	654	1,650	621	102	165	558
6	745	1,561	597	86	186	117
7	577	3,299	1,144	85	163	349
8	655	1,876	725	77	123	142
9	514	772	694	176	187	408
Mean	583	1,726	919	117	164	336

[1] Results of paired t tests were as follows: norepinephrine level, baseline $\times$ exercise, t $= -4.44$ (p <0.005); baseline $\times$ speaking, t $= -2.28$ (p <0.1); exercise $\times$ speaking, t $= 3.90$ (p <0.01); epinephrine level, baseline $\times$ exercise, t $= -3.68$ (p < 0.01); baseline $\times$ speaking, t $= -5.37$ (p < 0.001); exercise $\times$ speaking, t $= -3.42$ (p < 0.025).

Comment

It is of interest to note that the norepinephrine and the epinephrine response are not parallel; thus, it is an oversimplification to speak in terms of *a* 'sympathetic nervous system response' when in fact there may be an adrenal medullary response that is distinct from a sympathetic nervous system response.

In another study, we examined the time course of the response to public speaking more closely [8]. Figure 2 plots the epinephrine levels obtained in subjects at baseline, during the initial 3 min of their public speaking, and during the middle moments of public speaking (minutes 15 through 18). As can be seen from figure 2, epinephrine pursues a pulsatile course, peaking very rapidly and then falling off towards baseline in the middle moments of speaking. The implications of this rapid secretion of epinephrine are important for future studies of catecholamine response to stress. Let us imagine that a hypothetical investigator was interested in examining the plasma catecholamine response to public speaking. If he had chosen as his public speaking measure the plasma sample obtained during the middle moments of public speaking and then contrasted that sample with the baseline sample, he would have failed to discern an increase in plasma epinephrine levels in public

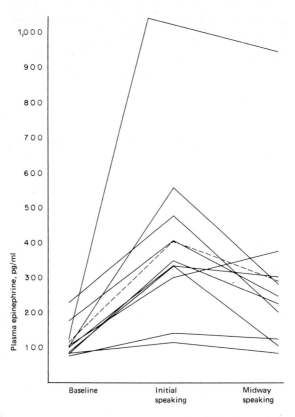

Fig. 2. Impact of sample timing on epinephrine levels during emotional stress [from ref. 8]. Each line represents one subject; the dotted line indicates the mean response.

speaking. In contrast, had he chosen the initial moments of public speaking to compare with a baseline measure, his conclusions would have been very different; public speaking leads to profound elevations of plasma epinephrine (table III). Thus, careful specification of sample timing vis-à-vis the stress event is crucial.

Conclusion

In this brief paper, I have tried to discuss another way of examining the pathophysiological impact of type A personality and other forms of emotional arousal that may convey risk to the heart. Between the availability of

Table III. Effect of sample timing on observing changes in plasma epinephrine during speaking compared with a baseline measure [from ref. 8]

	Mean epinephrine, pg/ml
Baseline	117
Initial moments	406
Paired t (d.f.)	−3.7 (9)
Significance	p < 0.005
Baseline	117
Midway moments	289
Paired t (d.f.)	−2.2 (9)
Significance	n.s.

sensitive plasma assays and the new ambulatory blood withdrawal pumps, a window has been opened for closer observation on the neuroendocrine response of individudals under stress. Given the methodological considerations that I have discussed, such a technique is readily applied and considerable information obtained from studies of individuals during vigorous physical exercise and also individuals in the throes of readily appreciated emotional stress.

References

1   Blumenthal, J.; Williams, R.; Kong, Y.; et al.: Type A behavior pattern and coronary atherosclerosis. Circulation *58:* 634–639 (1978).
2   Carruthers, M.; Taggart, P.; Conway, N.; Bates, D.; Somerville, W.: Validity of plasma catecholamine estimation. Lancet *July 11:* 62–67 (1970).
3   Cooper, T.; Detre, T.; Weiss, S. (eds): Coronary-prone behavior and coronary disease: a critical review. Circulation *63:* 1199–1215 (1981).
4   Dimsdale, J.; Hackett, T.; Block, P.; Hutter, A.: Emotional correlates of type A behavior pattern. Psychosom. Med. *40:* 580–583 (1978).
5   Dimsdale, J.; Hackett, T.; Catanzano, D.; White, P.: The relationship between diverse measures for type A personality and coronary angiographic findings. J. psychosom. Res. *23:* 289–293 (1979).
6   Dimsdale, J.; Hackett, T.; Hutter, A.; Block, P.: The risk of type A mediated coronary artery disease in different populations. Psychosom. Med. *42:* 55–62 (1980).
7   Dimsdale, J.; Moss, J.: Plasma catecholamines in stress and exercise. J. Am. med. Ass. *243:* 340–342 (1980).
8   Dimsdale, J.; Moss, J.: Short-term catecholamine response to psychological stress. Psychosom. Med. *42:* 493–497 (1980).
9   Engel, R.; Muller, F.; Munch, U.; Ackenheil, M.: Plasma catecholamine response and

autonomic functions during short-time psychological stress. Proc. 2nd Int. Symp. on Catecholamines and Stress, Smoleniche Castle 1979.

10   Frank, K.; Heller, S.; Kornfeld, D.; Sporn, A.; Weiss, M.: Type A behavior and coronary angiographic findings. J. Am. med. Ass. *240:* 761–763 (1978).

11   Frankenhaeuser, M.: Experimental approaches to the study of catecholamines and emotions; in Levi, Emotions – their parameters and measurement (Raven Press, New York 1975).

12   Glass, D.: Behavior patterns, stress, and coronary disease (Lea, Hillsdale 1977).

13   Glass, D.; Krakoff, L.; Contrada, R.; et al.: Effect of harassment and competition upon cardiovascular and plasma catecholamine responses in type A and type B individuals. Psychophysiology *17:* 453–463 (1980).

14   Jenkins, C.: A comparative review of the interview and questionnaire methods in the assessment of the coronary-prone behavior pattern; in Dembroski, Weiss, Shields, Haynes, Feinlieb, Coronary prone behavior (Springer, New York 1978).

15   LeBlanc, J.; Cote, J.; Jobin, M.; Labrie, A.: Plasma catecholamines and cardiovascular responses to cold and mental activity. J. appl. Physiol. *47:* 1207–1211 (1979).

16   Mason, J.: Emotions as reflected in patterns of endocrine integration; in Levi, Emotions – their parameters and measurement (Raven Press, New York 1975).

17   ·Matthews, K.: Assessment issues in coronary-prone behavior. Proc. German Conf. on Coronary-Prone Behavior, Altenberg 1981 (see *Matthews*, this volume).

18   Mefford, I.; Ward, M.; Miles, L.; Taylor, B.; Chesney, M.; Keegan, D.; Barchas, J.: Determination of plasma catecholamines and free 3,4-dihydroxyphenylacetic acid in continuously collected human plasma by high performance HPLC with electrochemical detection. Life Sci *28:* 477–483 (1981).

19   Moss, A.; Wynar, B.: Tachycardia in house officers presenting at grand rounds. Annls intern. Med. *72:* 255–256 (1970).

20   Rose, R.; Jenkins, C.; Hurst, M.: Air Traffic Controller Health Change Study (Boston University School of Medicine, Boston 1978).

21   Rosenman, R.; Brand, R.; Jenkins, C.; Friedman, M.; Strauss, R.; Wurm, M.: Coronary heart disease in the Western Collaborative Group study: final follow-up experience of 8½ years. J. Am. med. Ass. *233:* 872–877 (1975).

22   Taggart, P.; Carruthers, M.; Somerville, W.: Electrocardiograms, plasma catecholamines, and lipids, and their modification by oxprenalol when speaking before an audience. Lancet *August 18:* 341–346 (1973).

23   Taggart, P.; Hedworth-Whitty, R.; Carruthers, M.; Gordon, P.: Observation on electrocardiogram and plasma catecholamines during dental procedures: the forgotten vagus. Br. med. J. *ii:* 787–789 (1976).

24   Tang, S.; Stancer, H.; Takahashi, S.; Shephard, R.; Warsh, J.: Controlled exercise elevates plasma but not urinary MHPG and VMA. Psychiat. Res. *4:* 13–20 (1981).

25   Whitby, L.; Axelrod, J.; Weil-Malherbe, H.: The fate of H_3-norepinephrine in animals. J. Pharmac. exp. Ther. *132:* 192–201 (1961).

26   Williams, R.: Correlates of angiographic findings. Proc. German Conf. on Coronary-Prone Behavior, Altenberg 1981.

27   Young, L.; Barboriak, J.; Anderson, A.; Hoffmann, R.: Attitudinal and behavioral correlates of coronary heart disease. J. psychosom. Res. *24:* 311–318 (1980).

28   Zyzanski, S.; Jenkins, C.; Ryan, C.; et al.: Psychological correlates of coronary angiographic findings. Archs intern. Med. *136:* 1234–1237 (1976).

11 Coronary-Prone Behavior and Blood Pressure Reactivity in Laboratory and Life Stress[1]

Heinz Rüddel, E. Gogolin, G. Friedrich, H. Neus, W. Schulte

Background and Introduction

The mechanism of blood pressure (BP) regulation and the problems of cardiovascular reactivity have already been discussed in prior chapters. In our work, we emphasize not only the importance of stress, catecholamines, behavior and cardiovascular reactivity, but also consider a variety of psychosocial influences on BP regulation wherever an interaction with BP regulating processes might be involved (cortex, limbic system, central or peripheral receptors, etc.).

It is a well-known clinical phenomenon that BP becomes elevated when one is angry. However, it is important to also gain information about the prevailing individual mood at the time of BP elevation and about individual history of coping mechanisms, personality traits, and psychosocial determinants. The prediction of BP reactivity of a given individual in different situations is the central theme of our work.

In the early 1930s *Alexander* postulated a connection between hostility and BP. As a result of clinical observation from his psychoanalytic background he concluded that: 'The early fluctuating phase of essential hypertension is the manifestation of a psychoneurotic condition based on excessive and inhibited hostile impulse...' [1]. Since then, related hypotheses have been discussed on and off in the literature. However, at this point in time, no convincing answer has yet emerged [3].

In our studies, we also failed to demonstrate clinically important associations between personality traits and casual BP in healthy normotensive males and females. The observed correlations which were found between suppressed hostility and neuroticism on the one hand, and BP on the other, are difficult to interpret, because of the high intercorrelation between these personality scales and the 'social approval or lie' scale.

[1] This study was supported by Grant 68501 of the Ministry of Youth, Family and Welfare, FRG.

With regard to personality, we must keep in mind that in well-controlled studies, there is no association between resting BP and personality characteristics [5, 14, 18]. In this regard, many of the reported associations between BP and psychosocial characteristics can be explained by sampling procedures.

In our investigation of cardiovascular reactivity to mental stress testing situations we tried to find an association between psychosocial characteristics and BP reactivity. We examined 165 healthy male and female subjects from a random population in Bonn, West Germany. BP and heart rate (HR) were measured at rest and during mental arithmetic in conjunction with noise. Personality traits were examined by means of questionnaires designed to measure neuroticism, extroversion, hostility, anxiety, and others. *Jacksons* [12] Personality Research Form (PRF) was included in our questionnaires to obtain information on personal need for abasement, achievement, affiliation, aggression, autonomy, change, cognitive structure, dependence, dominance, endurance, exhibition, harm avoidance, impulsivity, nurturance, order, play, sentience, social recognition, succorance, and understanding. There was no significant association between personality characteristics and BP reactivity that was consistent except for the following findings in males: psychosocial stress $r = 0.25$ (systolic BP), $r = 0.36$ (diastolic BP); reactive aggression $r = 0.24$ (systolic BP), $r = 0.26$ (diastolic BP); anxiety $r = -0.29$ (systolic BP), $r = -0.40$ (diastolic BP); dominance $r = -0.28$ (systolic BP), $r = -0.28$ (diastolic BP).

A high BP reactivity was found to be associated with more pronounced psychosocial discomfort, more reactive hostility, less anxiety, and less dominance. The often discussed relationship between casual BP and hostility or neuroticism was not confirmed for BP reactivity.

We concluded that it is difficult, if not impossible, to find an association between general personality traits as presently assessed and reactivity of the autonomic nervous system especially for BP variation. However, a concept of state behavior may be more suitable for predicting BP reactions in stress testing situations. High achievement motivation and good performance during a reaction time task and a concentration task are associated with HR reactivity in mental stress testing ($r = 0.40$), and casual BP ($r = 0.25$), as well as BP reactivity ($r = 0.26$) and BP at rest ($r = 0.30$) [16]. Also keep in mind, that there are many intercorrelations between personality traits in such designs. Personality traits also correlate with age as well as infrequency or desirability in answering questions (PRF scale 21 and 22). The infrequency and desirability scales were included to uncover lying or social approval motivation, which is common in response to questions about neuroticism and hostility. Problems in assessing behavioral characteristics due to differences between state and trait variables, effects of sampling, and inappropriate scales, could all be important sources of error in predicting reactivity of individuals during stress testing.

In the last decades, however, it was not the resting or casual BP, but BP reactivity, that has been examined most intensively. BP hyperreactivity is said to precede hypertension in most cases. *Barnett* et al. [2] found that a pathological reaction to cold stress could be replicated 27 years later. 31 subjects, who were hyperreactors in 1934, were still hyperreactive in 1961. Of the 40 subjects that were hyperreactive in 1934, 4 became hypertensive, compared to none of the 167 normal reactors.

Franz [11] examined patients with borderline hypertension, who had an elevated systolic BP of more than 200 mm Hg during an ergometric exercise test in a supine position with a work load of 100 W. Of 26 'hyperreacting' patients with borderline hypertension, 25 were hypertensive 3.8 years later. Of the 19 'normoreacting' control patients with borderline hypertension, only 6 became hypertensive. In an earlier study, we reported that normotensives and patients with borderline hypertension did not differ in resting BP. However, those with borderline hypertension had the same increase in systolic and diastolic BP during mental stress as patients with stage I essential hypertension (WHO classification) [7]. We consider increases of more than 25/12 mm Hg during mental stress testing, 50/20 mm Hg during physical exercise, and of more than 35/30 mm Hg during the type A interview to be pathological. These upper limits of BP reactivity in stress testing were set by adding 1.5 standard deviations to the mean of a representative sample of 165 healthy subjects from Bonn [8].

In the study presented here, we have chosen a real life stressor – preparing for a final examination – as well as different stress testing situations in the laboratory, including mental arithmetic during noise, physical exercise testing, and the type A interview. We asked: (1) Can BP reactivity during stress testing in the laboratory predict casual BP and range of BP variation in healthy normotensive students during a 6-week observation period? (2) Are there any consistent modulating effects on BP by personality traits, the type A behavior pattern, or metabolism?

The time prior to a final examination was chosen because *von Eiff* [7] demonstrated that medical students showed a mean increase of 15 mm Hg, both in systolic and diastolic BP, 2 weeks before their first examination. During this period, however, each individual student showed large variations in BP. Thus, some decreased their BP, some increased their BP and many showed no systematic changes at all. *Francis* [10] reported repeated testing

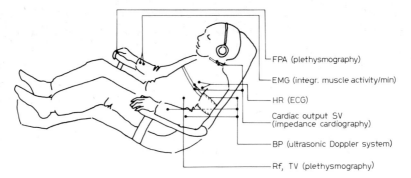

Fig. 1. Assessment of physiological data in the laboratory.

of 20 young physical therapy students during the winter academic quarter, in a longitudinal design. Correlations were reported between moods and feelings of anxiety, depression, and hostility, and serum indicators of stress, namely uric acid, cortisol, and cholesterol. There were three peak periods of observable elevation in stress during the course of the quarter. During the first two peak periods, the observed changes in serum cortisol were highly correlated with changes in anxiety and depression. The ratio of high-density lipoproteins (HDL) to total cholesterol was significantly depressed twice during the academic quarter, each time following a peak period of stress. We pursued a similar course of study.

Methods

54 male students, all non-smokers, were screened for physical health problems and examined weekly for 6 weeks. Half of them (n = 26) had no final examinations after the obervation period and served as a control group. BP was always measured twice in a sitting position with a 5-min rest in between using a random zero sphygmomanometer. HR was determined by measuring pulse rate for 30 s. Blood was taken for the following biochemical analyses: cortisol, uric acid, kidney function, lipoprotein metabolism, electrolytes, and liver function parameters. Questionnaires dealing with nutrition, physical activity, sleep, stress, psychosocial problems, and alcoholic beverages were collected weekly. All the blood samples were taken between 7:30 and 9:00 a.m., with all subjects fasting. The students were examined in the laboratory in an isolated room at the same time of the day prior to the observation period. They were placed in a semi-recumbent position in a reclining chair (fig. 1). Both at rest and during mental arithmetic, BP was recorded every minute by an ultrasonic Doppler system. HR was recorded continuously by ECG, cardiac output and stroke volume (SV) via impedance cardiography, muscle activity (EMG) by electromyography, respiratory frequency (Rf), tidal volume (TV) and finger pulse amplitude (FPA) by plethysmography.

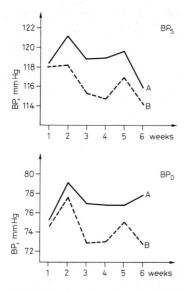

Fig. 2. Blood pressure (systolic and diastolic BP) during the observation period (group A, examination; group B, without examination).

The type A interview was conducted by a trained coworker in the laboratory. All interviews were tape-recorded and scored by two trained persons. For the physical exercise test, the students rode a bicycle in a semi-recumbent position while BP and HR were monitored. The work load was 80–100 W, depending on body size [17].

Hemodynamic parameters during the type A interview and during physical exercise could not be assessed by impedance cardiography due to insufficient artifact control caused by movement.

Results

BP during the Observation Period

There was no increase in BP prior to final examinations in this particular sample. During the weekly recordings of BP, there was no statistically significant difference between students preparing for an examination and those in the control group, although the data were in the predicted direction (fig. 2).

BP Reactivity in Three Different Stress Testing Situations

During mental arithmetic we observed an increase in BP of about $16 \pm 7 / 12 \pm 5$ mm Hg. During the type A interview the increase was $14 \pm 6 / 12 \pm 6$ mm Hg and during physical exercise it increased $42 \pm 11 / 14 \pm 7$

Table I. Correlations between increase in systolic blood pressure (BP) during mental arithmetic, the type A interview, physical exercise and different resting, casual and stress BP readings (mean of two readings) (n = 54)

Correlations	$\triangle$ Systolic BP		
	mental stress	type A	exercise
Casual systolic BP	0.31*	0.20	0.20
Systolic BP at rest	~0.50***	~0.20	~0.10
Mental stress $\triangle$ systolic BP	–	0.50**	0.11
Type A $\triangle$ systolic BP	0.50**	–	0.12
Exercise $\triangle$ systolic BP	0.12	0.12	–

* p < 0.01; ** p < 0.005; *** p < 0.001.

Table II. Correlations between increase in heart rate (HR) during mental stress, the type A interview, physical exercise and different resting, casual and stress BP readings

Correlations	$\triangle$ HR		
	mental stress	type A	exercise
Casual systolic BP	0.28	0.31	0.27
Systolic BP at rest	0.50***	0.10	0.32
Mental stress $\triangle$ systolic BP	0.78***	0.25	0.44**
Type A $\triangle$ systolic BP	0.16	0.17	0.00
Exercise $\triangle$ systolic BP	0.03	0.13	0.27*

* p < 0.01; ** p < 0.005; *** p < 0.001.

Table III. Correlations between increase in systolic blood pressure during mental arithmetic, the type A interview, ergometry and the weekly mean value of two systolic BP readings (see also Methods)

Correlations	Observation period, weeks						N[1]
	1	2	3	4	5	6	
Mental arithmetic	0.14	0.26*	0.33*	0.19	0.31*	0.43*	47
Type A interview	0.35*	0.29	0.06	0.34*	0.16	0.21	27
Ergometry	0.27*	0.27*	0.20	0.14	0.25*	0.11	50

[1] All data valid.

mm Hg. BP reactivity was not different between the two groups during the three testing situations (see table I for intercorrelations).

During mental arithmetic the increase of systolic BP was significantly correlated with the increase of HR (r = 0.78), and cardiac output (r = 0.40). Rf increased parallel to the reaction of systolic BP (r = 0.36) and TV decreased reciprocally (r = 0.33).

During the type A interview, HR reactivity was less than that during mental arithmetic (17.2 ± 9.0 bpm in contrast to 6.8 ± 5.5 bpm). There was no correlation between BP reactivity and reaction of HR during the interview (table II).

During exercise testing an increase in systolic BP was correlated with change in HR (r = 0.27). We also found a correlation between HR reactivity during exercise testing and increase in systolic BP during mental arithmetic testing (r = 0.44).

BP reactivity during mental arithmetic, the type A interview and physical exercise testing was only partially correlated with casual BP during the 6-week observation period (table III). BP reactivity was not correlated with range of BP variability during the observation period (mental arithmetic: r = 0.17, type A interview: r = 0.17, exercise testing: r = 0.29).

Moderating Effects of Personality Characteristics

A consistent association between personality traits and cardiovascular reactivity was not found. A significant correlation between a personality trait and BP reactivity found in one stress situation was never confirmed in the other two test conditions. Because of current discussions in the literature, however, which consider hostility to be crucial for the development of hypertension or coronary heart disease (CHD), a second look at our hostility indices was necessary. We used three different scales in our questionnaires and in scoring the type A interview [15]: (1) The aggression questionnaire (FAF), which is based on a theory of aggression as a learned trait, and factor-analyzed for suppressed hostility, anger, etc. (2) Need for aggression (PRF, scale No. 4). (3) In scoring components of the type A behavior pattern, hostility and verbal competition are rated on Likert-like scales from 1 to 5, 5 indicating pertinent hostile behavior during the interview (6).

In table IV Pearson correlation coefficients are summarized for the different scores of hostility and cardiovascular reactivity during mental stress, the type A interview and physical exercise. Only during the high challenge interpersonal interview situation is an association between reactivity and hostility evident. The pattern of correlations between hostility and BP

Table IV. Correlations between cardiovascular reactivity and different hostility scales (n=54)

	Mental stress			Type A			Exercise		
	△ syst.	△ diast.	△ HR	△ syst.	△ diast.	△ HR	△ syst.	△ diast.	△ HR
Type A									
Hostility	0.16	0.21	−0.01	0.48**	0.22	−0.36*	−0.06	0.31*	0.08
Verbal competition	0.09	−0.01	−0.06	0.57**	−0.07	−0.35*	0.25	0.40*	−0.16
FAF									
Suppressed aggression	−0.01	−0.09	0.17	−0.35*	−0.29	0.03	−0.04	0.16	0.01
Aggression	−0.11	−0.16	0.06	−0.17	−0.29	−0.07	−0.20	−0.02	−0.26*
PRF									
Aggression	0.08	−0.01	0.02	0.14	−0.07	0.08	−0.23	−0.24	−0.16

* $p < 0.01$; ** $p < 0.005$; *** $p < 0.001$.

changes is not uniform. The more general personality traits or basic needs fail to be associated to BP reactivity. Only the hostility and verbal competition components of the type A interview are correlated to increases in BP.

Moderating Effects of Metabolism

As is the case for psychosocial characteristics, the modulating effects of metabolism on cardiovascular reactivity were not uniform in different stress testing situations. There was a high correlation between lipoprotein metabolism, represented in HDL cholesterol, total serum cholesterol, and triglycerides and increase of systolic BP during the type A interview, but not with BP reactivity during mental arithmetic and ergometric exercise (table V).

There was no association between lipoprotein metabolism and resting or casual BP. The results presented here can be summarized as follows: (1) Systolic BP reactivity in mental stress is associated with an increase in HR and cardiac output. (2) A consistent association between personality traits or behavior patterns and cardiovascular reactivity in different stress testing situations was not found. (3) Lipoprotein metabolism is correlated with an increase in systolic BP during the type A interview. (4) Casual BP during the 6-week observation period is only partially correlated with systolic BP reactivity in stress testing (mental arithmetic, the type A interview, and ergometry).

Table V. Correlations between increase in systolic BP during mental stress, the type A interview, physical exercise and lipoprotein metabolism (fasting blood samples, n=54)

Correlations	$\triangle$ Systolic BP		
	mental stress	type A	exercise
HDL	0.16	0.53**	−0.08
Total serum cholesterol	0.07	0.44*	−0.12
Triglycerides	0.01	0.37*	−0.03

* $p < 0.01$; ** $p < 0.005$.

Discussion

In this study we failed to demonstrate a *consistent* pattern of cardiovascular reactivity for all of the different stress testing situations. The increase of systolic BP during mental arithmetic and the type A interview were correlated. There were no significant correlations between BP reactivity during either mental stress testing or the type A interview and during physical exercise testing. Non-homogeneity of the study population could have influenced this however, because one half of the subjects were working for a final examination and their cortisol samples were relatively high [15]. The mean increase of systolic BP of 16.5 mm Hg during mental arithmetic is somewhat higher than previously observed in groups of normotensive patients [8, 9]. Physical exercise work load in our protocol [17] might not be sufficient in this young, healthy population to reveal significant correlations between mental stress testing and physical exercise testing. However, we can also consider the influence of the physiological mechanisms involved in BP reactions during mental arithmetic, physical exercise and during the type A interview. Despite the vasodilatation caused by submaximal exercise testing, the reactivity of systolic BP in ergometry as well as in mental arithmetic is primarily associated with changes in HR, and consequently by an increase in cardiac output. BP reactivity during the type A interview is not associated with changes in HR; preliminary data suggest that it is essentially determined by an increase in peripheral resistance.

The type A interview seems to be representative of a high-challenge interpersonal interaction where overt hostility and competition is provoked [6]. We know that in some populations the maximum systolic BP during the type A interview is higher in type A subjects than in type B subjects [6]. Both large increases in BP and changes in metabolism (noradrenalin, adrenalin, cholesterol, cortisol) could be the pathophysiological pathway to atherosclerosis and CHD. We must keep in mind, however, that BP reactivity during the type A interview is primarily correlated to HDL cholesterol and HDL is regarded as protecting vessels from atherosclerosis.

Our results indicate that we must be careful in generalizing from cardiovascular reactivity during the type A interview, to BP reactivity during all other stress testing situations, to casual BP, BP at rest or BP measurements during an observation period. There is, however, an association between BP reactions during the type A interview and mental arithmetic. BP reactivity during mental arithmetic is related to casual BP, BP at rest, and to changes in HR during stress testing. BP reactivity during mental arithmetic is also correlated with four of the six casual BP readings taken during the 6-week observation period. Possibly, mental arithmetic plus noise is fairly comparable to daily life situations and gives a possible pathophysiological model of a typical stress situation with increased cardiac output. When considering the pathophysiological mechanism, the hemodynamic pattern during mental arithmetic represents quite a good model for cardiovascular reactivity in the early stage of essential hypertension, characterized by increased cardiac output [4]. The prognostic value of mental stress testing and exercise testing in the diagnosis of hypertension remains presently unresolved, but data emerging in the last few years are encouraging [8, 11].

Although some of our findings were consistent with past findings in the type A area, we were not able to confirm all of the observations of *Dembroski* et al. [6], who found type A subjects to be hyperreactive during different situations, such as the type A interview, a quiz on American history or a pong game at least under appropriately challenging conditions. The different challenge of stress testing in Bonn compared to the setting in Florida could perhaps explain this. But some of our findings represent cross-cultural replication of the findings of *Dembroski* et al. [6].

The current methods used to assess personality traits seem as yet inappropriate in psychophysiological studies. Our three different scales for hostility all had a different association to reactivity indices. Only overt hostility and verbal competition (as measured in the type A interview) were significantly correlated with BP activity during the type A interview. Hostility was only marginally correlated with BP reactivity in the other tasks. Personality traits assessed by questionnaire do not seem to explain much of the variance in cardiovascular reactivity during stress testing. State rather than trait descriptions or assessment of coping strategies will perhaps explain more of the individual variation in reaction to different stimuli. In fact, the hostility observed during the type A interview may be considered a state rather than a trait variable.

In this study we failed to observe an increase in BP during the preparation for a final examination. We followed the students for only 6 weeks, whereas *von Eiff* [7] did so for nearly 6 months. In our sample, only non-smokers were admitted, and these were highly motivated to participate, even though they had to spend a lot of time to complete all the psychophysiological testing and to fill out the daily nutrition sheets. Our control group was not a genuine control group inasmuch as these students reported a rather intensive work load for other examinations (3 h daily compared to 5 h daily in the 'examination' group). Both groups had a relatively high level of plasma cortisol during the 6-week observation period, which indicates a generally high level of stimulation of the hypothalamic-hypophyseal-adrenal system. Possibly, we failed to demonstrate an increase in BP because our observation period was too short and we had no real control group.

The partial correlations observed between BP reactivity during stress testing and during the 6-week observation period is promising, but more systematic studies comparing laboratory reactivity indices with variations of BP and HR in daily life are necessary to explain the inconsistent findings.

References

1 Alexander, F.: Emotional factors in essential hypertension. Psychosom. Med. *1:* 173–179 (1939).
2 Barnett, P.H.; Hines, G.A.; Schirger, A.; Gage, R.R.: Blood pressure and vascular reactivity to the cold pressor test. J. Am. med. Ass. *183:* 845–848 (1963).
3 Bauer, M.: Blutdruck und Persönlichkeit. Zusammenhanganalyse von psychologischen Testdaten und physiologischen Messergebnissen; unpublished doct. diss., Bonn (1981).
4 Brod, J.; Cachovan, M.; Bahlmann, J.; Bauer, G.E.; Celsen, B.; Sippel, R.; Hundeshagen, H.; Feldmann, U.; Rienhoff, O.: Haemodynamic changes during acute emotional stress in man with special reference to the capacitance vessels. Klin. Wschr. *57:* 555–565 (1979).
5 Cochrane, R.: Neuroticism and the discovery of high blood pressure. J. psychosom. Res. *13:* 22–25 (1969).
6 Dembroski, T.M.; MacDougall, J.M.; Shields, J.L.; Pettito, J.; Lushene, R.: Components of the type A coronary-prone behavior pattern and cardiovascular responses to psychomotor performance challenge. J. behav. Med. *1:* 159–176 (1978).
7 Eiff, A.W. von: Das vegetative Nervensystem; in Heilmeyer, Lehrbuch der speziellen pathologischen Physiologie (Fischer, Stuttgart 1968).
8 Eiff, A.W. von; Friedrich, G.; Langewitz, W.; Neus, H.; Rüddel, H.; Schirmer, G.; Schulte, W.: Verkehrslärm und Hypertonierisiko. Hypothalamustheorie der essentiellen Hypertonie. 2. Mitteilung. Münch. med. Wschr. *123:* 420–424 (1981).

9 Eiff, A.W. von; Neus, H.; Schulte, W.: Stressreagibilität als Charakteristikum von Blut-druckgruppen. Verh. dt. Ges. inn. Med. *84:* 792–795 (1978).

10 Francis, K.T.: Psychologic correlates of serum indicators of stress in man: a longitudinal study. Psychosom. Med. *41:* 617–628 (1979).

11 Franz, I.W.: Ergometrische Untersuchungen zur Beurteilung der Grenzwerthypertonie. Therapiewoche *30:* 7858 (1980).

12 Jackson, D.N.: Personality research form manual. (Research Psychologists Press, New York 1967).

13 Langosch, W.; Rüddel, H.; Schmidt, T.H.: Die deutschsprachige Form des strukturierten Interviews zur Verhaltenstyp-A-Diagnostik (unpublished manuscript).

14 Ostfeld, A.M.; Shekelle, R.B.: Psychological variables and blood pressure. Psychosom. Med. *35:* 321–331 (1973).

15 Rüddel, H.; Gogolin, E.; Neus, H.: Einfluss von Stress auf Lipoproteine. Unpublished report to the Minister of Youth, Family, and Welfare, Bonn 1981.

16 Rüddel, H.; Neus, H.; Schulte, W.: Beziehungen zwischen Leistung und Blutdruckverhal-ten. Med. Welt *29:* 1131–1135 (1981).

17 Schulte, W.; Neus, H.; Rüddel, H.; Schirmer, G.; Eiff, A.W. von: Ein ergometrisches Ver-fahren zur Bestimmung der Blutdruckreagibilität. Angiocardiology *2:* 320–328 (1979).

18 Spelmann, M.S.; Ley, P.: Psychological correlates of blood pressure. Med. J. Aust. *53:* 1130–1140 (1966).

12 Psychophysiological Testing of Postinfarction Patients
A Study Determining the Cardiological Importance of Psychophysiological Variables
W. Langosch, G. Brodner, F. Foerster[1]

Psychophysiological studies in humans and animals suggest that it is possible to change nearly every physiological parameter (i.e. heart rate (HR), blood pressure (BP), lipid metabolism, carbohydrate metabolism, catecholamine and corticoid metabolism) by means of psychological or physical stressors. Nevertheless, the results of these studies can hardly be generalized to everyday life situations for the following reasons: (1) In daily life, the patient is confronted with multidimensional, chronic and intensive psychophysiological stressors, whereas the stressors used in most laboratory studies are not only considerably limited in regard to their duration and intensity, but are relatively simple compared to the complexity of occupational demands [17]. (2) Whether a marked increase in physiological parameters under laboratory challenge indicates pathophysiological processes is uncertain, since it is unknown whether the observed physiological functions are reversible or irreversible.

To reduce, to some extent, the uncertainty experienced by postinfarction patients concerning the meaning of physiological reactivity induced by laboratory stressors, it is important to determine which of the many physiological parameters recorded during psychophysiological testing are empirically associated with medical findings essential to the long-term outcome of intervention given to postinfarction patients.

Due to the small covariation between different physiological variables – except for those variables belonging to the same physiologic, functional system [15] – it is indispensable to record many physiological variables that depict different physiologic, functional systems [13]. In general, postinfarction patients show a complex pattern of physiological reactivity, which is not uniform for the entire subject group, although in individual cases systematic correlations between physiological variables can be found [25]. According to

[1] The authors would like to express their gratitude to cand. phil. *M. W. Greenlee* for rendering this work into an idiomatic form.

these findings, multivariate physiological testing is required; i.e. it is not sufficient to record only variables like HR and BP, because these variables cannot be regarded as representative of the overall pattern of physiological reactivity.

The results of several studies conducted with myocardial infarction (MI) patients and type A subjects emphasize the importance of psychophysiological testing in a cardiological rehabilitation program. In a study by *Tänzer* et al. [42] 36 coronary heart disease (CHD) patients were challenged in an experimental condition involving time pressure. The authors report a marked increase in HR and BP for all subjects and for 17% of subjects the occurrence of ECG signs of ischemia, for 33% the occurrence of extrasystoles and for 25% changes in T wave amplitude. *Theorell* [43] also observed that postinfarction patients showed extrasystoles under emotional stress, which had not been found during exercise testing. In a study of *Valek* et al. [44] MI patients reacted to a psychological stressor with greater increases in diastolic (DBP) and systolic BP (SBP) compared to a control group of ill patients. Furthermore, *Dembroski* et al. [6] point out that in MI patients systolic BP increases more than in normal controls. Comparing type A with type B subjects, *Dembroski* et al. [7, 8] demonstrated that type A subjects are characterized by a more pronounced increase of SBP and HR under challenging conditions and by a greater variability in HR during rest, whereby there was no difference between the groups in the frequency of galvanic skin responses for several task conditions.

In summary, in psychophysiological studies with CHD patients and type A subjects, some ECG parameters and SBP and DBP as well have proved to be reliable indicators of physiological arousal under psychological challenge. It is, however, still unknown whether these physiological activation variables are associated with essential cardiological findings. Therefore, it remains quite equivocal whether even a marked increase in these variables is of any clinical importance to postinfarction patients.

Furthermore, in the above-mentioned studies activation and constitutional variables are not systematically differentiated. Whereas *activation variables* indicate *changes* in physiological functions under challenging psychophysiological conditions, most often expressed as difference scores between rest and task scores [15], *constitutional variables* are regarded as physiological traits allowing for a differentiation between subjects at rest as well as under challenge. While the efficiency to discriminate physiologically between rest and challenging conditions, and perhaps between different types of environmental challenge, is most important to activation variables, constitutional variables are primarily characterized by a high situational stability, i.e. the physiological interindividual differences remain stable across several periods of rest and tasks. From the findings of the above-mentioned studies it appears that HR and SBP should be regarded as activation variables, whereas HR variability may be interpreted as a constitutional variable. In psychophysiological studies with type A subjects, the recording of activation variables seems especially useful, because the type A behavior pattern has been conceptualized as the result of an interaction between personality and environmental challenges and not as a cluster of personality traits alone [37]. Psychophysiological testing with postinfarction patients should allow a prognosis that estimates how far the confrontation with psychophysiological challenges can be tolerated without negative cardiological consequences. Therefore, activation variables as well as constitutional variables must be recorded, since both types of physiological variables characterize different aspects of the psychophysiological reactivity pattern related to cardiological findings.

Although in type A studies, electrodermal activity (EDA) parameters have not proved to be very useful [7, 8], psychophysiological activation research has clearly shown that parameters of ECG, BP, respiration and EDA are of equal importance in the description of psychophysiological reactivity [15]. Based upon the results of several studies, these authors conclude that psychophysiological activation is quite a heterogeneous process that can best be described by means of a profile consisting of the most important activation variables that belong to several different physiologic, functional systems. Consequently, it is not possible to generalize from the values of a few physiological variables, for example HR and SBP, to the entire reactivity pattern, since it has been demonstrated that the individual change scores of an activation variable in one physiological system cannot be predicted from the change values of an activation variable in another physiological system [15]. Therefore, in psychophysiological testing a multivariate procedure is necessary, which demands the recording not only of several physiological variables belonging to the same physiologic, functional system, e.g. HR, frequence of extrasystoles, T wave amplitude, etc., but also the recording of variables appropriate for describing the physiological changes which occur in different physiologic functional systems.

In psychophysiological studies conducted with postinfarction patients, it has been found that in addition to the low correlations between physiological variables belonging to different physiologic, functional systems, the relationship between physiological and psychological variables is also negligible [22, 25]. Therefore, in testing the psychophysiological reactivity of postinfarction patients, the procedure used must be multivariate and as such should consider the following data levels: (1) several physiological variables most important for describing the reactivity occurring in a particular physiologic, functional system; (2) several physiologic, functional systems, most important for describing the complexity of the reactivity pattern; (3) several physiological variables useful in describing the activation process and/or in clarifying constitutional differences; (4) several psychological variables deemed important in describing subjective aspects on the state and/or trait level as well as behavioral and performance aspects, and (5) several psychological and physiological variables that – in addition to the above-mentioned requirements – are in fact related to essential cardiological findings.

Although *Dembroski* et al. [5] emphasize that self-rating scales used in the context of psychophysiological testing do not discriminate between type A and type B subjects and, additionally, that these psychological scores are not significantly correlated with physiological values, these results do not justify the exclusion of psychological variables in psychophysiological studies with type A subjects or with postinfarction patients altogether. *Myrtek* [34], on the other hand, stresses the necessity of analyzing psychologically the often pronounced discrepancies between self-ratings and physiological data, instead of assuming that there is, in general, an unequivocal psychophysiological covariation.

The pattern of psychophysiological reactivity depends not only on the type and intensity of challenging stimuli [5, 22], but also on physiological and psychological characteristics, conceived here as intervening variables, i.e. mediators, that relate stimuli input to reactivity output. For postinfarction patients, physiological mediators are, for example, the severity of atherosclerosis or extent of left ventricular dysfunction; psychological mediators seem to be: (1) personality traits like degree of irritability, unsociability, emotional lability and hypochondria [22–24]; (2) some aspects of vocational demands perceived as stressful, such as degree of extraneous control over work success, and degree of satisfaction with occupational activity [23], and (3) type A behavior pattern [6].

In summary, the psychophysiological testing of postinfarction patients requires the selection of a challenging stimuli input that simulates some aspects of the pattern of daily life stressors often confronted by postinfarction patients, the determination of physiological and psychological mediators, the selection of physiological and psychological variables appropriate in comprehensively describing the complexity of the psychophysiological reactivity pattern and the determination of the cardiological importance of those vari-

ables that have been evaluated as useful in describing the psychophysiological reactivity pattern.

The present study has considered aspects of psychophysiological
research related to the selection of those psychological and physiological
variables that should be taken into account in describing the psychophysiological reactivity pattern of postinfarction patients and the determination of
the cardiological importance that these variables possess.

The procedure is composed of two successive steps: (1) the stepwise
statistical evaluation of physiological and psychological variables in regard
to their usefulness as constitutional or activation variables, and (2) the empirical, criterion-oriented evaluation of the selected psychological and physiological variables regarding their ability to predict essential aspects regarding
the success of rehabilitation.

Psychophysiological Methods

In our standardized psychophysiological examination of postinfarction
patients below the age of 40 [23, 25], three types of stressors are used for simu-
lating aspects of everyday stress in the laboratory: (1) continuous concentration under disturbing environmental conditions combined with perfor-
mance-dependent frustration; (2) pronounced striving for a large quantity as
well as high quality of performance while having control over time pressure
compared to having no control over a time pressure that approaches the
upper limit of the individual's performance level; (3) emotional arousal
induced by thinking over the answers to three aversive, but very important,
topics and emotional arousal while having to give the answer to all three
questions in a 2-min period.

The psychophysiological examination is composed of five stressor
periods and six rest periods. Every task period has been preceded and followed by a rest period. All periods are limited to 2 min, except the task 'mental preparation', which had to be limited to 30 s, because otherwise the psychophysiological reactivity decreases. During the stressor period 'self-controlled time pressure', the exposition time per stimulus (five variously
coloured dots and two different tones) was exclusively controlled by the subject himself, who had been informed of this schedule. During the stressor
period 'extraneously imposed time pressure' the exposition time per stimulus
was 20% shorter than during the preceding stressor period for every subject.
Again, the subject was informed about the schedule. At the beginning of each

stressor period, the subject was urged to work as quickly as possible, but to avoid mistakes and to do his very best.

While BP was manually recorded at the beginning and the end of each period, ECG, EDA and respiration are recorded on a continuous basis. These physiological data have been analyzed by specific computer programs, which had been developed by the 'Forschungsgruppe Psychophysiologie Freiburg'. For further details concerning these computer programs, see *Walschburger* [45] and *Fahrenberg* et al. [15].

After every experimental period, the patient was asked to rate his actual psychological state in respect of the two dimensions 'degree of relaxation' and 'degree of feeling well' with references to his ratings in the initial rest period. Additionally, subjects were asked to rate their degree of satisfaction with their performance. To evaluate the subjects' performance level on a more objective basis, several performance scores, which refer specifically to each stressor period, are also taken into account. Furthermore, an experienced clinical psychologist rated the behavior of the subject on several aspects following each stressor period as well as after the conclusion of the entire examination. The rating scales used differed for each type of challenging stimuli. In summary, the initial set of psychophysiological data is composed of the following:

Physiological Variables. 21 ECG parameters for each of the 11 periods; 20 EDA parameters for each of the 11 periods; 6 respiration parameters for each of the 11 periods; 2 BP parameters for each of the 11 periods. Accordingly, 49 physiological variables are recorded at each period.

Psychological Variables (Self-Ratings and Behavioral Ratings). 2 self-ratings concerning the subjects' actual psychological state (relaxed and well-being) for each of the 11 periods, i.e. 22 scores across the whole psychophysiological examination; 1 self-rating concerning the degree of satisfaction with one's own performance after each of 4 tasks (this rating was not done after the stressor period 'mental preparation of answers'), i.e. 4 scores across the whole psychophysiological examination; 3 behavioral ratings concerning the patient's behavior while confronted with the tasks 'continuous concentration', 'self-controlled time pressure', 'extraneously imposed time pressure', i.e. 9 behavioral ratings across the whole psychophysiological examination; 4 behavioral ratings concerning the patient's behavior while confronted with the task 'answering to three aversive questions within a 2-min period'; 2 behavioral ratings concerning the patient's behavior while confronted with the task 'mental preparation of the answers'; 4 behavioral ratings of the patient's behavior during the entire psychophysiological examination. Accordingly, 45 psychological variables are recorded across the entire psychophysiological examination.

Performance Scores. 3 scores referring to patient's performance at the task 'continuous concentration'; 4 scores related to patient's performance of the task 'self-controlled time pressure' and 4 scores related to patient's performance of the task 'extraneously imposed time pressure'. Accordingly, 11 performance scores are recorded across the entire psychophysiological examination.

Stepwise Statistical Analysis

The stepwise statistical evaluation relies upon the data of a sample of male postinfarction patients under the age of 40 at the time of their infarction (n = 144).

The statistical selection has been performed in two steps: (1) all data were tested according to fundamental statistical standards, and (2) the retained variables were classified as either constitutional or activation variables or both. These selection steps were separately performed for physiological variables on the one hand and psychological variables and performance scores on the other hand.

Required statistical standards for physiological variables included: no significant deviation from normal distribution (skewness $\leq$ 6, kurtosis $\leq$ 10) during stressor periods; only small redundance ($r < 0.80$) of one variable in comparison with another variable; in the case of redundance, the variable is excluded that deviates more from normal distribution and/or has been more often evaluated to be of minor importance in psychophysiological research, and large range without ceiling effects.

Criteria for physiological activation variables were as follows: marked increase from preceding rest period to task period in at least four of the five stressor periods according to significant t-tests ($p < 0.05$); significant situation effect in a two-way analysis of variance (mixed model) with the factors 'periods' (one rest period, five stressor periods) and 'subjects' (VC_{sit}: $p < 0.01$); marked increase from preceding rest period to task period according to significant Scheffé tests in at least three of the five stressor periods ($p \leq 0.05$), and error variance $\leq$ 50% of total variance in a two-way analysis of variance (mixed model) with the factors 'six periods' and 'subjects'.

Criteria for physiological constitutional variables included: high stability across rest periods ($r_{tt} \geq 0.60$); significant interindividual differences according to a two-way analysis of variance (random model) with the factors 'subjects' and 'six rest periods' ($VC_{pat} \geq 50\%$), and no significant differences between several rest periods (VC_{rest}: $p \geq 0.01$).

Required statistical standards for psychological variables and performance scores were: no significant deviation from normal distribution (skewness ≤ 6, kurtosis ≤ 10) during stressor periods, and only small redundance (r > 0.80) of one variable in comparison with another variable; in the case of redundance, the variable is excluded that deviates more from normal distribution and/or has been more often evaluated to be of minor importance in psychophysiological research.

Criteria for psychological activation variables: Such self-ratings and behavioral ratings were selected which concern the subjects' actual psychological state or behavior during each of the five stressor periods.

Criteria for psychological constitutional variables: Of the self-ratings those variables were selected, which concern the subjects psychological state during the initial rest period, since these self-ratings were used as a frame of reference. Of the behavioral ratings, those variables were selected which concern the subjects' behavior during the entire psychophysiological examination.

Criteria for performance scores: All of these variables are defined as activation variables, since they only refer to the subjects' performance during stress periods.

According to these criteria the following physiological variables, psychological data, and performance scores have been selected as appropriate:

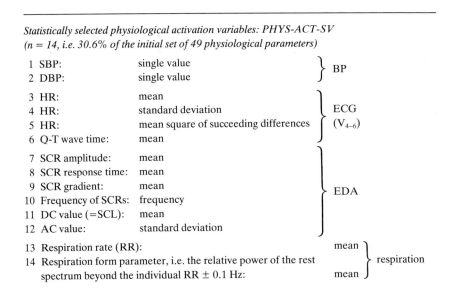

Statistically selected physiological activation variables: PHYS-ACT-SV
(n = 14, i.e. 30.6% of the initial set of 49 physiological parameters)

1 SBP:	single value	} BP
2 DBP:	single value	
3 HR:	mean	
4 HR:	standard deviation	ECG
5 HR:	mean square of succeeding differences	(V$_{4-6}$)
6 Q-T wave time:	mean	
7 SCR amplitude:	mean	
8 SCR response time:	mean	
9 SCR gradient:	mean	EDA
10 Frequency of SCRs:	frequency	
11 DC value (=SCL):	mean	
12 AC value:	standard deviation	
13 Respiration rate (RR):		mean	respiration
14 Respiration form parameter, i.e. the relative power of the rest spectrum beyond the individual RR ± 0.1 Hz:		mean	

Statistically selected physiological constitutional variables: PHYS-CON-SV
(n = 20, i.e. 40.8% of the initial set of 49 physiological parameters)

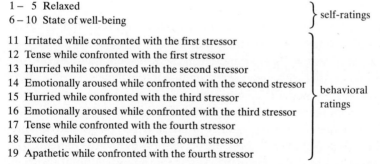

  1 SBP: single value
  2 DBP: single value
} BP

  3 Extrasystoles: frequency
  4 HR: mean
  5 HR: mean square of succeeding differences
  6 R wave amplitude: mean
  7 P wave amplitude: mean
  8 Q wave amplitude: mean
  9 Q-R wave amplitude: mean
} ECG (V_{4-6})

 10 P wave gradient: mean
 11 P-Q wave time: mean
 12 T wave amplitude: mean
 13 Q-T wave time: mean
} ECG (V_{4-6})

 14 Spectrum of amplitudes III (14–19)
 15 Spectrum of phases I (1,3)
 16 Spectrum of phases II (4, 6, 6, 11, 13)
 17 Spectrum of phases III (5, 10, 12, 14, 17, 19)
} using a unit of 1.95 Hz in each case

 18 SCR integral (amplitude *frequency):   mean
 19 DC-value (SCL):   mean
} EDA

 20 Estimated volume of respiration
     (i.e. square root of the total power):   mean   respiration

Statistically selected psychological activation variables: PSYCH-ACT-SV
(n = 2 self-ratings related to each of the five stressor periods and 9 behavioral ratings
= 2 × 5 + 9 = 19, i.e. 42.2% of the initial set of psychological variables)

 1 – 5 Relaxed
 6 – 10 State of well-being
} self-ratings

 11 Irritated while confronted with the first stressor
 12 Tense while confronted with the first stressor
 13 Hurried while confronted with the second stressor
 14 Emotionally aroused while confronted with the second stressor
 15 Hurried while confronted with the third stressor
 16 Emotionally aroused while confronted with the third stressor
 17 Tense while confronted with the fourth stressor
 18 Excited while confronted with the fourth stressor
 19 Apathetic while confronted with the fourth stressor
} behavioral ratings

Statistically selected psychological constitutional variables: PSYCH-CON-SV
(n = 5, i.e. 11.1% of the initial set of psychological variables)

 1 Relaxed during initial rest phase
 2 State of well-being during initial rest phase
} self-ratings

3 Shy during the entire psychophysiological examination ⎫
4 Apathetic during the entire psychophysiological examination ⎬ behavioral
5 Active during the entire psychophysiological examination ⎭ ratings

Statistically selected performance scores: PER-ACT-SV
(n = 7, i.e. 63.6% of the initial set of performance scores)

1 Number of errors during the first stressor phase
2 Number of correct responses during the second stressor phase
3 Work tempo achieved during the second stressor phase
4 Number of correct reactions during the third stressor phase
5 Number of latent responses during the third stressor phase
6 Number of incorrect responses during the third stressor phase
7 Work tempo achieved during the third stressor phase

Subsequently, for each of the selected 14 *activation variables*, the difference scores between stressor conditions and preceding rest phases have been calculated; this procedure was performed separately for each of the five stressor periods. These 14 change scores for each stressor period have also been tested for deviations from the normal distribution (criteria: skewness ≤ 6, kurtosis ≤ 10).

Only the change scores of the variables, HR (mean square of succeeding differences), SCR amplitude (mean), and AC value (standard deviation) deviated from normal distribution in respect of kurtosis in some (maximum: 3) of the five stressor conditions.

In testing the 14 activation variables in respect to the law of initial values [46], it has been found that 10 activation variables are positively and only two activation variables (Q-T wave time: mean; SCR response time: mean) are negatively associated with their corresponding initial values, i.e. the values in the preceding rest periods. This majority of antilaws of initial values corresponds well with the results of *Myrtek* et al. [35] and *Myrtek* [34], who have already questioned the general validity of this law. The positive covariation between task values and rest values means that postinfarction patients with high initial values are rather inclined to react more intensively to stressor conditions, even after the a (a-b) effect (a = rest value; b = task value) has been statistically controlled [34, 35]. In the further criterion oriented analysis change scores (difference between stressor phase and preceding rest phase values) have been applied for the physiological activation variables.

Each of the 20 *constitutional* variables has been averaged across all 11 phases for each subject, resulting in 20 habitual physiological values for each patient. Only the variable, P wave amplitude (mean), deviates from the normal distribution in respect of skewness and kurtosis, whereas the variables, frequency of extrasystoles, R wave amplitude, Q wave amplitude, Q-R wave amplitude, P wave amplitude and P wave increase, are only characterized by marked kurtosis.

In summary, the stepwise statistical analysis has resulted in a set of 14 physiological activation variables and 20 physiological constitutional variables. Concerning the activation variables, the law of initial values could only be confirmed for two variables and the corresponding change scores generally meet fundamental statistical standards. The constitutional values characterize the patient's physiological reactivity across periods of rest and challenge. While the set of activation variables is composed of variables belonging to different physiologic functional systems, ECG parameters prevail in the set of constitutional variables. Additionally, a set of 31 psychological variables and performance scores has been evaluated to meet fundamental statistical standards.

Empirical, Criteria-Oriented Analysis

The empirical, criteria-oriented analysis should select psychophysiological variables that are significantly related to essential aspects of rehabilitation success. Based on the notion that psychophysiological reactivity is best described by a multivariate pattern, it has been concluded that the association of a single physiological or psychological variable with a specific aspect of rehabilitation success is not of importance in itself, but rather the covariation between a set of physiological and psychological variables and a set of rehabilitation success aspects should have priority.

Next it seems important to determine which aspects of the process of rehabilitation should be utilized as criteria in the regression analysis that employs psychophysiological variables as predictors. Various cardiological parameters and vocational aspects shall be selected for describing the success of rehabilitation, since these appear to be also of legal interest. According to paragraph 184a RVO of the German National Medical Insurance, the patient's present need for treatment is an essential criterion, whereas for social security the decrement of occupational capability due to an anomal, pathological state of health is decisive [14]. These authors have also emphasized psychological findings, and correctly so, as criteria of the success of a comprehensive rehabilitation program [14]. Their importance has been substantiated by various follow-up studies conducted with postinfarction patients that have employed scales assessing subjective state, mood, personality and behavioral aspects [26–28]. Nevertheless, the criteria selection shall be limited to cardiological and vocational findings, since these variables are, first, objectively assessable and, second, have received high priority as criteria for the success of treatment.

The cardiological parameters have been selected based on the following two perspectives: first, only parameters that have proved their significance in cardiological longitudinal prognoses of young MI patients [38, 41]; second, only those parameters shall be employed that according to theoretical considerations are at least partially under autonomic control and as such are related in some way to subjective appraisal processes or coping strategies on the behavioral level. Consequently, the amount of scar tissue is not selected, since there is no empirical or theoretical indication that this cardiological variable is in any way associated with the psychophysiological variables of reactivity or activation. Contrarily, a relationship between the intensity or duration of a response that is subjected to autonomic control that may lead to atherosclerosis or sudden death seems more probable [2]. Various authors contend that type A individuals have a higher risk of suffering from MI due to autonomic hyperreactivity [4, 18–20]. *Schaefer and Blohmke* [39] assess a high tonic level of the sympathetic nervous system as a primary risk factor for MI. *Siegrist* [40] suggests a relationship between vocational ambition and stress, life-changing events and coping strategies on the one hand, and a long-term, continuous pathological development in the coronary vessels due to disorders of the adrenomedullary system, on the other hand. The results of investigations dealing with the relationship between the type A behavior pattern and the degree of coronary atherosclerosis suggest a close connection, although the findings are not completely unequivocal [1, 9, 16, 25, 49]. Also in these studies, the relationship between behavior and coronary sclerosis is generally accounted for by enhanced reactivity of the autonomic nervous system. Since coronary sclerosis is assumed to be the most frequent cause of MI [21], such cardiological findings are selected as criteria, especially those that describe the degree of atherosclerosis in the postinfarction patient. Accordingly, the results of coronary angiography and floating catheter examination, which is an indicator of coronary insufficiency, are considered.

Since the results of coronary angiographic and floating catheter examinations provide various aspects of the patient's condition subsequent to MI,

Table I. Intercorrelations of aspects of rehabilitation success (n = 51)

	1	2	3	4	5	6
1 Severity of atherosclerosis	1.00					
2 ST segment depression	0.29	1.00				
3 PCP increase	0.29	0.15	1.00			
4 Degree of angina pectoris	0.28	0.67	0.30	1.00		
5 Exercise-induced ischemia	0.07	0.40	0.38	0.63	1.00	
6 Vocational reintegration	0.21	0.17	0.14	0.63	0.52	1.00

differential statements may be made as to whether psychophysiological data predict more precisely morphologic or functional cardiological findings.

The criterion describing vocational reintegration, namely the item 're-tired' vs 'not retired', has also been chosen. As to the legal decision whether a patient is capable of working again or not, cardiological findings remain in highest priority. The 'psychophysical fitness' of the postinfarction patient, as measured in psychophysiological studies, contributes, however, to the assessment of the illness behavior [3] exhibited by the patient [see also ref. 33 regarding the discrepancy between 'objective impairments' and the 'frequency of patients' complaints'], which may influence return-to-work. According to these considerations, the following cardiological and vocational variables have been selected as criteria:

Cardiological Findings. Morphology of the coronary vessels (coronary angiographic results): severity of atherosclerosis: 0, 1, 2, 3 (luminal occlusion of each vessel $\geq$ 50%). Coronary insufficiency (floating catheter examination): ST segment depression; increase in pulmonary capillary pressure; clinical diagnosis from physician concerning the intensity of angina pectoris; clinical diagnosis from physician concerning the intensity of the exercise-induced ischemia.

Vocational Reintegration. Patients receiving pension funds at the time of the investigation were classified as 'retired'; all others were classified as 'not retired'.

Since none of the cardiological criteria was found to be redundant based on correlation analysis (table I), all cardiological variables were employed. The variable 'vocational reintegration' describes a further independent aspect of the rehabilitation and as such is used as a criterion.

The basis of the criteria-oriented selection is the extent to which the psychophysiological variables can more or less predict these six criteria that are viewed as important to the long-term success of rehabilitation. In light of the relatively independent nature of the various criteria, it may be expected that on the one hand the exactness of prediction shall be very considerable, and on the other hand that the single psychophysiological variables or variable groups that contribute to the prediction should not be the same for each criterion. Since the results of regression analyses will be the basis of this selection, a further test as to which groups of psychophysiological parameters or single variables prove to be the best predictors for the essential aspects of the success of rehabilitation should be made. This general question may be subdivided into the following:

(1) Is the formation of psychophysiological indices meaningful, which consist of the following variables:

Constitutional, physiological variables (PHYS-CON-SV)
Constitutional, psychological variables (PSYCH-CON-SV)
Physiological activation variables (PHYS-ACT-SV)
Psychological activation variables (PSYCH-ACT-SV)
Performance parameters (PER-ACT-SV)

Since each index consists of various single variables, the single scores are transformed into T scores. Accordingly, each variable group is characterized by an index (T sum score). Furthermore, it should be emphasized that the indices consist of variables that were considered adequate in the first selection phase, i.e., the complete set of psychophysiological variables ordered in subgroups has been employed. The basis for this step is found in the assumption that a single-component model, depicted in a one-dimensional, unspecific psychophysical activation [10, 30], is deemed as inadequate for the description of psychophysical reactivity or activation [15]. Here, a multicomponent model has been chosen, whereby each component is represented in an index. Fahrenberg et al. [15] have, however, warned against use of such indices, since the presentation of T scores from various strain phases and/or activation variables may lead to a considerable reduction of variance and as such provides little intersubject discrimination. Furthermore, such a presentation is questionable since stimulus-specific response patterns may be active. In light of these objections, only low regression coefficients should be expected. Therefore, if the predictions made show sufficient exactness, the constitutional, as well as the activation indices should prove their individual contributions to the predictions, thus demonstrating their individual value.

(2) May a data set be obtainable, which is selected according to general theoretical and statistical considerations from each of the five variable subgroups, and which is superior over the exactness of prediction provided for by the entire set of psychophysiological variables? This selection has served primarily in the reduction of the variable set.

Therefore, a relatively high precision of prediction is expected for this reduced data set, since a well-defined selection of the theoretically relevant and statistically most satisfying physiological variables should screen out variables that are either irrelevant for the prediction, or that due to suboptimal parametric extraction lead to an impairment of predictive validity.

Consequently, the reduction of total variance due to the formation of indices, subsequent to a reduced selection of averaged variables, should not be as considerable, i.e. the discriminating value of the data should be less impaired. The strict selection of variables has been conducted for each variable group separately. In the following, these selected variables shall be referred to as type 1 variables.

(3) Which of the type 1 activation variables are especially important for the prognosis of the various criteria? Since such a differentiation of type 1 variables according to the amount of the variance accounted for by the type 1 single variables for the various criteria is desired, thoroughly situative independence of the single activation parameter is strived for here. The corresponding values of each type 1 activation variable assessed over the five challenge phases are summarized in an individual index (T sum score). This index should characterize situationally independent change in state of the respective activation variable. Since the psychophysical activation is a heterogeneous process that is best described by a profile of the various marker variables of the different functional subsystems [15], it is expected that the psychophysiological activation variables of the cardiovascular system should prove to be the best predictors of cardiological criteria.

(4) To which extent are sufficient prognoses possible that are singly based on the activation variable scores derived in a single challenge phase, instead of being based on the value collected over an entire experiment? Of the challenge conditions, the stressor is selected that evokes the most substantial change in arousal on the various, important parameters of different physiological subsystems. The following parameters, determined in psychophysiological research as 'marker variables' have been employed in the selection of stressors [15], HR mean (HR-$\bar{x}$), respiration form parameter (RFO), frequency of SCR (SCR-f). In addition SBP has been considered, since it has

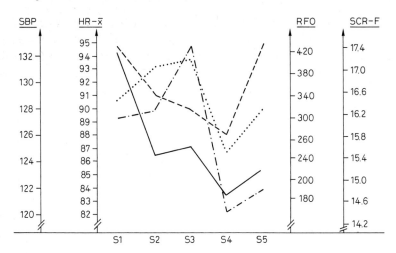

Fig. 1. Mean values of heart rate: mean (HR-x̄, ——), respiration form parameter (RFO, ·······), frequency of SCR (SCR-f, –·–·–), and systolic blood pressure (SBP – – –) in the various stressor conditions of psychophysiological investigation.

been shown that in postinfarction patients SBP is an essential activation parameter [6].

As may be seen in figure 1, the stressor phase 'continuous concentration' evokes the most substantial change in arousal state. Accordingly, this challenge phase has been selected as the best stressor. As predictors, the type 1 activation variables were used that were registered during this stressor phase.

Consequently, the subsequent prognosis in this case is based on the variables that are the 'best psychophysiological activation variables monitored in the best challenge phase'. Furthermore, since the relative contribution of each type 1 activation variable is to be determined, the raw scores of these variables have been employed. It is expected, therefore, that the precision of prediction provided for by this predictor set should prove to be superior to a prediction based on the type 1 activation indices over the entire experiment. Furthermore, cardiovascular variables should provide the highest contribution to the prediction. This hypothesis is inferred from the conclusions made by *Fahrenberg* et al. [15], namely that activation processes may be better represented by means of a profile of the important activation variables than by a multicomponent model. Additionally, the finding that correlations between variables of the same functional subsystems are considerably higher than those found between different subsystems [15] adds support to this hypothesis.

(5) Is the predictive character of the best psychophysiological activation variables essentially dependent on the respective stressor phase or are the various stressor phases unimportant? According to the 'stimulus-specific response patterns' (SSR) found in earlier psychophysiological research, a stimulus or situation can evoke a hyperreaction in a single physiological subsystem or a similar response pattern [11, 15]. The portion of variance accounted for by the SSR principle has been estimated at roughly 6%. Results of the type A research indicate further the importance of such situation-specific response patterns [6]. Since lack of patience has always been emphasized in the description of the type A behavior pattern [36], and since this type A component provides a relatively good predictor for the occurrence of CHD [32] it is expected that the two stressor phases in which a distinct time pressure is presented as the strain condition are especially important for the prediction of the degree of coronary atherosclerosis. In the regression analyses, the various type 1 activation variables have been summarized for each respective stressor phase in the form of an index (T sum score), so that each index characterizes a situation-specific activation pattern.

(6) Is a sufficient prognosis of important criteria depicting the process of rehabilitation possible in the application of exclusively habitual parameters? In order to answer this question, constitutional type 1 variables shall be applied as predictors after various forms of activation indices have already been analyzed regarding their contribution to the variance of the various criteria. Since these constitutional variables per definition refer to the entire investigation, and also considering the fact that the relative weight of the constitutional variables should be determined, the raw values shall be applied as predictors.

According to these six above-listed questions, six various psychophysiological predictor groups shall be applied in the prognosis of six criteria:

First Predictor Group. Multicomponent model consisting of stepwise, statistically selected variables (M-SV): For each psychophysiological subgroup (i.e. physiological and psychological constitutional variables, physiological and psychological activation variables, performance parameters) an index (T sum score) is formed in which all variables retained in the stepwise statistical selection are applied (table II).

Second Predictor Group. Multicomponent model consisting of stepwise statistically selected variables of the type 1 (M-SV1): For each psychophysiological variable group an index (T sum score) is formed consisting of the best psychophysiological single variables, i.e. type 1 variables. Within each of these variable groups the following single variables have been selected as type 1 variables:

PHYS-ACT-SV1 (n = 25 single variables)
  BP   SBP (1–5)
  ECG   HR ($\bar{x}$) (6–10)
                         HR (MQSD) (11–15)
  EDA   SCR integral measure (16–20)
  Respiration   respiratory form parameter (21–25)
  EDA   SCR integral measure (16–20)
  Respiration   respiratory form parameter (21–25)

For each stressor phase, five physiological type 1 activation variables have been found; therefore this index is based on 25 single variables (5 variables × 5 stressor phases = 25 scores)

PSYCH-ACT-SV1 (n = 8 single variables)
  Self-rating   degree of subjective relaxation in each of the five stressor
                           phases (1–5)
  Behavioral ratings   tense during the first stressor phase (6)
                         hurried during the second and third stressor phase (7–8)

PER-ACT-SV1 (n = 3 single variables)
  Number of errors in performance during the first stressor phase (1)
  Response time during the second stressor phase (2)
  Number of latent responses during the third stressor phase (3)

PHYS-CON-SV1 (n = 5 single variables)
  BP   SBP (1)
  ECG   HR ($\bar{x}$) (2)
                         HR (MQSD) (3)
  EDA   SCR integral measure (4)
  Respiration   respiratory volume estimate (5)

PSYCH-CON-SV1 (n = 5 single variables)
  Self-ratings   degree of subjective relaxation in the initial rest phase (1)
  Behavioral ratings   active behavior during the entire experiment (2)

The second predictor group consists of the variables presented in table III.

Third Predictor Group. Stepwise statistically selected type 1 activation variables over all five stressor phases (ACT-SV1): For each of the type 1 activation variables monitored over all five phases, a score over all experimental phases has been made in the form of an index (T sum score). Consequently, performance parameters and behavioral ratings could not be considered specifically for the respective experimental phases (table IV).

Fourth Predictor Group. Stepwise statistically selected type 1 activation variables monitored during the first stressor phase (ACT-SV1-S1): As predictors all psychophysiological activation variables of the type 1 have been used, that were monitored during the first stressor phase (table V).

Table II. Variables in the first predictor group (M-SV) listed according to name of predictor, method of selection, type of variable, number of single variables, and the experimental phase in which data on variables were collected

Predictor group	Method of selection	Type	Number of single variables	Experimental phase
1 PHYS-ACT	stepwise stat.	index (T sum)	70	5 stressor phases
2 PSYCH-ACT	stepwise stat.	index (T sum)	19	5 stressor phases
3 PER-ACT	stepwise stat.	index (T sum)	7	3 stressor phases
4 PHYS-CON	stepwise stat.	index (T sum)	20	entire exp.
5 PSYCH-CON	stepwise stat.	index (T sum)	5	entire exp.

Table III. Variables in the second predictor group (M-SV1) listed according to name of predictor, method of selection, type of variable, number of single variables, and the experimental phase in which data on variables were collected

Predictor group	Method of selection	Type	Number of single variables	Experimental phase
1 PHYS-ACT	stepwise and type 1	index (T sum)	25	5 stressor phases
2 PSYCH-ACT	stepwise and type 1	index (T sum)	8	5 stressor phases (2nd and 3rd)
3 PER-ACT	stepwise and type 1	index (T sum)	3	1st, 2nd, 3rd stressor phase
4 PHYS-CON	stepwise and type 1	index (T sum)	5	entire exp.
5 PSYCH-CON	stepwise and type 1	index (T sum)	2	1st rest phase

Table IV. Variables in the third predictor group (ACT-SV1) listed according to name of predictor, method of selection, type of variable, the experimental phase in which data on variables were collected, and the variable group to which it belongs

Predictor	Method of selection	Type	Experimental phase	Variable group
1 SBP	stepwise and type 1	index (T score)	S1–S5[1]	PHYS-ACT
2 HR ($\bar{x}$)	stepwise and type 1	index (T score)	S1–S5	PHYS-ACT
3 HR (MQSD)	stepwise and type 1	index (T score)	S1–S5	PHYS-ACT
4 SCR frequency	stepwise and type 1	index (T score)	S1–S5	PHYS-ACT
5 Respiratory form parameter	stepwise and type 1	index (T score)	S1–S5	PHYS-ACT
6 Subjective report of relaxed state	stepwise and type 1	index (T score)	S1–S5	PSYCH-ACT

[1] S1–S5 represents the different stressor phases.

Table V. Variables in the fourth predictor group (ACT-SV1-S1) listed according to the name of the predictor, method of selection, type of variable, the experimental phase in which the data on the variable were collected, and the variable group to which it belongs

Predictor	Method of selection	Type	Experimental phase	Variable group
1 SBP	stepwise and type 1	raw scores	S1[1]	PHYS-ACT
2 HR ($\bar{x}$)	stepwise and type 1	raw scores	S1	PHYS-ACT
3 HR (MQSD)	stepwise and type 1	raw scores	S1	PHYS-ACT
4 SCR frequency	stepwise and type 1	raw scores	S1	PHYS-ACT
5 Respiratory form parameter	stepwise and type 1	raw scores	S1	PHYS-ACT
6 Subjective report of relaxed state	stepwise and type 1	raw scores	S1	PHYS-ACT
7 Tense behavior	stepwise and type 1	raw scores	S1	PSYCH-ACT
8 Number of errors	stepwise and type 1	raw scores	S1	PER-ACT

[1] S1 represents the first stressor phase (continuous concentraction).

Table VI. Variables in the fourth predictor group (S-ACT-SV1) aggregated into an index for the respective stressor phases: name of predictor (i.e. stressor phase), method of selection, type of variable, number of variables monitored, and variable group

Predictor	Method of selection	Type	Number of single variables	Variable group
First stressor phase	stepwise and type 1	index (T score)	5	PHYS-ACT
			2	PSYCH-ACT
			1	PER-ACT
Second stressor phase	stepwise and type 1	index (T score)	5	PHYS-ACT
			2	PSYCH-ACT
			1	PER-ACT
Third stressor phase	stepwise and type 1	index (T score)	5	PHYS-ACT
			2	PSYCH-ACT
			1	PER-ACT
Fourth stressor phase	stepwise and type 1	index (T score)	5	PHYS-ACT
			1	PSYCH-ACT
Fifth stressor phase	stepwise and type 1	index (T score)	5	PHYS-ACT
			1	PSYCH-ACT

Table VII. Variables in the sixth predictor group (CON-SV1) listed according to name of predictor, method of selection, type of variable, the experimental phase in which data were collected and the variable group

Predictor	Method of selection	Type	Experimental phase	Variable group
1 SBP	stepwise and type 1	raw scores	entire experiment	PHYS-CON
2 HR ($\bar{x}$)	stepwise and type 1	raw scores	entire experiment	PHYS-CON
3 HR (MQSD)	stepwise and type 1	raw scores	entire experiment	PHYS-CON
4 SCR integral	stepwise and type 1	raw scores	entire experiment	PHYS-CON
5 Respiratory volume estimate	stepwise and type 1	raw scores	entire experiment	PHYS-CON
6 Subjective report of relaxed state	stepwise and type 1	raw scores	entire experiment	PSYCH-CON
7 Active behavior	stepwise and type 1	raw scores	entire experiment	PSYCH-CON

Fifth Predictor Group. Stepwise statistically selected type 1 activation variables over the five stressor phases (S-ACT-SV1): All type 1 variables have been specially aggregated for each stressor phase into an index (T sum score). Since each index should describe the change of state evoked by the respective phase, only activation variables have been considered in the extraction of each stressor parameter (table VI).

Sixth Predictor Group. Stepwise statistically selected constitutional variables of type 1 (CON-SV1): Here, the various constitutional, physiological and psychological variables have been applied as predictors (table VII).

The predictive precision of the six predictor groups for each of the six criteria is calculated by means of multiple regression analysis. Based on the findings derived from a subject sample (n = 51) of young postinfarction patients, who were examined for the first time on psychophysiological parameters 4.0 years subsequent to their first stay at the rehabilitation center in Bad Krozingen, W. Germany, these regression analyses have been conducted. Since the independent and dependent variables were measured at the same time, the predictive precision of the psychophysiological predictor groups must be estimated by means of the determination of the concurrent validity. It cannot be ruled out, however, that such a method may well lead to an overestimate of the predictive precision compared to that that would be found in a second follow-up study. The regression analyses produced the results, regarding the experimental hypotheses, listed in table VIII.

The present results suggest the following conclusions: (1) The predictive precision of the predictor group (M-SV) in which index variables have been applied consisting of all statistically selected parameters derived from different psychophysiological functional subsystems, the values of which

Table VIII. Predictive precision of the six psychophysiological predictor groups for the essential criteria regarding the success of rehabilitation in postinfarction patients

Predictor group		Morphology: severity of athero- sclerosis		Coronary insufficiency								Vocational reintegration: retired	
				PCP		ST		EI		AP			
name	n	R	p	R	p	R	p	R	p	R	p	R	p
1 M-SV	5	0.28	n.s.	0.35	n.s.	0.28	n.s.	0.44	0.07	0.46	0.05	0.36	n.s.
2 M-SV1	5	0.39	n.s.	0.54	0.01	0.28	n.s.	0.45	0.06	0.51	0.02	0.44	0.08
3 ACT-SV1	6	0.37	n.s.	0.38	n.s.	0.50	0.04	0.47	0.09	0.57	0.01	0.42	n.s.
4 ACT-SV1-S1	8	0.32	n.s.	0.41	n.s.	0.60	0.02	0.33	n.s.	0.46	n.s.	0.36	n.s.
5 S-ACT-SV1	5	0.45	0.07	0.33	n.s.	0.29	n.s.	0.33	n.s.	0.30	n.s.	0.28	n.s.
6 CON-SV1	7	0.30	n.s.	0.65	0.00	0.30	n.s.	0.39	n.s.	0.34	n.s.	0.35	n.s.

n = Number of predictors; PCP = increase in pulmonary capillary pressure; ST = ST segment depression; EI = intensity of exercise-induced ischemia; AP = intensity of angina pectoris; R = multiple regression coefficient; p = level of significance; n.s. = $p \geq 0.11$.

were obtained in various stressor phases, can be improved by rigorously selecting 'marker variables' for the various psychophysiological, functional subsystems, thereby reducing the heterogenity of the psychophysiological data set (M-SV1). (2) Only by means of the predictor group (S-ACT-SV1) that depicts the situationally specific nature of psychophysiological reactivity the predictive precision of the number of stenotic coronary arteries approaches significance ($p < 0.10$). (3) The predictor group consisting of the constitutional marker variables (CON-SV1) produces on the one hand the relatively best single prognosis, but otherwise the predictive precision of the predictor groups consisting of psychophysiological activation parameters is superior. (4) The predictor group consisting of situationally independent psychophysiological activation variables (ACT-SV1) most precisely predicts the two clinical diagnoses 'exercise-induced ischemia' and 'intensity of angina pectoris'. (5) The clinical diagnosis 'intensity of angina pectoris' is significantly predicted by three various predictor groups (M-SV, M-SV1, ACT-SV1). Furthermore, the prediction of the degree of exercise-induced ischemia by the same three predictor groups approaches statistical significance ($p < 0.10$). (6) The criterion 'successful vocational reintegration' is predicted by the predictor group M-SV1 with a precision that approaches statistical significance ($p < 0.10$).

The results further show that no predictor group produces a prognosis of sufficient precision for all six criteria.

Five of the six predictor groups are assessed as being adequate for the prediction of the various criteria; the predictor group M-SV has not been considered here, since compared with the predictor groups ACT-SV1 and M-SV1 it proved to give lower predictive precision. Three of the five remaining predictor groups consist exclusively of type 1 activation variables (ACT-SV1, ACT-SV1-S1, S-ACT-SV1) that not only contain physiological parameters but also subjective reports and performance parameters. The fourth predictor group, CON-SV1, only consists of constitutional variables and combines physiological and self-report parameters; the fifth predictor group, M-SV1, that has predicted four criteria with sufficient precision, however, consists of constitutional and activation indices which had been seperately for physiological and psychological parameters aggregated into indices.

In the next step of the analysis, the relative contribution of the single predictors belonging to these five predictor groups shall be determined from the prediction of the various criteria used here. To the extent that only one significant multiple regression coefficient resulted for a single criterion, the individual predictors of the corresponding predictor group have been rank-ordered according to the magnitude of the coefficients, whereby all variables below the median have been discarded. Whenever more than one significant multiple regression coefficient was found for the same criterion, the predictor group is selected that indicates the coefficient with the lower error probability.

The following psychophysiological parameters have by the above-described means been assessed as particularly important for the prognoses of individual criteria:

Criterion: Severity of Atherosclerosis
Index consisting of all type 1 activation variables monitored during the third stressor phase: S3-ACT-SV1. Index consisting of all type 1 activation variables monitored in the second stressor phase: S2-ACT-SV1.

Criterion Group: Coronary Insufficiency
Criterion: Pulmonary Capillary Pressure. SBP during the entire investigation: CON-SBP. Respiratory volume during the entire experiment: CON-RVO2. HR variability during the entire experiment: CON-HR (MQSD).

Criterion: ST Segment Depression. SBP during the first stressor phase: SBP-S1. Mean HR during the first stressor phase: HR ($\bar{x}$)-S1. Number of errors during the first stressor phase: NE-S1. HR variability during the first stressor phase: HR (MQSD)-S1.

Criterion: Clinical Diagnosis of Exercise-Induced Ischemia. Index consisting of the best psychological activation variables during all stressor phases: PSYCH-ACT-SV1. Index consisting of the best psychological, constitutional variables: PSYCH-CON-SV1.

Criterion: Clinical Diagnosis of Angina pectoris. Index consisting of the changes in mean HR during all five stressor phases: ACT-HR ($\bar{x}$). Index consisting of the change in HR variability during all five stressor phases: ACT-HR (MQSD). Index consisting of changes in respiratory form during all five stressor phases: ACT-RFO. Index consisting of the changes in SBP during all five stressor phases: ACT-SBP.

Criterion: Vocational Reintegration
Index consisting of the best physiological activation variables during all stressor phases: PHYS-ACT-SV1. Index consisting of the best psychological, constitutional variables: PSYCH-CON-SV1.

These results suggest the following conclusions:

(1) The psychophysiological changes induced by means of considerable time pressure provide the relatively best contribution for the prediction of stenotic coronary arteries.

(2) Exclusively, the multicomponent model consisting of the best psychophysiological single variables proved meaningful for the prognosis of 'successful vocational reintegration'. In addition, the physiological activation index and the psychological, constitutional index are given the relatively highest rank-order position for the prediction of this criterion.

(3) The pulmonary capillary pressure is best predicted by constitutional, physiological parameters, among which the cardiovascular variables are superior.

(4) The ST segment depression induced by ischemia may be primarily predicted by physiological activation variables of the cardiovascular system monitored during the 'continuous concentration' challenge condition.

(5) The clinical diagnosis 'angina pectoris' is predicted best by various physiological activation variables that characterize functions of the cardiovascular system; in contrast, the clinical diagnosis 'exercise-induced ischemia' is best predicted by psychological indices.

(6) Parameters of EDA are obviously of minor importance for the prediction of the various criteria.

The results of the criterion-oriented selection of variables suggest the presence of a substantial heterogeneity in the activation process, indicated by the relatively worst prognoses produced by the predictor group (M-SV) that was based on a multicomponent model that consisted of all psychophysiological variables that met fundamental statistical standards. Note, however, that this multicomponent model is merely a variation of a dual-component model that consists of a psychological and physiological principle component, even if a differentiation between activation processes and constitutional traits are made for each of these principle components, thus subdividing each component into two parts. Nevertheless, this concept remains less differentiated than that put forth by *Fahrenberg* et al. [15], namely a five-component model consisting of a psychological dimension (subjective state) and four primarily functionally oriented physiological scales (cardiovascular, EEG, sensor motor skills, EDA). This differentiated version of the dual-component model failed, however, in the investigation conducted by *Fahrenberg* et al. [15], to provide sufficient predictive precision.

The adequacy of a component model in depicting psychophysiological activation processes may, therefore, be generally criticized, especially if the problems of specificity are considered (response-specific, situation-specific, and motivational-specific response patterns). Consequently, *Fahrenberg* [12] argues that the assumption that a throughly proportional change in the individual activation variables or functional subsystems exists is no longer viable. These authors put forth the notion that the variety of activation processes may be more adequately predicted by a profile consisting of the scores on psychophysiological 'marker variables', i.e. type 1 variables. Since five different psychophysiological variable groups have proved to be the best predictor groups for the six criteria investigated here, and additionally, for those predictor groups to which more than one criterion has been assigned, the relative importance of psychophysiological indices changes in dependence on the respective criterion, it may be assumed that, first, we are dealing with a substantial heterogeneity in psychophysiological activation processes and, second, a considerable criterion-oriented specificity of psychophysiological activation patterns is evident. It follows, therefore, that clinical psychophysiological activation diagnosis must specify the criteria involved, since otherwise variables or indices may be used that are irrelevant for the prediction of the criteria of interest. Consequently, different psychophysiological variables and indices are to be applied, for example, if the hypothesis is to be tested that type A subjects are more readily disposed to developing substantial coronary atherosclerosis than are type B subjects, compared to testing the hypothesis putting forth that type A individuals exhibit relatively greater increase in pulmonary capillary pressure under strain than do type B subjects. Such a criterion specificity demands that differences must be evident among the psychophysiological variables that have been depicted as important in predicting the given criterion.

The analysis of the best individual predictors for the various criteria has confirmed our hypothesis that among the best psychophysiological variables, those variables are dominant that are identical to, or at least closely associated with, the functional system from which the criterion of interest stems. Moreover, the finding that the marker variables of EDA do not prove to be important individual predictors for the cardiological criteria further supports this conjecture. Accordingly, in the case that no empirical studies are present in the literature that have produced corresponding, criterion-oriented results, an a priori selection of variables can be made for the prognosis of a certain criterion by limiting itself to the marker variables of the psychophysiological, functional subsystems for that given criterion.

As expected, the limitation of a reduced data set consisting of psychophysiological variables proved to be advantageous for the enhancement of predictive precision. In limiting the data set to marker variables for each of the respective subsystems (ECG, BP, respiration, EDA, subjective state, behavior, performance), as well as to activation variables or constitutional variables, the heterogenity of the activation processes is reduced, i.e. the variety of changes occurring within a single functional subsystem is considerably limited, thereby increasing the discriminatory value of the various criteria between subjects. Since this concept assumes that the selected 'best' variables actually adequately depict the changes in functional systems and thus may be referred to as marker variables, and in light of the 'individual-response principle', the statistical method used in the present variable selection should be specially conducted for each patient sample that differs in relevant variables from the present patient sample. Moreover, according to the principle of symptom specificity, already formulated by *Malmo* et al. [31], the possibility not only exists for hyperreactivity within a single functional system depicted by the symptoms to occur, but also the assumption is suggested that within a single functional system the rank-order for the relatively 'best' variables for each patient group may vary. It should be emphasized, here again, that the profile of the marker variables not only depicts physiological functional subsystems but also psychological processes, evident in that all five predictor groups considered useful contain psychological parameters. Thus, the principle of complementarity of psychological and physiological functional systems [15] is further supported by the present findings.

The question as to whether change scores are to be preferred over steady-state values, or vice versa, cannot be answered here based on the present results. As of yet, the three predictor groups consisting exclusively of activation scores (i.e. change scores) have proved to be the best predictor groups for three of the six criteria considered here. It should, however, be noted that the pulmonary capillary pressure is best predicted by constitutional variables (i.e. steady-state scores). It remains for future research to determine whether or not one of these two variable types (i.e. activation or constitutional) should be discarded. Even if theoretical considerations suggest applying one of these types, e.g. activation scores in type A research, the prognostic utility of these two variable types obviously remains criterion-dependent and thus the predictive superiority of one over the other must first be proved for the given criterion. This conclusion implies for present application that the psychophysiological investigation in cardiological and type A research must be so designed that the statistical analysis of rest values, change scores, and strain scores can be conducted.

The results presented here suggest, however, not only the necessity of monitoring and analyzing the responses, i.e. psychophysiological variables, with sufficient differentiation, but also suggest the need for sufficient complexity of the stressors themselves. The various stressors viewed as representative for different stimulus classes must be applied in inducing psychophysiological activation processes. Although psychophysiological variables monitored in the 'best' stressor phase have proved to be the best predictor group for one criterion, predictors for other criteria are necessary that are based on activation processes or steady-state values determined in various challenge situations.

Especially in type A research, the conditions in the experiment should consist of various stressors, since the occurrence for the type A behavior pattern is dependent on the demands of the environment [37]. Assuming that there is an association between the degree of type A behavior pattern and the severity of coronary atherosclerosis [1, 16, 47, 48], the present finding that the frequency of stenotic coronary arteries may be best predicted by situationally specific psychophysiological activation indices further supports this hypothesis. The special role of substantial time pressure evoking psychophysiological activation in the prediction of the frequency of stenotic coronary arteries corresponds well with the notion put forth by *Matthews* et al. [32], namely that type A individuals are often characterized by 'impatience' and 'irritability'. For the psychophysiological diagnosis in cardiological rehabilitation, these results also suggest the necessity of applying various stimulus classes as stressors to be able to predict the essential criteria of long-term success in cardiological rehabilitation.

Summarizing the above-listed results, the following findings from the present study appear to be of importance: (1) The stepwise statistical analysis of the variety of parameters derived from ECG, BP, respiration, EDA, subjective state, behavior and performance resulted in a reduced set of physiological and psychological data that fulfils fundamental statistical conditions. (2) Subsequently, the selection of 'marker variables' for each psychophysiological functional subsystem and for each of the two variable types, i.e. activation values and constitutional scores, from the selected data set was made. (3) The determination of the predictive precision of the various psychophysiological predictor groups for the important criteria for long-term success of cardiological rehabilitation was made. (4) The determination of the best psychophysiological individual predictors for each criterion was made.

The conclusions to be drawn that appear most important are as follows: (1) The inadequacy of a differentiated version of the dual-component model of arousal that consists of all statistically selected psychophysiological variables is evident. (2) The necessity of monitoring constitutional, as well as activation variables, appears evident. (3) The necessity of applying various stimulus classes in the psychophysiological experiment is obvious. (4) The relative importance of the close association of the criteria and predictors to the same or similar psychophysiological functional subsystem is evident. (5) The necessity of a multivariate description of the individual functional subsystems is supported. (6) The necessity of a complementary experimental design, i.e. monitoring psychological and physiological functional systems, is supported. (7) Considerable criterion-specific predictive precision for the various predictor groups is evident.

The above statements should be made with the following limitations: (1) Generally, the predictive precision of the psychophysiological predictor groups has not been determined, but rather as an estimate, multiple regression coefficients have been calculated indicating the degree of concurrent validity. (2) The present patient sample, the data from which have been applied in the calculation of multiple regression coefficients, is relatively small (n = 51). (3) Only some physiological functional systems have been included in the present investigation; biochemical parameters have been completely neglected in favor of biosignals. (4) For the psychological functional systems, the initial set of parameters is relatively small.

Although the present results must be replicated by further studies on samples of postinfarction patients, this approach however, appears promising, especially if the psychophysiological data set can be further enlarged with marker variables of other functional systems. The applied areas of cardiological rehabilitation and type A research should, therefore, find the present results, despite the limitations mentioned above, of significant interest.

References

1   Blumenthal, J.A.; Williams, R.B.; Kong, Y.; Schanberg, S.M.; Thompson, L.W.: Type A behavior and angiographically documented coronary disease. Circulation 58: 634 (1978).

2   Buell, J.C.; Elliot, R.S.: Psychosocial and behavior influences in the pathogenesis of aquired cardiovascular disease. Am. Heart J. 100: 723 (1980).

3   Cohen, F.: Personality, stress, and the development of physical illness; in Stone, Cohen, Adler, Health psychology, a handbook, p. 77 (Jossey-Bass, San Francisco 1979).

4   Dembroski, T.M.; MacDougall, J.M.; Buell, J.C.; Elliot, R.S.: Type A, stress and autonomic reactivity: considerations for a study of these factors in the work place; in Siegrist, Halhuber, Myocardial infarction and psychosocial risks, p. 89 (Springer, Berlin 1981).

5   Dembroski, T.M.; MacDougall, J.M.; Herd, J.A.; Shields, J.L.: Effect of level of challenge on pressor and heart rate responses in type A and B subjects. J. appl. soc. Psychol. 9: 209 (1979).

6   Dembroski, T.M.; MacDougall, J.M.; Lushene, R.: Interpersonal interaction and cardiovascular response in type A subjects and coronary patients. J. hum. Stress 5: 28 (1979).

7   Dembroski, T.M.; MacDougall, J.M.; Shields, J.L.; Pettito, J.; Lushene, R.: Components of the type A coronary-prone behavior pattern and cardiovascular responses to psychomotor performance challenge. J. behav. Med. 1: 159 (1978).

8   Dembroski, T.M.; MacDougall, J.M.; Shields, J.L.: Physiologic reactions to social challenge in persons evidencing the type A coronary-prone behavior pattern. J. hum. Stress 3: 2 (1977).

9   Dimsdale, J.E.; Hutter, A.M.; Gilbert, J.; Hackett, T.P.; Block, P.C.; Catanzano, D.M.: Predicting results of coronary angiography. Am. Heart J. 98: 281 (1979).

10   Duffy, E.: Emotion: an example of the need for reorientation in psychology. Psycholog. Rev. 41: 184 (1934).

11   Engel, B.T.: Response specifity; in Greenfield, Sternbach, Handbook of psychophysiology, p. 571 (Holt, Rinehart & Winston, New York 1979).

12   Fahrenberg, J.: Psychophysiologische Methodik; in Groffmann, Michel, Psychologische Diagnostik, Handbuch der Psychologie, Bd 6 (Hogrefe, Göttingen 1979).

13   Fahrenberg, J.: Zur Bedeutung der individualspezifischen Reaktionsmuster und der Labor-Feld-Vergleiche für die psychophysiologische Diagnostik; in Langosch, Psychosoziale Probleme und psychotherapeutische Interventionsmöglichkeiten bei Herzinfarktpatienten, p. 263 (Minerva, München 1980).

14   Fahrenberg, J.; Medert-Dornscheidt, G.; Wittman, W.W.; Knobloch, H.: Grundlagen einer Psychologischen Diagnostik- und Indikations-Hilfe im Hinblick auf die effektive Behandlung von Patienten mit psychosomatischen Krankheiten oder Störungen in stationären Heilverfahren, insbesondere mit psychotherapeutischen Massnahmen (Bundesversicherungsanstalt für Angestellte, Berlin 1978).

15   Fahrenberg, J.; Walschburger, P.; Foerster, F.; Myrtek, M.; Müller, W.: Psychophysiologische Aktivierungsforschung (Minerva, München 1979).

16   Frank, K.A.; Heller, S.S.; Kornfeld, O.S.; Sporn, A.A.; Weiss, M.B.: Type A behavior pattern and coronary angiography findings. J. Am. med. Ass. *240:* 761 (1978).
17   Frieling, E.: Zur Generalisierung der Wirkung von Laborstressoren auf berufliche Belastungen; in Langosch, Psychosoziale Probleme und psychotherapeutische Interventionsmöglichkeiten bei Herzinfarktpatienten, p. 271 (Minerva, München 1980).
18   Glass, C.D.: Stress, behavior patterns, and coronary disease. Am. Sci. *65:* 177 (1977).
19   Glass, C.D.: Type A behavior: mechanisms linking behavioral and pathophysiologic processes; in Siegrist, Halhuber, Myocardial infarction and psychosocial risks, p. 77 (Springer, Berlin 1981).
20   Halhuber, M.J.: Einführung in die Thematik aus der Sicht des kardiologischen Rehabilitationsklinikers; in Dembroski, Halhuber, Psychosozialer Stress und koronare Herzkrankheit, Bd 3, p. 1 (Springer, Berlin 1981).
21   Hort, W.: Kreislauforgane; in Eder, Gedigk, Lehrbuch der allgemeinen Pathologie und der pathologischen Anatomie, p. 297 (Springer, Berlin 1977).
22   Langosch, W.: Beiträge zu einer Diagnostik psychophysiologischer Reaktivität bei Herzinfarktpatienten; Phil. Diss., Feiburg (1977).
23   Langosch, W.: Diagnostik psychophysiologischer Reaktivität als Beitrag zu einer individualzentrierten Rehabilitation des jugendlichen Herzinfarktpatienten; in Langosch, Psychosoziale Probleme und psychotherapeutische Interventionsmöglichkeiten bei Herzinfarktpatienten, p. 281 (Minerva, München 1980).
24   Langosch, W.: Ergebnisse psychologischer Verlaufsstudien bei Herzinfarktpatienten (Ein- und Drei-Jahres-Katamnese); in Langosch, Psychosoziale Probleme und psychotherapeutische Interventionsmöglichkeiten bei Herzinfarktpatienten, p. 99 (Minerva, München 1980).
25   Langosch, W.: Psychosocial stressors in patients with premature myocardial infarction; in Siegrist, Halhuber, Myocardial infarction and psychosocial risks, p. 120 (Springer, Berlin 1981).
26   Langosch, W.; Brodner, G.: Ergebnisse einer psychologischen Verlaufsstudie an Herzinfarktpatienten. Z. klin. Psychol. *8:* 256 (1979).
27   Langosch, W.; Brodner, G.: Persönlichkeits- und Befindlichkeitsveränderungen von Herzinfarktpatienten in Abhängigkeit von Erkrankungsdauer und Untersuchungssetting im Vergleich zu einer Kontrollgruppe chronisch Kranker. Z. klin. Psychol. (in press, 1982).
28   Langosch, W.; Brodner, G.; Michallik-Herbein, U.: Psychological and vocational aspects in postinfarction patients below the age of 40; in Roskamm, Myocardial infarction of young age (Springer, Berlin 1981).
29   Langosch, W.; Prokoph, J.H.; Brodner, G.: Der psychologische Screeningbogen für Patienten mit Myocardinfarkt (PSM) bei verschiedenen Diagnosegruppen; in Fassbender, Mahler, Der Herzinfarkt als psychosomatische Erkrankung in der Rehabilitation, p. 89 (Boehringer, Mannheim 1980).
30   Lindsley, D.B.: Emotion; in Stevens, Handbook of experimental psychology (Wiley, New York 1951).
31   Malmo, R.B.; Shagas, C.; Davis, F.H.: Symptom specificity and bodily reactions during psychiatric interview. Psychosom. Med. *12:* 362 (1950).
32   Matthews, K.A.; Glass, D.C.; Rosenman, R.W.; Bortner, R.W.: Competitive drive, pattern A and coronary heart disease: a further analysis of some data from the Western Collaborative Group Study. J. chron. Dis. *30:* 489 (1977).

33   Mayou, R.; Foster, A.; Williamson, B.: Psychosocial adjustment in patients one year after myocardial infarction. J. psychosom. Res. *22:* 447 (1978).

34   Myrtek, M.: Psychophysiologische Konstitutionsforschung – ein Beitrag zur Psychosomatik (Hogrefe, Göttingen 1980).

35   Myrtek, M.; Foerster, F.; Wittmann, W.: Das Ausgangswertproblem. Theoretische Überlegungen und empirische Untersuchungen. Z. exp. angew. Psychol. *24:* 463 (1977).

36   Rosenman, R.H.: The interview method of assessment of the coronary-prone behavior pattern; in Dembroski, Weiss, Shields, Haynes, Feinleib, Coronary-prone behavior, p. 55 (Springer, Berlin 1978).

37   Rosenman, R.H.; Friedman, M.: Modyfying type A behavior pattern. J. psychosom. Res. *21:* 323 (1977).

38   Samek, L.; Spinder, M.; Müller, F.; Betz, P.; Schnellbacher, K.; Roskamm, H.: Occupational situation in postinfarction patients under the age of 40; in Roskamm, Myocardial infarction at young age, p. 174 (Springer, Berlin 1981).

39   Schaefer, H.; Blohmke, M.: Herzkrank durch psychosozialen Stress (Hüthig, Heidelberg 1977).

40   Siegrist, J.: Der Einfluss psychosozialer Risikokonstellationen auf den Ausbruch des ersten Myocardinfarkts; in Dembroski, Halhuber, Psychosozialer Stress und koronare Herzkrankheit, p. 112 (Springer, Berlin 1981).

41   Stürzenhofecker, P.; Samek, L.; Droste, C.; Gohlke, H.; Petersen, J.; Roskamm, H.: Prognosis of coronary heart disease and progression of coronary arteriosclerosis in postinfarction patients under the age of 40; in Roskamm, Myocardial infarction at young age, p. 82 (Springer, Berlin 1981).

42   Tänzer, J.; Weyhmann, J.; Zipp, H.; Hildebrandt, G.: Herz- und Kreislaufuntersuchungen bei Koronarkranken während dosierter psychovegetativer Belastung am Wiener Determinationsgerät. Herz/Kreisl. *6:* 249 (1974).

43   Theorell, T.: Psychosocial stressors and cardiovascular disease; in Stocksmeier, Psychological approach to the rehabilitation of coronary patients, p. 146 (Springer, Berlin 1976).

44   Valek, J.; Kühn, E.; Howzak, R.; Vavrinokova, H.: Emotions and personality of patients with ischaemic heart disease during shortlasting psychical laboratory stress. Cor Vasa *13:* 165 (1971).

45   Walschburger, P.: Zur Beschreibung von Aktivierungsprozessen; Phil. Diss., Freiburg (1976).

46   Wilder, J.: Stimulus and response: the law of initial value (Wright, Bristol 1967).

47   Williams, R.B.; Haney, T.; Gentry, W.D.; Kong, Y.: Relation between hostility and arteriographically documented coronary atherosclerosis. Psychosom. Med. *40:* 88 (1978).

48   Zyzanski, S.J.: Coronary-prone behavior pattern and coronary heart disease: epidemiological evidence; in Dembroski, Weiss, Shields, Haynes, Feinleib, Coronary-prone behavior, p. 25 (Springer, Berlin 1978).

49   Zyzanski, S.J.; Jenkins, C.D.; Ryan, T.J.; Flessas, A.; Everist, M.: Psychological correla' of coronary angiographic findings. Archs intern. Med. *136:* 1234 (1976).

13 Psychophysiological Risk Factors of Ischemic Heart Disease
A Primary Preventive Study in Czechoslovakia
M. Horváth, E. Frantík, A. Slabý

An important task of preventive medicine is to increase our knowledge of mechanisms contributing to the evolution of cardiovascular diseases, with the aim of devising new measures applicable in primary and secondary prevention. Among the risk factors participating in the multifactorial etiopathogenesis of ischemic heart disease, great attention is being given worldwide to psychosocial stress. From the point of view of active intervention, ever increasing interest is being devoted to the possibilities of increasing individual coping abilities and of favorably influencing the psychophysiological mechanisms which represent a connecting link to cardiovascular pathology. As a long-term social program, changes in psychosocial etiological factors, as well as in life-style, have to be persistently pursued.

The efforts of our working group concentrate on intervention of occupationally specific psychophysiological risk factors of ischemic heart disease in managerial and research personnel. In this communication, our preliminary experience will be presented. Since 1977, we have been following 780 men aged 30–59 who are responsible for research tasks in eight institutes of engineering. For comparison, we have examined the same psychosocial and personality parameters in a population-based group of 1,000 men of the same age who have been followed up in a district of Prague by the Epidemiological Department of the Institute of Clinical and Experimental Medicine, and in several occupationally selected groups studied by nine co-working centers.

The occupations requiring highly complex mental work do not involve traditional work hazards, but they have risk factors of their own. Single purpose of the work, lack of physical activity, and intense prolonged activation of higher nervous functions characterize the role. Since creative performance requires to maintain the central activation in narrow limits, the optimum level can easily be overstepped. A state of negative emotional tension will then be reached, which interferes with the ability of relaxation and unfavorably affects the autonomic regulatory mechanisms.

Our study comprises a multistage procedure. In the first stage, a screening examination is performed, directed at the standard risk factors of car-

diovascular disease. At the same time, several questionnaires are administered, including the Jenkins Activity Survey (JAS) and the Eysenck Personality Questionnaire. The second stage adds clinical and laboratory examinations and the type A structured interview. The third stage includes reactions
to laboratory maneuvers, among others a test of cardiovascular reactivity to
be described later in this chapter. In selected subsamples of high-risk subjects, monitoring of cardiovascular functions during the working day is
planned as the fourth stage of the project in order to gain information about
the sources of the occupational stress, and to ascertain the individual differences in cardiovascular reactivity in real-life conditions.

On the basis of the medical, psychological, and occupational explora-
tions, a comprehensive program of intervention has been started. From a
medical point of view, it was characteristic of the group of research workers
to show an overall morbidity rate that was lower than that in the sample from
the general population. However, analysis of absence due to sickness and of
health complaints in this professional group indicated a high incidence of
three types of difficulties, namely psychological, vertebrogenic, and cardiovascular. Considering six standard risk factors (i.e. hypertension, hyperlipidemia, positive glucose tolerance test, smoking of cigarettes, overweight,
and family history of ischemic heart disease), in about 60% of the group, two
or more of these risk factors were present.

Type A behavior pattern, as determined by the structured interview
and/or by the JAS, was found in two thirds of the sample. In one half of the
sample, the diagnosis by both methods was the same, and this subsample
included the greatest part of extraverted and labile subjects according to the
Eysenck Personality Questionnaire. These respondents scored higher in the
MHQ questionnaire, especially in the anxiety subscale, they had more pronounced tension, autonomic difficulties and poor ability for relaxation, and
they also consumed more coffee and cigarettes. Type A research workers
rated their institutes less favorably, had a lower scientific competence but a
higher scientific output.

About two thirds of respondents mentioned serious work problems
which in more than one half caused frequent or intensive feelings of tension.
In 80% of the entire group, symptoms of increased irritability were present,
indecision in 75%, vague bodily complaints and blunted emotions in 60%,
and mental fatigue in 50%. Except for mental fatigue, no obvious increase
in the intensity of symptoms over the years of research activity was observed.
This finding suggests that these symptoms reflect some psychopathological
deviations which are present in subjects who selected this type of occupation,

or which arise early in the primary adjustment to the requirements of mental work.

Five types of working life problems were identified in psychological consultations, which were performed in a selected subsample of problem subjects. First, an immature relationship to authority was observed in the form of surviving adolescent rebellious attitudes or of an extreme submissivity or of a combination of both, which was frequently accompanied by depressive and psychosomatic problems. On the other end of the age continuum, difficult adaptation to aging was associated with feelings of frustration. Underdeveloped cognitive needs as the specific motivation to research work lead to externally oriented dissatisfaction. An excessive dependence on success, pushing the essential motives of the research work to the background, dampened the production of original solutions and accentuated hostile and conflict-producing types of behavior. A defective regimen of work and relaxation, especially a systematic transfer of work tasks to leisure time, lack of physical activity and diminished close family relations and social contacts, strongly affected work and general life well-being. The last two types of problems are very near to the characteristics of type A behavior.

As to the concept of the coronary risk behavior, we share the opinion of other authors that some features may be useful for creative mental work, and that it is essential to discover those components which carry the cardiovascular risk, e.g. hostility, and to compensate for their effects.

Another important question in psychophysiological research is the relation of cardiovascular hyperreactivity to coronary risk. We are studying circulatory reactions to three standard stimuli. Laboratory examinations were performed at the same time in the morning, in a sound-proof room. Subjects were made familiar with the setting at a previous medical examination. The subject was examined resting semi-supine in a special chair. Heart rate (HR) was recorded continuously by a cardiotachometer, blood pressure (BP) was measured automatically at predetermined intervals using an indirect method (Physiomat). Changes in forearm blood flow were registered by means of occlusion plethysmography according to *Dohn* [1]. Blood flow was expressed in terms of milliliters per 100 ml of tissue volume per minute. The basal values were registered six times during a rest period of 20 min. Subsequently, orthostatic test (5 min), cold pressor test (1 min), and an emotional test (10 min) were performed, separated by periods of rest of sufficient duration to warrant a complete return of cardiovascular parameters to basal values. The emotional test consisted of two parts, i.e. the Stroop word/color conflict task (color naming, 3 min) immediately followed by a number-ranging test.

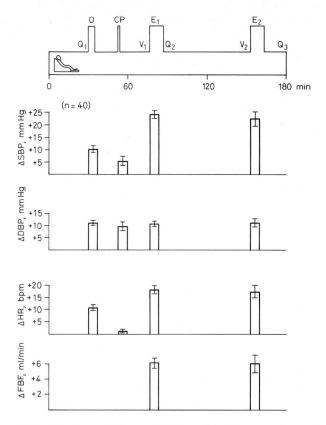

Fig. 1. Time-course of the examination and circulatory reactions to three standard stimuli (mean ± SD). O = orthostasis; CP = cold pressor test; E = emotional test; Q = Adjective Checklist and Scale of Tension; V = Valsalva maneuver; SBP = systolic blood pressure; DBP = diastolic blood pressure; HR = heart rate; FBF = forearm blood flow; $\triangle$ = difference from basal values.

The latter was selected because it elicits a similar cardiovascular response, being different from the usual tests of mental arithmetic. The emotional test was repeated after 60 min. In the course of the examination, the Mood Activity Checklist according to Lorr and a 100-point analogue relaxation scale were administered three times (Q_{1-3} in fig. 1). Figure 1 shows that the mild emotional stress used elicited substantial increases in systolic BP (SBP) and diastolic BP (DBP), HR, and forearm blood flow. When repeated after a placebo, the emotional test produced practically the same response. Inspection

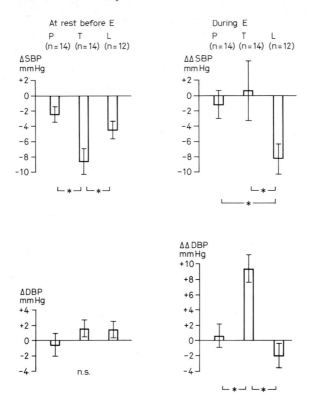

Fig. 2. Effect of β-adrenergic blockade on emotional changes in blood pressure. P= placebo; T= metipranolol (Trimepranol); L= metoprolol (Lopresor); △△ = difference in emotional changes between the second and first emotional tests; *p < 0.05. For other explanations see figure 1.

of correlations between the circulatory changes at the first and second emotional tests confirmed that the reactions were individually constant.

The cardiovascular responses to emotion were differentially influenced by a non-selective β-adrenoceptor antagonist metipranolol (Trimepranol) in a single dose of 10 mg, and by a cardioselective antagonist metoprolol (Lopresor) in a clinically equieffective dose of 50 mg. While the non-selective blockade failed to mitigate the emotional increases in SBP, the increases in DBP were even greater than after placebo. The cardioselective blockade did diminish the emotional pressor reaction (fig. 2). Trimepranol, in comparison with Lopresor, caused a greater decrease in HR, both at rest and during the second emotional test. Both β-blockers caused a significant reduction of the

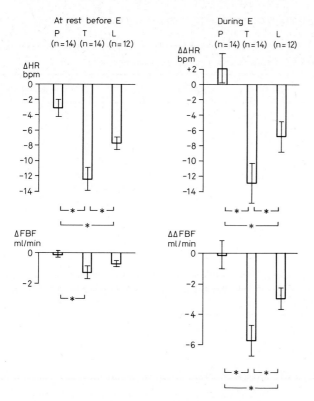

Fig. 3. Effect of β-adrenergic blockade on emotional changes in heart rate and forearm blood flow. For explanation of symbols see figures 1 and 2.

emotional increases in forearm blood flow (fig. 3). Trimepranol, but not Lopresor, significantly diminished the subjective feeling of tension.

Some significant correlations were found between the resting values of circulatory characteristics, and the cardiovascular responses to standard tests used (table I). The reported associations between the resting BP values, represented by medians of at least four previous measurements, and the circulatory responses seem to suggest that the acute emotional pressor reactions (such as those that occur many times in the course of 24 h) bear relation to long-term regulatory mechanisms of BP.

Only a few significant correlations were found between the personality characteristics and the circulatory reactions. A positive correlation was found

Table I. Significant correlations (r) between acute changes and basal values of some cardio-vascular characteristics

Cardiovascular reactions		Cardiovascular characteristics at rest				
		SBP	DBP	HR	SBP × HR	FBF
Upright	△ SBP	0.359*				
	△ DBP					0.321*
Valsalva	△ HR (during)			0.421**	0.343*	0.387*
	△ HR (after)			− 0.440**		
Emotion	△ SBP	0.323*			0.327*	
	△ HR			− 0.402**		
	△ FBF				0.319*	
	△ FVR			0.524**		
After	△ DBP					0.420*
emotion	△ FBF	− 0.404**	− 0.434**			

DBP = Diastolic blood pressure; FBF = forearm blood flow; FVR = forearm vascular resistance; HR = heart rate; SBP = systolic blood pressure; △ = difference from basal values; * p < 0.05; ** p < 0.01.

between JAS scores and increases in HR during the emotion test, as well as between JAS scores and the lasting increases in systolic pressure after emotion. Smokers had a greater increase in forearm vascular resistance during emotion than non-smokers (table II). On the whole, results of this analysis confirm the conclusions of our pilot study [2] that personality characteristics and cardiovascular responses to acute stimuli are mostly uncorrelated. This holds for the non-specific emotional stress we are using, and does not exclude the possibility that higher responses can be elicited in type A subjects by specifically challenging situations.

Many significant correlations were found between the characteristics describing the actual mood state, and the circulatory reactions (table III). The higher the tension before the examination, the higher the increases in DBP caused by cold stress and increases in forearm blood flow during emotion. The opposite was true for comfort and activation. The reactions which correlated with tension seem to have a common mechanism in sympathoadrenergic activation. In our experience, increases in forearm blood flow can be used as an indicator of enhanced tension, and of reduced comfort and activation.

Table II. Significant correlations (r) between cardiovascular reactions and some personality characteristics

Cardiovascular reactions	Personality characteristics			
	JAS	P	L	smoking
Emotion △ SBP		− 0.449**		
△ HR	0.390*			
△ FBF				− 0,376*
△ FVR			0.480**	0.445**
After △ SBP	0.319*			
emotion				

JAS = Jenkins Activity Survey; P, L = scores in Eysenck Personality Questionnaire; for other abbreviations see table I.

Table III. Significant correlations (r) between cardiovascular reactions and some characteristics of actual mood state

Cardiovascular reactions	Mood at rest		
	comfort	activation	tension
Cold △ DBP	− 0.492**	− 0.439**	0.599**
Valsalva △ HR (after)	0.361*	0.408*	− 0.348*
Emotion △ DBP			0.317*
△ FBF	− 0.392*		0.478**
After △ FBF			− 0.467**
emotion			

For abbreviations see table I.

The following conclusion can be drawn from these results. With the exception of HR and lasting SBP, no overall cardiovascular hyperreactivity was found in type A subjects, and therefore no long-term pharmacological suppression of cardiovascular reactivity appears to be indicated just because someone happens to be a type A. On the other hand, the actual mood state highly influences cardiovascular reactions elicited by challenging situations. Specific measures of intervention may be required to mitigate circulatory reactions elicited by emotional stressors under prevailing tension in some individuals, and here pharmacological means may be needed in some cases.

In our further work, we shall concentrate on the relationships between various components of the coronary-prone behavior pattern and the circulatory responses to emotional stress, to obtain additional clues for psychophysiological intervention.

References

1   Dohn, K.: Plethysmography during functional states for investigation of the peripheral circulation. Proc. 2nd Int. Congr. of Physical Medicine, Copenhagen 1965, p. 51.
2   Slabý, A.; Horváth, M.; Frantík, E.: Cardiovascular responses in stress testing related to some personality characteristics. Activitas nerv. sup. *23:* 64–66 (1981).

14 Behavior and the Pathophysiology of Coronary Heart Disease in Humans

James C. Buell, Robert S. Eliot

The purpose of the Coronary Prone Behavior Review Panel [7] was to address five major issues. These were: (1) What was the specific evidence that suggested causal links between coronary-prone behavior and coronary heart disease (CHD)? (2) How was the coronary-prone behavior pattern assessed? (3) What were the mechanisms that translated the behavior pattern into CHD? (4) How did coronary-prone behavior originate? (5) What could be done to alter coronary-prone behavior.

The results ot the Review Panel validated the fact that type A behavior is correlated with a significant increase in the incidence of CHD and is a valid risk factor in an epidemiologic sense. In essence, the Review Panel reported that the available body of scientific evidence demonstrates that type A behavior, as defined by the structured interview used in the Western Collaborative Group Study (WCGS), the Jenkins Activity Survey (JAS) and the Framingham Type A Behavioral Scale, is associated with an increased risk of clinically apparent CHD in middle-aged US citizens. This risk is found to be beyond that imposed by age, elevated systolic blood pressure (SBP), serum cholesterol or cigarette smoking, and appears to be of at least the same order of magnitude as the relative risks associated with the latter three of these factors. Clearly the gold standard in the available tests for assessment of type A behavior is the structured interview (SI) of *Friedman* and *Rosenman*. No behavioral test, however, was considered satisfactory with regard to prognostic sensitivity, specificity, and selectivity in predicting the advent of CHD.

Type A behavior may be described as an aroused state superimposed on a *complex* substrate of interrelated factors. Metaphorically, it can be viewed as an iceberg with a small portion apparent above the surface. Unfortunately, situational or environmental determinants, individual perceptive or cognitive differences and other psychological components such as anxiety, depression, psychosocial problems, physiological variations, pathophysiological aging mechanisms, and genetic susceptibility are not easily assessed.

The mechanisms through which type A behavior operates as a risk factor and by which it facilitates the progression of CHD remain conjectural, a weakness shared with all risk factors until the pathogenesis of CHD is fully understood. However, the prevalence of certain biochemical and physiological phenomena are highly associated with fully developed type A behavior [9]. These include elevated serum cholesterol levels, elevated preprandial and postprandial triglycerides, enhanced platelet aggregation, faster clotting time, higher excretion of norepinephrine particularly when provoked by emotional challenge, a higher average serum level of corticotropin, a greater insulinemic response to glucose, a decreased growth hormone response to arginine, and greater lability and magnitude of blood pressure (BP) response under time-demand tasks [17].

We believe it is important to make a distinction between type A behavior, which is a well-defined entity, and the ill-defined but constantly evolving concept of coronary-prone behavior. For example, cultural determinants are likely to be important modifiers. The cross-cultural study of *Cohen* et al. [5] of the type A/CHD relationship among Japanese Americans living in Hawaii demonstrated that men who were culturally mobile and type A had a 2- to 3-times greater risk of CHD than men with either characteristic alone. Whether one speaks of type A behavior or a disruption of social roots, the way one behaves in terms of adaptation to life carries with it certain health consequences.

Vaillant [37] has published a 40-year prospective study of 95 healthy young men which looked at modes of adaptation. He found that maturity of defensive style was powerfully inversely correlated with somatic illness per se. 80% of the 25 men who deployed predominantly mature defenses before age 47 remained in excellent health after age 55. In contrast, only a third of the 31 men who characteristically deployed immature defenses prior to the age of 47 are still in excellent health at age 55. 11 have died or have become disabled by chronic illness, i.e. congestive heart failure and multiple sclerosis. Even when the contributions of smoking, suicide, alcohol use, obesity, and age at death of parents and grandparents have been controlled for, correlations between the mode of psychological defense and physical health remain significant. The most mature defense mechanisms include humor, altruism, sublimation and suppression. When confronted with stressful stimuli, these mechanisms still distort and alter feelings, conscious relationships and reality. But they perform this task gracefully and flexibly.

Perhaps mature defenses like humor and art, while defending against stress, more closely approximate reality than do projection and fantasy. In addition, mature defenses are more socially acceptable and tend to bind people together and provide social supports. Social supports are correlated in important ways with health but the statistical correlation of social supports with good health may be merely part and parcel of behavioral phenomena representing flexible adaptation. *Henry and Stephens* [22] have also written about an effective cultural canon being protective against cardiovascular disease. Thus, while type A behavior represents an important risk factor, some individuals manifesting type A behavior will survive unscathed into old age attending the funerals of their younger type B counterparts. After all, it is not surprising that the association is incomplete. It is obvious that genetic, perceptive, and other coping factors likely operate to counterbalance predisposing behavioral effects in many individuals. Furthermore, it appears that only certain components of type A behavior correlate with CHD and the cognitive integrative aspects of behavior and their link to pathophysiologic responses remains largely unknown.

If, by behavior, one means the actions or reactions of man or animals under specified circumstances, the study by *Dembroski* et al. [8] illustrates one distinction between behavior in coronary patients and in noncoronary control patients. During the type A structured interview and an American history quiz, the investigators noted increases in SBP during the history quiz in type B coronary patients but not in type B controls. Indeed, the greatest increment of BP change in either type A or B groups was evoked in type B myocardial infarction (MI) patients during the American history quiz. Such observations suggest that we must attempt to examine and integrate the multifaceted aspects of overt psychomotor behavior with those of cognition and physiologic behavior and translate these into physiologic mechanisms if we are to gain further understanding of how behavioral facets translate into coronary proneness.

The major manifestations of CHD are considered to be angina pectoris, MI, and sudden cardiac death. While a considerable overlap exists among all three of these entities, it is clear that sudden cardiac death and acute MI are not necessarily synonymous. In addition, although coronary atherosclerosis is usually found at autopsy in either MI or sudden cardiac death, either condition can occur in the absence of coronary atherosclerosis. Indeed, a renaissance of interest in coronary spasm [4, 6, 23] testifies to the dynamic and capricious nature of CHD not easily understood by those who focus exclusively on plumbing and plaques as the total explanation. It is ironic that both new items of interest and research in CHD today, namely spasm and coronary-prone behavior, were expounded upon by *Osler* [28] at the turn of the century. Suffice it to say that since exactly how the traditional risk factors participate in the pathogenesis of atherosclerosis remains unknown and the correlation between degree of coronary obstruction and incidence of angina, infarction or sudden death is also less than perfectly clear, commentary on the role of behavior and the pathophysiology of CHD must represent an intelligent but speculative hypothesis rather than a dogmatic pronouncement.

At the present state of our understanding, it appears that the atherosclerotic process involves injury and proliferation of intimal smooth cells with subsequent alteration in permeability and/or metabolism and tends to occur at bifurcating or originating sites of vessel branches. With the progressive insudation of lipid material, hemodynamic impairment of flow eventually results. The site of lesion formation suggests that hydrodynamic stress and sheer forces participate in the process and that the higher and more frequent the kinetic energy trauma to the vessels at these points of turbulence, the more rapid the evolution of the lesion. These findings are consistent with hypertension as a risk factor and it is generally accepted that elevated BP and increased sheering forces constitute an aggravating cause in the development of atherosclerosis. Hypertension also places an increased work load and oxygen demand upon the myocardium. These findings are also consistent with hypertension as a risk factor, but it is obvious that additional factores must be operative. Those individuals possessing the $C3^F$ gene in essential hypertension have a coronary risk rate nearly 7 times higher than those who are $C3^F$-negative [26]. Futhermore, epidemiologic studies in Japan suggest that in some populations the incidence of hypertension may be remarkably high without a concomitant increase in CHD [25]. Nevertheless, those centrally mediated neuroendocrine responses producing enhanced velocity of myocardial fiber shortening, augmented total systemic resistance, and a general increase in the hydrodynamic stress placed upon the cardiovascular system, likely foster and sustain endothelial injury factors and may precipitate clinical events in the critically jeopardized myocardium.

A variety of investigators have demonstrated that groups manifesting type A behavior tend to have higher challenge-induced mean values for BP, pulse pressure, and heart rate (HR), and greater lability of these values than do groups of type B individuals [8, 17, 27]. It appears reasonable to hypothesize that both excess magnitude and frequency of hydrodynamic trauma imparts a greater risk of endothelial injury as well as greater burdens upon left ventricular work and oxygen demand. Therefore, an overactive circulatory state may be one mechanism through which behavior translates into a pathophysiologic mechanism.

The second factor having obvious face validity is that enhanced lipid availability is an integral part of the atherosclerotic process. *Friedman* et al. [18] long ago reported the correlation between accountants' self-reports of stress and their cholesterol levels with minimal cholesterol values occurring during periods of minimal stress, all independent of the diet. *Troxler* et al. [35] have shown the high correlation between cortisol and angiographic evidence of atherosclerosis and others have demonstrated that high-density lipoprotein/low-density lipoprotein (HDL/LDL) ratios are consistently altered approximately 10 days after a reported stress [15]. The association between cortisol and atherosclerosis as well as cortisol and stress and cortisol and depression [32] is consistent with *Glass's* [19] observations that those manifesting type A behavior may be vulnerable to depression. His findings are also in accord with the studies by *Thomas* et al. [34] of physicians with MI who readily became depressed even as students. Likewise, the results of a study by *Bruhn* et al. [3] of coronary-prone individuals showed them to be effort-oriented people whose achievements gave them little satisfaction. The pathophysiologic mechanisms linking behavior and atherosclerosis constitute a full separate paper by *Herd* and others [this volume], but it is likely that those who perceive the environment about them as stressful may also elicit those mechanisms which are lipogenic and atherogenic.

The work by *Theorell* et al. [33] on personality traits and psychophysiological reactions in twins with varying degrees of CHD indicates that measures of those traits associated with early onset of CHD (type A behavior, impulsiveness and muscle tension) are genetically influenced. Despite relatively high correlation coefficients in the monozygotic series, however, genetic influence never explained more than 46%. Nevertheless, genetic influence on BP, peripheral vasoconstriction, and serum growth hormone levels is of greater importance during interview than at rest. The subjects of these authors were all twin pairs who had grown up together. Comparisons between series of monozygotic pair members grown up together and series of monozygotic pairs grown up apart have indicated that the concordance within pairs of personalty measures is greater among those grown up apart than among those grown up together [30]. Twins growing up together may be assumed to try to accentuate their own identities by behaving differently as compared to their partner. Such a tendency would create a bias against observable genetic influences in *Theorell's* studies, if anything. However, because *Theorell* et al. [33] could study less healthy and more healthy twin pairs, it is interesting that very marked increases in stroke volume, as reflected by ballistocardiography during interview, belonged to the less healthy group.

Thus, whereas neurophysiologic and neuroendocrine activation patterns have significant genetic components, behavioral factors appear to be important in orchestrating the timetable for disease development. Again, the mechanisms appear to involve a heightened physiologic reactivity involving neuroendocrine patterns of excessive sympathetic adrenal medullary activity and adrenal cortical activity.

Panin and Sokolov [29] studied psychophysiological and biochemical factors in Soviet polar regions and also found that subjects suffering from CHD tended to show elevated serum 11-hydroxycorticosteroid levels, whereas arterial hypertension subjects showed higher free fatty acid levels which they interpreted to imply activation of the sympathoadrenal medullary system. As alluded to earlier, many of these mechanisms are consistent with findings in type A behavior patterns. However, the association is obviously modified by genetic factors and it is unreasonable to expect that overt behavior would unequivocally mirror neuroendocrine and physiologic responses in all cases. Thus, while a style of overt behavior to environmental circumstances may provide clues, a style of covert physiologic and neuroendocrine behavior is probably closer to providing answers.

An additional link to be considered in the pathophysiological chain of events is the role of platelets and thrombosis. If smooth muscle cell proliferation, lipid accumulation and thrombosis are parts of the atherosclerotic mosaic, clotting and platelet function must be suspected as potentially culpable agents in the process. The recent discovery of platelet-dervived growth factor in the alpha granules of platelets indicates that platelets contain a potent stimulator of smooth muscle proliferation [24]. Increased platelet activity in vitro has been reported in patients with familial hypercholesterolemia [20], but it is necessary to determine whether the decreased survival is a direct effect of cholesterol or lipoproteins upon the platelets or is a manifestation of increased platelet consumption by exposed subendothelial surfaces. Platelet-derived growth factor is primarily carried through the circulation in the alpha granules of the platelet and, while in this cryptic state, it cannot stimulate cell replication. However, this arrangement provides a remarkably specific delivery system for this polypeptide hormone which initiates the replication of arterial smooth muscle cells in vitro and is suspected of doing so in vivo. Thus, one suspected mechanism for platelet involvement is that a fundamental response to some form of injury to the endothelium may be platelet mediated intimal smooth muscle proliferation.

In addition, when vascular damage leads to platelet deposition in the endothelial wall, liberation of the vasoconstrictor thromboxane A_2 tends to propagate the platelet aggregation process and perhaps contributes to the development of coronary spasm [13, 20]. Using coronary angiography, *De Wood* et al. [10] have demonstrated total coronary occlusion in 87% of 126 acute MI patients who were evaluated within 4 h of the onset of symptoms. The proportion manifesting total occlusion decreased significantly to 65% when patients were studied 12–24 h after the onset of symptoms. Thus, this study suggests that total coronary occlusion is frequently seen during the early hours of transmural infarction and that coronary spasm or thrombus formation or both may be important in the evolution of infarction. Whereas the absolute incidence of acute thrombosis and/or spasm remains debatable, increased platelet aggregation is a very real pathophysiological phenomenon of significant consequence. A variety of studies have demonstrated the ability of catecholamines to enhance platelet stickiness and aggregation, while other studies have demonstrated increased platelet aggregation and consumption under a variety of situations both emotional and physical, broadly referred to as 'stress' [14, 21]. As mentioned earlier, enhanced platelet aggregation and rapid clotting times are more frequently seen in subjects evidencing type A behavior. Indeed, recognizing that the plasma free fatty acid levels are known to be increased in all types of stress, *Altura* [1] postulates that type A arousal induces increased free fatty acid levels which reduce free ionized levels of magnesium in the blood thus promoting the development of coronary vasospasm. This is predicated on the observation that magnesium deficiency enhances basal tone in arteries and veins in vitro [36]. Thus, a variety of behaviorally related biochemical and neuroendocrine mechanisms appear potentially operative.

Most of the behaviorally mediated risk mechanisms appear to operate through the sympathetic adrenal medullary system with catecholamine surges and/or through the pituitary adrenocortical axis with release of glucocorticoids. Catecholamines promote platelet adhesiveness and aggregation, promote arrhythmias, lower the threshold to arrhythmia generation, and increase secretion of glucagon, thyroxin, calcitonin, parathormone, renin, erythropoietin, and gastrin. Catecholamines diminish insulin secretion.

Glucocorticoids convert protein into carbohydrate and fat, have a minor antagonistic effect on insulin, promote the development of diabetes, foster hyperlipidemia and hypercholesterolamia, enhance water diuresis, diminish circulating lymphocytes, reduce leukocytosis and polycythemia, increase platelet counts with an enhancement of clotting tendencies, lower the electrical excitation threshold of the brain, increase gastric acidity and pepsin production, block growth hormone secretion, decrease calcium absorption, enhance angiotensinogen production, sensitize arterioles to the pressor effects of catecholamines, and decrease the inflammatory response. A clinical model for pure catecholamine excess is pheochromocytoma with its known sequelae of hypertensive crises, MI with or without coronary disease, arrhythmias, and catecholamine myocarditis. The clinical model of pure glucocorticoid excess is Cushing's syndrome with its well-known sequelae of hypertension and accelerated atherosclerosis.

The sequelae of CHD include angina pectoris, MI, and sudden cardiac death. Any of these phenomena can occur in the absence of coronary atherosclerosis and conversely asymptomatic normal life spans also occur in the presence of marked coronary atherosclerosis. Yet, these oftentimes dramatic sequelae of CHD are far from random and chance occurrences. Engrafted upon a genetic substrate of physiological and biochemical predispositions and some environmental risks such as diet and smoking lies a wealth of centrally mediated pathophysiologic mechanisms. These include platelet aggregation, lipid mobilization, adrenergically mediated vasospasm and positive inotropic arousals which may inexorably strangle the vulnerable subendocardium in a hemodynamic vise.

If we have learned anything, it is that many pathophysiological roads converge in CHD. Among the major risk factors of CHD are those of hypertension, elevated serum cholesterol, cigarette smoking, age, sex, and diabetes. Recently, type A behavior has been added to this group, but upon reflection it is obvious that many of the traditional risk factors are themselves behaviors, or behaviorally mediated. Certainly, smoking a cigarette is a behavior. Yet, despite the powerful physiologic effects of tobacco smoke, the Seven Country Study [25] demonstrated that there was not an immutable relationship with CHD in all populations, cultures, and societies. Indeed, cigarette smoking is a sociocultural behavior and perhaps when examining smoking as a risk factor, the sociocultural and motivational aspects of the habit should be examined in addition to its prevalence.

Although type A behavior has been validated by the WCGS [31], the association with coronary disease is noticeably affected by age, sex, and occupation. There are many different pathophysiological sites whereby a psychosocial factor may engender risk. However, the site that has received the most attention is the coronary arteries as seen on angiography. Some investigators [2, 16, 38] have found a relationship between type A behavior and the angiographic extent of coronary disease and some have not [11, 12]. Be that as it may, if we are to talk about risk factors as phenomena which may accelerate the biologic timetable for a degenerative process, psychosocial and behavioral factors provide a unifying link between epidemiologic and patho-physiologic mechanisms. Although type A behavior constitutes an important behavioral association in CHD, it probably only represents one of many styles of behavior conveying risk. Also, some may question the diagnostic utility of a risk factor as ubiquitous as type A behavior.

The undisputed value of the type A concept is that for the first time a central nervous system function has been statistically linked to the develop-ment of CHD. This has opened up exploration of the ways in which the cen-tral nervous system controls metabolic functions and a variety of patho-physiological processes. For example, the role of the central nervous system in arrhythmogenesis and sudden cardiac death is an important and scientifi-cally well-validated research topic. Yet, these clinical victims of sudden death do not necessarily manifest a uniform overt style of behavior. However, the subset of psychological trigger patients all manifest rhythm disturbances under emotional stress. As the link between cognitive integrative functions and physiologic responses to environmental circumstances becomes better understood, we will gain a better understanding of which components of behavior, both overt and covert impart coronary proneness.

A distinguished Review Panel [7] focused on type A behavior and recog-nized it as a valid coronary-prone behavior. It is important for us to recognize that it does not represent the only aspect of behavior conferring coronary proneness. Other cognitive and behavioral elements must also be explored. Type A behavior is an important keystone in the historical developments by which central nervous system influences have become scientifically accepted as valid participants in the epidemiologic mosaic of CHD. It is time, however, to move beyond the type A construct to more intensely explore the relation-ship between overt behavior, cognitive processes and sociocultural support systems and their mechanistic links to styles of covert physiologic and neuroendocrine behavior. It is through integrating behavioral facets with physiologic and metabolic pathways that we can best advance our under-standing of behavior and the pathophysiology of CHD.

References

1   Altura, B.T.: Type A behavior and coronary vasospasm: a possible role of hypomagne-semia. Med. Hypotheses 6: 753–757 (1980).
2   Blumenthal, J.; Williams, R.; Cong, Y.; et. al.: Type A behavior pattern and coronary ath-erosclerosis. Circulation 58: 634–639 (1978).

3   Bruhn, J.G.; Paredes, A.; Adsett, C.A.; Wolf, S.: Psychological predictors of sudden death in myocardial infarction. J. psychosom. Res. *18:* 187–191 (1974).

4   Coffman, J.D.; Cohen, R.A.: Vasospasm-ubiquitous? New Engl. J. Med. *304:* 780–782 (1981).

5   Cohen, J.B.; Syme, S.L.; Jenkins, C.D.; et. al.: The cultural context of type A behavior and the risk of coronary heart disease. Am. J. Epidem. *102:* 434 (1975).

6   Conti, C.R.; Curry, R.C.: Coronary artery spasm and myocardial ischemia. Mod. Concepts cardiovasc. Dis. *49:* 1–6 (1980).

7   Weiss, S.M.: Coronary-prone behavior and coronary heart disease: a critical review. Proc. of a review panel sponsored by NHLBI. Circulation *63:* 1199–1215 (1981).

8   Dembroski, T.M.; MacDougall, J.M.; Lushene, R.: Interpersonal interaction and cardiovascular response in type A subjects and coronary patients. J. hum. Stress *5:* 28–36 (1979).

9   Dembroski, T.M.; MacDougall, J.M.; Shields, J.L.: Physiologic reaction to social challenge in persons evidencing the type A coronary-prone behavior pattern. J. hum. Stress *3:* 2–9 (1977).

10   DeWood, M.A.; Spores, J.; Notske, R.; Mouser, L.T.; Burroughs, R.; Golden, M.S.; Lang, H.T.: Prevalence of total coronary occlusion during the early hours of transmural myocardial infarction. New Engl. J. Med. *303:* 897–902 (1980).

11   Dimsdale, J.; Hackett, T.; Hutter, A.; Block, P.; Catanzano, D.: Type A personality and the extent of coronary atherosclerosis. Am. J. Cardiol. *42:* 583–586 (1978).

12   Dimsdale, J.; Hackett, T.; Hutter, A.; Block, P.; Catanzano, D.; White, P.: Type A behavior and angiographic findings. J. psychosom. Res. *23:* 273–276 (1979).

13   Dusting, G.J.; Moncada, S.; Vane, J.R.: Prostaglandins, their intermediates and precursors. Cardiovascular actions and regulatory roles in normal and abnormal circulatory systems. Prog. cardiovasc. Dis. *21:* 405–430 (1979).

14   Fleischman, A.I.; Bierenbaum, M.L.; Stier, A.: Effect of stress due to anticipated minor surgery upon in vivo platelet aggregation in humans. J. hum. Stress *2:* 33–37 (1976).

15   Francis, K.T.: Psychologic correlates of serum indicators of stress in man: a longitudinal study. Psychosom. Med. *41:* 617–628 (1979).

16   Frank, K.; Heller, S.; Kornfeld, D.; Sporn, A.; Weiss, M.: Type A behavior pattern and coronary angiographic findings. J. Am. med. Ass. *240:* 761–763 (1978).

17   Friedman, M.; Byers, S.O.; Diamant, J.; Rosenman, R.H.: Plasma catecholamine response of coronary-prone subjects (type A) to a specific challenge. Metabolism *24:* 205–210 (1975).

18   Friedman, M.; Rosenman, R.H.; Carroll, V.: Changes in the serum cholesterol and blood clotting time in men subjected to cyclic variation of occupational stress. Circulation *17:* 852–861 (1958).

19   Glass, D.C.: Behavior patterns, stress and coronary disease (Erlbaum, Hillsdale 1977).

20   Haft, J.I.: Role of blood platelets in coronary artery disease. Am. J. Cardiol. *43:* 1197–1206 (1979).

21   Haft, J.I.; Arkel, Y.S.: Effect of emotional stress on platelet aggregation in humans. Chest *70:* 501–505 (1976).

22   Henry, J.P.; Stephens, P.M.: Stress, health, and the social environment (Springer, New York 1977).

23   Hillis, L.D.; Braunwald, E.: Coronary artery spasm. New Engl. J. Med. *299:* 695–702 (1978).

24   Kaplan, D.R.; Chao, F.C.; Stiles, C.D.; Antoniades, H.N.; Scher, C.D.: Platelet alpha granules contain a growth factor for fibroblasts. Blood *53:* 1043–1052 (1979).

25   Keys, A.; Aravanis, C.; Blackburn, H.W.; et al.: Epidemiological studies related to coronary heart disease. Characteristics of men aged 40–59 in seven countries. Acta med. scand. suppl. *460:* 1 (1967).

26   Kristensen, B.O.; Petersen, G.B.: Association between coronary heart disease and the C3^F gene in essential hypertension. Circulation *58:* 622–625 (1978).

27   Manuck, S.B.; Carft, S.; Gold, K.J.: Coronary-prone behavior pattern and cardiovascular response. Psychophysiology *15:* 403–411 (1978).

28   Osler, W.: Lectures on angina pectoris and allied states. N.Y. med. J. *64:* 177–183 (1896).

29   Panin, L.Y.; Sokolov, V.P.: Psychophysiological and biochemical factors in the development of coronary heart disease and arterial hypertension in a non-resident population of the Asiatic North. J. psychosom. Res. *24:* 39–44 (1980).

30   Plomin, R.; Willerman, L.; Leohlin, J.C.: Resemblance in appearance and the equal environments assumption in twin studies of personality traits. Behav. Genet. *6:* 43 (1976).

31   Rosenman, R.H.; Brand, R.J.; Jenkins, C.D.; et al.: Coronary heart disease in the Western Collaborative Group Study. Final follow-up experience of 8½ years. J. Am. med. Ass. *233:* 872–877 (1976).

32   Starkman, M.N.; Schteingart, D.E.; Schork, M.A.: Depressed mood and other psychiatric manifestations of Cushing's syndrome: relationship to hormone levels. Psychosom. Med. *43:* 3–18 (1981).

33   Theorell, T.; Faire, U. de; Schalling, D.; Adamson, U.; Askevold, F.: Personality traits and psychophysiological reactions to a stressful interview in twins with varying degress of coronary heart disease. J. psychosom. Res. *23:* 89–99 (1979).

34   Thomas, C.B.; Ross, D.C.; Duszynski, K.R.: Youthful hypercholesterolemia: its associated characteristics and role in premature myocardial infarction. Johns Hopkins med. J. *136:* 193–208 (1975).

35   Troxler, R.G.; Sprague, E.A.; Albanese, R.A.; Fuchs, R.; Thompson, A.J.: The association of elevated plasma cortisol and early atherosclerosis as demonstrated by coronary angiography. Atherosclerosis *26:* 151–162 (1977).

36   Turlapaty, P.D.M.V.; Altura, B.M.: Magnesium deficiency produces spasms of coronary arteries: relationship to etiology of sudden death ischemic heart disease. Science *208:* 198–200 (1980).

37   Vaillant, G.E.: Natural history of male psychologic health. Effect of mental health on physical health. New Engl. J. Med. *301:* 1249–1254 (1979).

38   Zyzanski, S.; Jenkins, C.; Ryan, C.; et al.: Psychological correlates of coronary angiographic findings. Archs. intern. Med. *136:* 1234–1237 (1976).

15 Physiological Basis for Behavioral Influences in Arteriosclerosis

J. Alan Herd

The concept underlying the neuroendocrine correlates of behavioral processes arose with *Cannon* [8] and was elaborated by *Selye* [38]. The original concept was one of a general physiological response including adrenal medullary, adrenal cortical, and sympathetic nervous system (SNS) responses to physical and psychological stimuli. Refinements of the original concept have included identification of different physiological and behavioral responses to acute and chronic conditions and different responses to anticipated and current stimulation [32]. *Mason* [29, 30], in reviewing the results of neuroendocrine research on the pituitary-adrenal-cortical system, concluded that most studies of acute anticipated stimulations showed an increase in cortisol levels. However, physiological and behavioral responses to chronic conditions are more variable than responses to acute stimulation [4, 17, 29].

Psychologic stress research in humans has developed a large body of evidence indicating that the anticipation of personal injury may lead to important changes not only in thought, feeling, and action, but also in endocrine and autonomic processes, and hence in a wide variety of visceral functions. Much work in this field has centered on the changes in adrenocortical functioning that occur in association with emotional distress. Investigators have generally found the adrenal cortex to be stimulated via the brain under environmental conditions perceived by a person as threatening to him. Usually such personally threatening conditions precipitate clearly detectable emotional distress. In some studies, it has been possible systematically to correlate the extent of emotional distress with plasma and urinary corticosteroids assessed independently. Similar studies relying upon biochemical methods of measurement of epinephrine, norepinephrine, and aldosterone under conditions of emotional distress have yielded similar results. Moreover, experimental approaches in monkeys and humans have generated substantial data indicating a linkage between emotional responses and adrenal function [21]. Overall, the evidence clearly indicates that emotional distress in humans is associated with elevated blood levels and urinary excretion of adrenal hormones.

The physiological responses to physical and psychological stressors are similar in that several neurogenic, endocrine, and metabolic effects are elicited by both types of stressors. The neurogenic effects include alterations in central integrative mechanisms, an increase in SNS activity and a decrease in parasympathetic activity. The endocrine effects include increased rates of secretion and increased circulating levels of epinephrine, norepinephrine, cortisol, growth hormone, plasma renin activity, and angiotensin II. The metabolic effects include increased rates at which glucose is released from glycogen, increased rates at which free fatty acids (FFA) are released from adipose tissue, increased rates at which amino acids are produced from protein, reduced sensitivity to insulin, increased utilization of glucose and FFA and increase relative rates at which FFA are utilized as well as an increase in metabolic rate. All of these physiological responses are useful in preparing for vigorous physical activity.

The physiological responses to physical stressors such as exercise are dominated by activity of the SNS in conjunction with musculoskeletal activity [22, 44]. With moderate amounts of exercise, the predominant endocrine response is an increase in circulating levels of norepinephrine and the predominant metabolic response is increased utilization of both glucose and FFA. Levels of these metabolic substrates in blood may actually fall especially during prolonged exercise. With severe amounts of exercise, the endocrine response includes increases in circulating levels of epinephrine and cortisol [2] as well as norepinephrine. The predominant metabolic responses in severe exercise are marked increases in the utilization of FFA and the production of lactic acid. Increased plasma renin activity also occurs during severe exercise. The transition between response to moderate physical stressors and response to severe prolonged physical stressors of several types is marked by the increased secretion of epinephrine, cortisol, and plasma renin activity.

The physiological responses to psychological stressors are more similar to the responses to severe physical stressors than the responses to moderate ones [13, 32]. Even mild psychological stressors such as mental arithmetic [25, 27] elicit an increase in secretion of epinephrine and cortisol as well as an increase in norepinephrine. The result is an increase in circulating levels of glucose and FFA, reduced sensitivity to insulin, a relative increase in utilization of FFA, and a moderate increase in metabolic rate.

SNS activity stimulates adipose tissue to release FFA, stimulates liver to release glucose, stimulates kidney to decrease excretion of sodium and water and to release renin, stimulates heart to increase rate and force of contraction, stimulates arterioles to increase peripheral vascular resistance and veins to increase venous return, and stimulates adrenal medulla to release epinephrine and norepinephrine.

FFA released by lipolysis apparently play an important role in cardiovascular and metabolic function. Catecholamines are probably the most important factors promoting lipid mobilization [23]. They are effective in mobilizing lipid from adipose tissue [33] by their liberation from noradrenergic nerve terminals in adipose tissue through the circulation [23]. Also, glucocorticoids promote lipid mobilization [23] and insulin opposes it [20]. Thus, lipid mobilization is promoted by sympathetic adrenomedullary (SAM) stimulation of adipose tissue, especially when levels of glucocorticoids in the blood are rising and levels of insulin are falling.

When triglyceride stores in adipose tissue are mobilized, they are hydrolyzed to FFA and glycerol [23]. These FFA are utilized by skeletal muscles and myocardium in the production of energy [50]. They both are stored in these tissues as triglycerides and are used directly. The FFA not stored or utilized in the production of energy are eventually taken up by the adipose tissues or by the liver [40]. FFA taken up by the liver are formed into triglycerides and secreted as a component of very low-density lipoproteins (VLDL) [37].

The rate at which the liver secretes VLDL is determined partly by the rate it synthesizes FFA from carbohydrates and partly by the rate it receives FFA in the blood. In the fasting state, the secretion of VLDL by the liver is determined principally by the levels of FFA in the blood [1]. These levels, in turn, are determined principally by the effects of catecholamines on adipose tissue and rates of energy production.

The effects of neuroendocrine factors on cardiovascular diseases involve many components and mechanisms. Pathophysiological mechanisms leading to atherosclerosis include damage to vascular endothelium and proliferation of vascular smooth muscle cells [35]. Damage to vascular endothelium may be the result of hemodynamic factors such as high levels of arterial blood pressure (BP) or turbulence at bifurcations in large arteries. It also may be the result of chemical factors such as high blood levels of VLDL or other circulating substances [36]. Proliferation of vascular smooth muscle also may be influenced by several different factors. Tissue cultures of vascular smooth muscle cells proliferate most readily in the presence of VLDL [34]. Proliferation in vitro also is enhanced by the presence of insulin in the culture medium [24, 43]. These results from laboratory studies of atherogenic factors suggest mechanisms whereby physiological processes associated with neuroendocrine and metabolic factors may influence atherogenesis in humans and experimental animals [18].

The association between neuroendocrine processes and arteriosclerosis is suggested by several clinical and experimental studies. *Troxler* et al. [47] found a significant correlation between elevated serial morning plasma cortisol levels and moderate to severe coronary arteriosclerosis. This association was noted in asymptomatic male subjects who had coronary angiography as part of their evaluation at the USAF School of Aerospace Medicine. In these men, plasma cortisol was second only to serum cholesterol as a discriminator between coronary disease and non-diseased individuals. Corticosteroids are reported to accelerate coronary atherosclerosis in patients with lupus erythematosus [5, 26] and patients with rheumatoid arthritis. Finally, *Friedman* et al. [16] have reported that plasma corticotropin (ACTH) levels were significantly higher in type A subjects than in type B subjects.

Eliot [14] and *Buell and Eliot* [3] have suggested links between risk factor behavior and underlying mechanisms: (1) hypertension increases local vascular turbulence with special hydrodynamic impact at vascular branching sites and thus tends to induce mechanical trauma; (2) serum lipids, both from diet and mobilized from body stores by neuroendocrine processes, foster smooth muscle cell proliferation, and become incorporated in the proliferative and necrotic lesions; (3) smoking behavior, through its nicotine effects on catecholamines and also the effects of carbon monoxide upon vascular permeability, tends to promote processes contributing to atherogenesis; (4) platelet mobilization and aggregation in areas of endothelial trauma release a platelet-derived growth factor and the vasospastic agent, thromboxane A_2, contributing to smooth muscle cell proliferation in combination with vasoactive constriction. Catecholamines appear to be significantly involved at several points in these pathophysiologic processes. Their secretion is heavily influenced by the central nervous system and linked to behavior.

In addition to evidence supporting the involvement of chronic psychosocial forces in the initiation and progression of arteriosclerotic cardiovascular diseases, there is a role for highly stressful experience in the precipitation of acute clinical events, including fatal arrhythmias [15, 28]. It is hypothesized that such events as the unexpected death of a loved person can cause such a massive outpouring of catecholamines that coagulative myocytolysis occurs, with concomitant vasospasm or myocardial infarction (MI). The

study of possible behavioral and neuroendocrine events in sudden death is
of special interest [12].

The influence of cortisol on development of atherosclerosis was tested
experimentally in cynomolgus monkeys. *Sprague* et al. [42] administered cortisol orally to monkeys each day in doses which significantly diminished the
diurnal variations of serum cholesterol without elevating daily peak cortisol
concentrations. Animals which were fed a high cholesterol diet and received
cortisol daily had a significantly greater involvement of aortic intimal surface
area with atherosclerotic lesions compared to animals receiving a high
cholesterol diet only. This atherogenic effect occurred independently of any
effect of cortisol on serum lipoprotein cholesterol concentrations.

A number of studies have been undertaken in attempts to identify psychophysiological and neuroendocrine mechanisms which might account for
the increased coronary heart disease (CHD) rates observed among type A
persons [11]. When challenged to perform a variety of behavioral tasks, type
As are observed to show greater increases in heart rate, BP, and catecholamine secretion [10]. Among those psychological characteristics which have
been implicated in the tendency to display overt type A behavior under challenge are increased need for control [19] and increased levels of hostility.

The most reasonable interpretation of these elevations is that they reflect
increased secretion of its principal hormones by the adrenal gland, involving
both the cortex and the medulla. These increases are associated with a wide
variety of stressful conditions and emotional responses; not only with stresses
that directly threaten the physical survival of the person but also with stresses
that threaten self-respect or crucial human relationships. These responses
appear to be part of a complex set of metabolic and cardiovascular adjustments in anticipation of vigorous action; a vital feature of adaption over the
long course of human evolution. With respect to the metabolic events, the
adrenal surge not only facilitates mobilization of carbohydrate but mobilization of fat as well. Epinephrine and cortisol act cooperatively in accomplish-
ing fat mobilization [48, 49]. The well-established effect of epinephrine in
raising circulating concentrations of plasma lipids (notably cholesterol, FFA,
and phospholipids) is dependent upon an intact adrenal cortex. The effect
of injected epinephrine can be experimentally abolished by adrenalectomy
and restored by injection of cortisol [39]. Moreover, chronic low-grade injection of epinephrine to normal dogs produces relatively chronic elevation
of cholesterol and phospholipids; administration of cortisone to normal
dogs further accentuates the plasma lipid response to injected epinephrine.
These experiments are similar to common psychological stress situations

in which chronic, low-grade elevations in secretion of adrenal hormones occur.

We may summarize several major trends of the evidence on adrenal function under conditions of psychological stress as follows: (1) there is an important set of brain regulatory functions acting upon the adrenal, particularly through brain structures in the hypothalamus and limbic system; (2) elevations in plasma and urinary adrenal compounds are regularly observed under difficult circumstances perceived by the individual as threatening; (3) there is a positive correlation between the degree of distress experienced by the individual and the tendency toward hormone elevation; (4) consistent individual differences have been observed both in the range within which a person's adrenal hormone level fluctuates under ordinary circumstances and in the extent of adrenal response to a difficult, disturbing experience.

Results obtained recently from several laboratories also suggest that FFA may play an important role in the pathogenesis of cardiovascular disease. FFA may predispose to development of atherosclerosis and they may precipitate cardiac arrhythmias. Therefore, individuals who maintain high levels of FFA [31] may be at high risk for developing cardiovascular disease.

FFA levels in plasma have at least two important physiological effects. Increases in FFA levels increase intensity of platelet aggregation [7]. Since platelet aggregation plays a major role in evolution of atheroma, it influences the basic disease process. Increases in FFA levels also increase myocardial oxygen requirements [41]. Catecholamines sensitize the heart of FFA in such a way that FFA account for a major part of the increased myocardial oxygen requirement during SAM stimulation. In the presence of coronary artery disease, increases in FFA and increases in myocardial oxygen requirement or decreases in myocardial oxygen supply frequently may cause serious ventricular arrhythmias.

The physiological mechanisms linking behavioral factors to cardiovascular diseases are worthy of further research. The hypothesis is that intense SAM activity elicited by behavioral factors is a cause of hypertension, MI, and sudden death. However, SAM activity is essential for normal physiological function. It is the excess SAM activity above that required for normal function that predisposes to cardiovascular disease and precipitates clinical manifestations.

The persistence of physiological responses to psychological stressors parallels the individual's inability to cope effectively with the stressor. Some individuals who remain anxious or depressed for long periods of time continue to have elevated levels of urinary epinephrine [45, 46] and 17-OH corticosteroids [6, 9], with reduced circadian variation. As normal individuals develop a coping strategy which reduces the psychological impact of the stressor, the neuroendocrine response abates along with corresponding adjustments in physical, psychological, social, and behavioral variables.

Although the neurobiologic links between behavioral processes and arteriosclerosis are still unknown, a general concept is emerging. Physiological and psychological stimuli which are aversive modify both adrenal medullary and adrenal cortical activity through secretion of neuropeptides as well as by direct neural influences. These neuropeptides also modify behavior and may be conditioned by environmental stimuli to be secreted even in the absence of painful stimuli.

Adrenal medullary and adrenal cortical secretions appear to influence the development of arteriosclerosis and precipitation of complications. However, the pathophysiological mechanisms influencing arteriosclerosis under these conditions are still largely unknown.

References

1   Basso, L.V.; Havel, R.J.: Hepatic metabolism of free fatty acids in normal and diabetic dogs. J. clin. Invest. *49:* 537–547 (1970).

2   Brandenberger, G.; Follenius, M.: Influence of timing and intensity of muscular exercise on temporal patterns of plasma cortisol levels. J. clin. Endocr. Metab. *40:* 845–849 (1975).

3   Buell, J.C.; Eliot, R.S.: The role of emotional stress in the development of heart disease. J. Am. med. Ass. *242:* 365–368 (1979).

4   Bourne, P.G.; Rose, R.M.; Mason, J.W.: Urinary 17-OCHS levels. Data on seven helicopter ambulance medics in combat. Archs gen. Psychiat. *17:* 104–110 (1967).

5   Bulkley, B.H.; Roberts, W.C.: The heart in systemic lupus erythematosis and the changes induced in it by corticosteroid therapy. Am. J. Med. *58:* 243–264 (1975).

6   Burchfield, S.R.; Woods, S.C.; Elich, M.S.: Pituitary adrenocortical response to chronic intermittent stress. Physiol. Behav. *24:* 297–302 (1980).

7   Burstein, Y.; Berns, L.; Heldenberg, D.; Kahn, Y.; Werbin, B.Z.; Kamir, I.: Increase in platelet aggregation following a rise in plasma free fatty acids. Am. J. Hematol. *4:* 17–22 (1978).

8   Cannon, W.B.: The role of emotion in disease. Ann. intern. Med. *9:* 1453–1465 (1936).

9   Caplan, R.D.; Cobb, S.; French, J.R.P., Jr.: White collar work load and cortisol. Disruption of a circadian rhythm by job stress? J. psychosom. Res. *23:* 181–192 (1979).

10 Dembroski, T.M.: Environmentally induced cardiovascular response in type A and B individuals; in Weiss, Herd, Fox, Perspectives on behavioral medicine (Academic Press, New York 1981).

11 Dembroski, T.M.; Weiss, S.M.; Shields, J.L.; Haynes, S.G.; Feinleib, M. (eds): Coronary-prone behavior (Springer, New York 1978).

12 Dews, P. (Chairman): Institute of Medicine, National Academy of Sciences: Conf. on Biobehavioral Factors in Sudden Cardiac Death, 1980.

13 Dimsdale, J.E.; Moss, J.: Plasma catecholamines in stress and exercise. J. Am. med. Ass. *243:* 340–342 (1980).

14 Eliot, R.S.: Stress and the major cardiovascular disorders (Futura, New York 1979).

15 Eliot, R.S.; Baroldi, G.; Leone, A.: Necropsy studies in myocardial infarction with minimal or no coronary luminal reduction due to atherosclerosis. Circulation *49:* 1127–1131 (1974).

16 Friedman, M.; Byers, S.O.; Rosenman, R.H.: Plasma ACTH and cortisol concentration of coronary-prone subjects. Proc. Soc. exp. Biol. Med. *140:* 681–684 (1972).

17 Friedman, S.B.; Mason, J.W.; Hamburg, D.A.: Urinary 17-hydroxycorticosteroid levels in parents of children with neoplastic disease: a study of chronic psychological stress. Psychosom. Med. *25:* 364–376 (1963).

18 George, R.; Ramasarma, T.: Nature of the stimulation of biogenesis of cholesterol in the liver by noradrenaline. Biochem. J. *162:* 493–499 (1977).

19 Glass, D.C.: Behavior patterns, stress and coronary disease (Erlbaum, Hillsdale 1977).

20 Gutstein, W.H.; Harrison, J.; Parl, F.; Kiu, G.; Avitable, M.: Neural factors contribute to atherogenesis. Science *199:* 449–451 (1978).

21 Hamburg, D.: Genetics of adrenocortical hormone metabolism in relation to psychological stress; in Hirsch, Behavior-genetic analysis, pp. 154–175 (McGraw-Hill, New York 1967).

22 Hartley, L.H.; Mason, J.W.; Hogan, R.P.; Hones, L.G.; Kotchen, T.A.; Mongey, E.H.; Wherry, F.E.; Pennington, L.L.; Rickets, P.T.: Multiple hormonal responses to prolonged exercise in relation to physical training. J. appl. Physiol. *33:* 607–610 (1972).

23 Heindel, J.J.; Orci, L.; Jeanrenaud, B.: Fat mobilization and its regulation by hormones and drugs in white adipose tissue; in Masoro, International encyclopedia of pharmacology and therapeutics. Pharmacology of lipid transport and atherosclerotic processes, sect. 24, pp. 175–373 (Pergamon Press, Oxford 1975).

24 Huttner, J.J.; Gwebu, E.T.; Panganamala, R.V.; Milo, G.E.; Cornwell, D.G.: Fatty acids and their prostaglandin derivatives: inhibitors of proliferation in aortic smooth muscle cells. Science *197:* 289–291 (1977).

25 Januszewicz, W.; Sznajderman, M.; Wocial, B.; Feltynowski, T.; Klonowicz, T.: The effect of mental stress on catecholamines, their metabolites and plasma renin activity in patients with essential hypertension and in healthy subjects. Clin. Sci. *57:* suppl. 5, pp. 229s–231s (1979).

26 Kalbak, K.: Incidence of arteriosclerosis in patients with rheumatoid arthritis receiving long-term corticosteroid therapy. Ann. rheum. Dis. *31:* 196–200 (1972).

27 LeBlanc, J.; Cote, J.; Jobin, M.; Labrie, A.: Plasma catecholamines and cardiovascular responses to cold and mental activity. J. appl. Physiol. *47:* 1207–1211 (1979).

28 Lown, B.; DeSilva, R.A.; Lenson, R.: Roles of psychologic stress and autonomic nervous system changes in provocation of ventricular premature complexes. Am. J. Cardiol. *41:* 979–985 (1978).

29 Mason, J.W.: Psychoendocrine approaches in stress research. Symp. on Medical Aspects of Stress in the Military Climate, pp. 375–421 (Walter Reed Army Institute of Research, Washington 1964).

30 Mason, J.W.: A review of psychoendocrine research on the pituitary-adrenal cortical system. Psychosom. Med. *30:* 576–607 (1968).

31   Nestel, P.J.; Ishikawa, T.; Goldrick, R.B.: Diminished plasma free fatty acid clearance in obese subjects. Metabolism 27: 589–597 (1978).

32   Rose, R.M.: Endocrine responses to stressful psychological events. Psychiat. Clins N. Am. 3: 251–276 (1980).

33   Rosell, S.; Belfrage, E.: Adrenergic receptors in adipose tissue and their relation to adrenergic innervation. Nature, Lond. 253: 738 (1975).

34   Ross, R.; Glomset, J.A.: Atherosclerosis and the arterial smooth muscle cell. Science 180: 1332–1339 (1973).

35   Ross, R.; Glomset, J.A.: The pathogenesis of atherosclerosis. New Engl. J. Med. 295: 369–377, 420–425 (1976).

36   Ross, R.; Harker, L.: Hyperlipidemia and atherosclerosis. Science 193: 1094–1100 (1976).

37   Schonfeld, G.; Pfleger, B.: Utilization of exogenous free fatty acids for the production of very low density lipoprotein triglyceride by livers of carbohydrate-fed rats. J. Lipid Res. 12: 614–621 (1971).

38   Selye, H.: The stress of life (McGraw-Hill, New York 1976).

39   Shafrir, E.; Steinberg, D.: The essential role of the adrenal cortex in the response of plasma free fatty acids, cholesterol, and phospholipids to epinephrine injection. J. clin. Invest. 39: 310–319 (1960).

40   Shapiro, B.: Triglyceride metabolism; in Renold, Cahill, Jr., Handbook of physiology, sect. 5, pp. 217–223 (Am. Physiological Society, Washington 1965).

41   Simonsen, S.; Kjekshus, J.K.: The effect of free fatty acids on oxygen consumption during atrial pacing and catecholamine infusion in men. Circulation 58: 484–491 (1978).

42   Sprague, E.A.; Troxler, R.G.; Peterson, D.F.; Schmidt, R.E.; Young, J.T.: Effect of cortisol on the development of atherosclerosis in cynomolgus monkeys; in Kalter, The use of non-human primates in cardiovascular diseases, pp. 261–264 (University of Texas Press, Austin 1980).

43   Stout, R.W.; Bierman, E.L.; Ross, R.: Effect of insulin on the proliferation of cultured primate arterial smooth muscle cells. Circulation Res. 36: 319–327 (1975).

44   Sutton, J.R.; Young, J.D.; Lazarus, L.; Hickie, J.B.; Maksvytis, J.: The hormonal response to physical exercise. Australas. Ann. Med. 18: 84–90 (1969).

45   Timio, M.; Gentili, S.: Adrenosympathetic overactivity under conditions of work stress. Br. J. prev. soc. Med. 30: 262–265 (1976).

46   Timio, M.; Gentili, S.; Pede, S.: Free adrenaline and noradrenaline excretion related to occupational stress. Br. Heart J. 42: 471–474 (1979).

47   Troxler, R.G.; Sprague, E.A.; Albanese, R.A.; Fuchs, R.; Thompson, A.J.: The association of elevated plasma cortisol and early atherosclerosis as demonstrated by coronary angiography. Atherosclerosis 26: 151–162 (1977).

48   Wool, I.G.; Goldstein, M.S.: Role of neurohumors in the action of the adrenal cortical steroids: mobilization of fat. Am. J. Physiol. 175: 303–306 (1953).

49   Wool, I.G.; Goldstein, M.S.; Ramey, E.R.; Levine, R.: Role of epinephrine in the physiology of fat mobilization. Am. J. Physiol. 178: 427–432 (1954).

50   Zierler, K.L.; Maseri, A.; Klassen, D.; Rabinowitz, D.; Burgess, J.: Muscle metabolism during exercise in man. Trans. Ass. Am. Physns 81: 266–273 (1968).

16 Role of the Central Nervous System in Sudden Cardiac Death

Robert S. Eliot, James C. Buell

Sudden cardiac death (SCD) is the most common cause of death in the industrialized world. In the USA alone, more than 1,200 people experience SCD per day. One study reported that 26% of sudden deaths occurred on Monday, suggesting that life-style, behavior, and stress play significant roles [38]. Better prediction of the individual at risk is thus dependent upon a better understanding of the multiple components that contribute to the overall risk in any given case. Awareness of the role of behavior and the central nervous system in this phenomenon is fundamental to the understanding of pathophysiologic mechanisms, the detection of the individual at risk, and ultimately the management and prevention of SCD. This paper will address itself to the impact of life-style, behavior, and stress in the genesis of SCD.

The World Health Organization criteria have defined SCD as that which occurs within 24 h and is related to cardiovascular disorders. Most die within 30 s to 1 h and their deaths are predominantly associated with rhythm disturbances [6, 18]. In those individuals who survive up to 24 h after the onset of cardiac signs or symptoms, it is more likely that myocardial infarction (MI) underlies or will ensue. Thus, the longer the interval between the onset of symptoms and death, the more likely classic MI is the cause. By contrast, the shorter the interval between the onset of symptoms and death, the more likely that an arrhythmia is the cause.

It is interesting to compare the clinical studies of *Cobb* et al. [4–6] with the pathological observations of *Baroldi* et al. [2, 3]. *Cobb* et al. [4–6] studied individuals who collapsed in the Seattle area and who were resuscitated and brought to the hospital. Two distinct groups were obvious. In the first group there was classic MI; in the second group, there was no evidence of infarction as measured by enzymatic or evolutionary electrocardiographic change. Recurrent episodes of SCD occurred in approximately 2% of the group manifesting MI. In the second group with no evidence of MI, recurrent SCD occurred at a rate of 20% per year. This difference of 10 fold suggests that not only are the clinical features different but also the pathophysiologic mechanisms are different.

Indeed, the studies of *Baroldi* et al. [2, 3] confirm this impression. In studying the pathology of 208 victims of witnessed SCD, they demonstrated that coagulation necrosis, the hallmark of typical MI, was present in only 17%. Overall, only 75% had one or more coronary vessels obstructed. Of these, only 15% demonstrated an acute occlusive thrombus. Remarkably, the heart weight was in excess of 500 g in more than 42% of cases.

Thus, it is obvious that one of the more troublesome phenomena to explain is that of the variation in anatomic degrees of obstruction to be found in victims of SCD. This is of equal concern in those who survive to old age in apparent good health. The studies of *Baroldi* et al. [3] demonstrate that in coroners' cases of victims who die of causes unrelated to cardiovascular disease there is a 38% incidence of one or more old coronary obstructions. We would indeed be wise were we able to understand the difference between those who have obstructive disease and good health and those who have obstructive disease and rampant clinical evidence of ischemic heart disease (IHD). We would be equally happy to know how it is that those with normal vessels can experience either good health or various manifestations of IHD including MI as well as SCD.

Of particular interest is the unique finding of coagulative myocytolysis in 72% of SCD victims. This lesion is a form of hyperfunctional necrosis generally considered to be mediated through outpourings of catecholamines. It is associated with an acidophilic clumping of myofibrillar material near the intercalated disc and total disruption of the normal Z band structure of the myofibril. This in no way relates to coagulation necrosis which is slower to develop and totally different in histopathologic features. An additional observation of importance was the presence of fibrosis of the myocardium in 81% of the cases reported by *Baroldi* et al. [2, 3]. As we review the findings of SCD and the role of the central nervous system, it is important to keep these clinical and pathological observations in mind as they relate strongly to previously accepted and recently discovered risk factors.

In developing an understanding of the mechanisms of SCD, it is helpful to realize that the pathophysiologic events result from the contributions of three separate spheres of risk: (1) coronary artery disease; (2) electrical instability of the heart, and (3) myocardial disorders. These factors develop over time in three classic stages: chronic, subacute, and acute. Ultimately, the three spheres can be brought together by behavioral influences mediated through the central nervous system and, if circumstances are appropriate, they may lead to SCD. Indeed, each of these biobehavioral spheres is strongly influenced by the role of the central nervous system. Let us begin with the coronary artery disease sphere.

Coronary Artery Disease

Elevated blood pressure (BP) has long been an established risk factor leading to coronary artery disease. Remarkably, there are some societies and nations in which elevated BP is relatively rare. Yet in the USA, more than 40 million Americans experience high BP. Animal studies have clearly demonstrated that crowded circumstances, frustrating reward systems, increased vigilance activity, and learned helplessness can lead to significant BP elevations. *Ostfeld and Shekelle* [35] stated it well: 'There has been an appreciable increase in uncertainty of human relations as man has gone from the relatively primitive and more rural to the urban and industrial. Contemporary man, in much of the world, is faced every day with people and with situations about which there is uncertainty of outcome, wherein appropriate behavior is not prescribed and validated by tradition, where the possibility of bodily or psychological harm exists, where running or fighting is inappropriate, and where mental vigilance is called for.'

Furthermore, BP elevation is not a static phenomenon. Sudden increases in systolic and diastolic BP frequently reflect marked increases in total systemic resistance (TSR). In our experience, TSR can double or triple with simple mathematical tests in the susceptible individual. Thus, hyperreactive physiologic states are a frequent feature of hypertensive and, indeed, even normotensive individuals. Unquestionably, hypertension can induce intimal damage on the basis of acute and chronic mechanical trauma, although there are other reasons as well.

Cigarette smoking is also a contributor and is a well-recognized factor in coronary artery disease. A major destructive factor is the disruption of the oxygen carrying capacity of blood. Oxygen is displaced by various quantities of carbon monoxyhemoglobin. In addition, cigarette smoking impacts on the adrenal medullary system through nicotine stimulation. These factors contribute to damage of the arterial intima, thus permitting the influx of atheromatous lipid material. In addition, cigarette smoking promotes chronic bronchitis which reduces respiratory efficiency. Under critical circumstances, this may be an important factor even in the absence of emphysema. Furthermore, cigarette smoking has many powerful behavioral components which make it extremely difficult for some individuals to discontinue the habit.

Surprisingly, in sudden cardiac death, hypercholesterolemia is not as significant a risk factor as hypertension and cigarette smoking. Indeed, it appears that hypercholesterolemia must exceed 250 mg/100 ml before it is of significance. Unquestionably, hypercholesterolemia contributes to coronary artery disease but it does so in a very complex manner.

Epidemiologic studies have demonstrated that hypercholesterolemia has actuarial significance in coronary disease and the relationship between coronary heart disease (CHD) and serum cholesterol elevations is statistically significant. Although appropriate for population studies, these observations are of lesser applicability in individual cases. Furthermore, the cause of cholesterol elevation is multifactorial. It is not the sole end product of dietary cholesterol or saturated fat. For example, cholesterol levels may be significantly elevated by stimulation of the central nervous system in certain animals [16, 17, 20]. In addition, cholesterol levels may be lowered by ablation of other portions of the brain [15].

Clinical studies have indicated it is possible to see very significant (100 mg/100 ml or more) elevations of serum cholesterol in individuals put through stressful environmental circumstances. These include following a certified public accountant from the first of January to the 15th of April (deadline for the income tax forms in the USA) [19] or a medical student during an examination [47]. Each of these phenomena suggests that human behavior is a powerful mediator of serum lipid levels. These observations do not exclude the importance of rare hereditary hyperlipidemias nor do they deny the importance of elevated serum cholesterol. Instead, they point toward the substantial interaction of factors which provoke these changes and are often dominated by the central nervous system. The relevance of these observations is obvious for large portions of the population.

Obesity is an interesting risk factor in that it contributes to coronary artery disease when any other risk factor exists. By itself, as a contributor to coronary artery disease, it does not appear to be very important. Of interest, by contrast, is its importance in SCD. In this case, isolated obesity is indeed a significant risk factor according to the studies of *Hinkle* [24]. To be significant, weight must exceed desirable body weight by 20%.

Diabetes mellitus is an additional risk factor well known to be associated with coronary artery disease. It, too, can become deranged under the influence of the central nervous system primarily through the stimulation of corticoids via the pituitary adrenal axis. This response is frequently provoked during chronic states of vigilance or depression. Excess cortisol is known to disrupt the balance in insulin-dependent diabetes in particular, but may also have more chronic effects leading toward atherosclerosis in the susceptible individual.

A variety of new factors have been found to be of considerable importance in coronary artery disease and, thus, in SCD. The Western Collaborative Group Study (WCGS) showed a definite relationship between type A behavior and the incidence of coronary artery disease [43]. Type A behavior has been reviewed by the First National Forum on Coronary-Prone Behavior [7] in St. Petersburg, Florida, in 1977 and by the Coronary-Prone Behavior Review Panel [51] at the Amelia Island, Florida, Conference in 1978. At the 1978 meeting, it was determined that type A behavior was a risk factor equal in importance to other major reported risk factors in coronary artery disease. It should be noted that coronary-prone behavior and type A behavior are not the same; i.e. only some type A behaviors may qualify as components of coronary-prone behavior. Moreover, all of the dimensions of coronary-prone behavior have not yet been revealed. Thus, we are seeing only a small part of a large puzzle. The statistical risk of type A behavior, in more mundane terms, is equal to the risk of not fastening one's automobile seatbelt. It is well to recall that type B behavior is associated with a lesser but very real incidence of coronary artery disease. Thus, the type B is certainly not excluded from CHD.

An additional factor found to be of increasing importance in the development of coronary artery disease is that of sedentary life-style [42]. The degree of its influence and its precise relationship to coronary artery disease remains to be delineated at this juncture. As with other risk factors, it is not universally applicable.

Family history is also known to be an important predictor of coronary artery disease. Whether the question is answered by nature or nurture remains a concern to be evaluated in a large number of twin studies in progress at this time. Certainly, one cannot deny the importance of genetics in the predisposition to coronary artery disease. On the other hand, it is important to note that those with good genetic backgrounds may show premature development of coronary artery disease independent of an apparently resistant family history.

Observations by *Lapin and Cherkovich* [28] point to a direct relationship between the central nervous system and hypertension. These investigators studied Hamadryas baboons who form very strong attachments to their mates and mate for life. After the original male was removed from the cage and placed in another cage in full view of his original habitat, a new male of the same age was moved into the original cage with the original female.

Without changing diet or any other component of the experiment, the original males were reported to have developed hypertension, coronary insufficiency or MI within 6 months to a year. A variety of other investigators [45, 46] have reported arterial intimal disruption in animal experiments as well as in animals in captivity; these disruptions appear related to central nervous system activity and support the observations of *Lapin and Cherkovich* [28].

Even when we look at the development of coronary thrombosis, it is possible to envision the role of the central nervous system. Platelet adhesiveness, for example, is markedly enhanced by conditions of anxiety which are transmitted through neurochemical processes to the platelet system [14, 22]. Increased platelet adhesiveness is well known to be associated with increased platelet consumption and is a demonstrable phenomenon in acute anxiety states. Platelets are most adhesive at the site of intimal wall injury. Indeed, the release of thromboxane A_2 from platelets after they have become adherent to the wall may induce coronary artery spasm [8, 21].

Coronary artery spasm is another factor in coronary artery obstruction, which is strongly linked to the central nervous system. This phenomenon may account for SCD in some individuals with normal coronary arteries. In those with the more classic forms of coronary obstruction, it may also account for the additional obstruction in series beyond or proximal to points of fixed obstruction. It thus may function as a precipitating factor in those with fixed obstruction or as an isolated entity.

In studies by *Nerem* [34] with rabbits placed on atherogenic diets, it was noted that animals in one cohort were not experiencing the predicted degree of coronary atherosclerosis and complications. Closer investigation revealed that the animals were being fondled by the caretaker. These studies have been replicated employing the same technique or utilizing diazepam. Results have demonstrated that although cholesterol levels may be the same, the degree and extent of atherosclerosis may be less in animals receiving affection than in those being treated in a more detached manner. These studies remind us that such factors are rarely considered in research experiments proclaiming the effects of atherogenic diets on animals in laboratory settings.

In both human and animal studies, depression or chronic vigilance activity is associated with perceived loss of environmental control. This is followed by elevation of cortisol and depression of gonadotropin levels among many other phenomena [33]. This is a result of pituitary adrenal cortical stimulation. It is of further interest that Cushing's syndrome is known to be associated with more extensive and severe atherosclerosis. In other studies on young Air Force pilots in whom both serum cortisol levels and cholesterol levels were elevated, the prediction of obstructed coronary vessels was in excess of 80% [48]. Central nervous system pathways, which elevate serum cholesterol, are apparently distinct from those that elevate cortisol. Clearly, elevated serum cortisol can contribute to elevated BP as well. This is well demonstrated in both man and animals. By contrast, the challenge to control, which is an aggressive response produces arousal and stimulation of the sympathetic adrenal medullary system. The release of catecholamines from this pathway may also be associated with elevation of BP which can become chronic if the alarm reaction persists.

Electrical Instability

The second sphere in SCD is electrical instability of the heart leading to fatal ventricular dysrhythmias or cardiac arrest. This subject has been well reviewed by a variety of authors. Among those who have contributed much to our understanding of this problem are *Lown* and colleagues. In their animal studies, the ventricular fibrillatory threshold was significantly lowered by restraining dogs in a sling [29]. This manipulation was also associated with significant elevations of epinephrine and norepinephrine. It is known that the likelihood of SCD is enhanced by marked increases in ectopic activity, persistent bradyarrhythmias/tachyarrhythmias, conduction defects, QT prolongation, and a family history of electrical instability. Of interest is that the arrhythmogenic potential of central nervous system stimulation may be unaccompanied by hemodynamic alterations. Nevertheless, increased sympathetic activity alone and under any circumstances predisposes to ventricular fibrillation. Protection in this instance is often achieved with surgical or pharmacologic denervation which reduces sympathetic tone [31].

Lown et al. [30, 32] have demonstrated in certain subjects that diverse stresses of various psychologic states provoke extensive ectopic ventricular activity. Furthermore, *Verrier* et al. [49] have clearly identified a link between the central nervous system and ventricular fibrillation. By stimulating the posterior hypothalamic area in dogs, the ventricular fibrillatory threshold was lowered. Approaching the problem from another angle, *Rabinowitz and Lown* [37] increased serotoninergic stores by injection of precursors and enzyme blockers. The rationale for such treatment was based upon its ability to diminish sympathetic activity. Indeed, this treatment produced significant elevations in the ventricular threshold for repetitive extrasystoles after exogenous stimulation.

It is also well known that voodoo death may be associated with marked bradyarrhythmias [12]. This suggests that there may be vasovagal phenomena. Marked slowing of heart rate reduces cardiac output to the point where coronary vessels can no longer be perfused leading to SCD. Indeed, *Hinkle* et al. [25] demonstrated that a constant slow heart rate in middle-aged men is by itself a risk factor for sudden death. *Engel* [13] has demonstrated that vagally mediated factors may lead to an imbalance between the sympathetic and parasympathetic systems. This in turn has a potential adverse effect. For example, it is possible for the cardiovascular system to collapse in the face of emotional arousal and psychological uncertainty when sympathomimetic activity is suppressed. An interesting study was conducted by *Schneider* [44] in post-MI patients. It was revealed that those with the greatest tendency to bradycardia in response to a startle had the poorest prognosis. *Kerzner* et al. [27] have demonstrated that vagal stimulation in the ischemic heart can precipitate ventricular tachycardia.

Thus, it is safe to conclude at this time that the mechanisms responsible for arrhythmic death often involve disturbances of the central nervous system circuitry that regulates the heart beat. Although many details of these underlying neural pathways and their mechanisms are understood, much remains to be clarified. Whereas bradyarrhythmias and tachyarrhythmias represent the electrophysiologic components and final pathway to sudden death, other factors may underlie the more superficial electrophysiologic components. These underlying mechanisms may also be neurohumorally mediated.

Myocardial Disorders

One of the most important and most neglected contributing spheres in SCD is that of myocardial disorders. A recent conference, to which we contributed, at the Institute of Medicine, National Academy of Sciences [26], has afforded a number of new and practical clinical observations in this area. Among the most significant is that of ethyl alcohol abuse.

The studies of *Regan* et al. [39, 40] have clearly revealed that coronary sinus enzymes become elevated during the ingestion of ethanol. This indicates that there is enzyme leakage from the myocardium related to alcohol ingestion. Additional studies have demonstrated a loss of contractility of the left ventricle in acute alcohol ingestion in susceptible individuals [1]. The loss of contractility is attended by increases in filling pressure in the left ventricle.

The resultant increased wall tension of left atrium or ventricle may foster the development of ventricular or supraventricular arrhythmias. A rapid tachycardia of any type, in the presence of coronary disease, can preclude adequate myocardial perfusion. This can be a fatal step toward the development of a vicious cycle leading to SCD.

On the other hand, it has been observed by some that small amounts of alcohol decrease the risk of CHD [23, 52]. Here, we are perhaps seeing the difference between therapeutic and toxic effects. Small amounts of alcohol, up to 8 ounces of wine or 2 ounces of hard liquor, may be beneficial and appropriate in this regard. Obviously, individual variation and susceptibility must be considered.

Another factor in SCD is left ventricular hypertrophy, which is often secondary to chronic hypertension. Left ventricular hypertrophy creates a larger mass to be innervated and perfused by a limited supply. Furthermore, the work of the heart is markedly increased from hypertrophy alone. In view of the fact that hypertension is the usual cause of left ventricular hypertrophy and that the total peripheral resistance is elevated, it is clear that the afterload of the left ventricle will be increased as well, which contributes markedly to the work of the heart.

Dilatation of the left ventricle has been observed by *Hinkle* [24] to be a major factor in the phenomenon of SCD and, surprisingly, is often unassociated with hypertension. The finding of dilatation of the left ventricle carried an ominous prognostic implication in his prospective series of more than 1,000 apparently healthy individuals followed for more than 5 years. Obviously, dilatation attends failure, and failure attends a decreased ejection fraction. Dyssynergy of the left ventricular contractile state may also be present. Each of these is a powerful prognostic indicator for potential SCD and in general reflects a diminished left ventricular reserve.

Among the most interesting and, perhaps, the most unrecognized features in SCD are those of coagulative myocytolysis and patchy fibrosis of the left ventricle. These conditions are deserving of some discussion. SCD is a rare event in the histologically normal heart, but the most frequent histologic abnormality is coagulative myocytolysis (anomalous contraction bands of an acidophilic staining character) [2, 3]. These contraction bands can be found within 5 min when boluses of catecholamines are injected into dogs in our controlled laboratory studies. Clearly, central nervous system overdrive can result in rapid neurohumoral changes which may lead to these changes as well. Such histologic and metabolic change results in a myocardium which is much more vulnerable to a final electrical catastrophe. These

acute histologic changes can set the stage for chaotic electrophysiologic circumstances leading to arrhythmia and sudden death.

Following investigation of the high incidence of sudden death at the
Kennedy Space Center, *Eliot* [9] began to investigate the role of sympathetic
arousal due to stress as an operating mechanism. Although the traditional
risk factors were no greater, psychoneuroticism was rampant and coagulative
myocytolysis was a common feature among the majority of those experiencing SCD [10, 41, 50]. Coronary obstruction alone rarely accounted for these
deaths. These observations have been enhanced by studies on dogs in our
laboratory. We demonstrated that β-adrenergic (isoproterenol and norepinephrine) administration increased left ventricular dP/dt and significantly
reduced the level of total high-energy phosphates [36]. It is interesting that
there was a preferential depletion of high-energy phosphates in the inner
third of the left ventricle. The associated histologic counterpart of these metabolic changes was coagulative myocytolysis with its typical contraction band
lesions [11].

Of further interest is that these lesions occurred within 5 min of isoproterenol infusions. If the animal was kept alive without fatal rhythm disturbance and sacrificed 24 h after the infusion, extensive evidence of empty sarcolemmal tubules suggested that myocytolysis was indeed an appropriate
eponym. There was no evidence of coagulation necrosis in the animals. In
those animals kept alive for 72 h or more, patchy fibrosis was demonstrated
throughout the left ventricle. It will be recalled that patchy left ventricular
fibrosis has been found in more than 80% of victims of sudden death as
reported by *Baroldi* et al. [3].

Thus progressive loss of myocardium might result from literally overdos-
ing on one's own catecholamines. This progressive myocytolysis with its
residual empty sarcolemmal cells and patchy fibrosis might deplete the
myofibrillar work force and result in left ventricular dilatation. It may be that
this phenomenon explains the clinical feature of dilatation of the left ventricle in the absence of hypertension. The dilatation may be the end product
of chronic intermittent catecholamine-induced necrosis.

It is of further interest that in those individuals who die suddenly and
have chest pain prior to death that coagulation necrosis is a more frequent
histopathologic feature. In those who experience sudden death without chest
pain, coagulative myocytolysis is the most frequent observation. In the latter,
it is unusual to find evidence of coagulation necrosis.

When discussing the myocardium, it is always important to recall that
the inner third of the left ventricle has an inordinate vulnerability to all forms

of necrosis, ischemic or otherwise. The reasons for this are complex but include the fact that the heart has the highest of all oxygen demands and the poorest oxygen supply of any organ in the body. The inner third of the left ventricle is more vulnerable to a reduction in the diastolic interval, since diastole is required for coronary perfusion. In the end, due to this and other factors, the myocardial tissue PO_2 is lowest in the inner third of the left ventricle. Thus, it is not surprising that the inner third of the left ventricle is the most frequent site in the body to undergo necrosis.

In setting the stage for myocardial disorders, the elevation of cortisol by central nervous system stimulation of the pituitary adrenal cortical axis in the presence of chronic vigilance or depression is of important note.

Synthesis

In considering the three major spheres of risk – (1) coronary artery disease; (2) electrical instability, and (3) myocardial disorders – leading to SCD, it is obvious that sudden death, although sudden, may not be unexpected. Atherogenesis is strongly influenced by central nervous system factors. Acute obstruction of the coronary vessels can be brought about either by coronary spasm or by thrombosis, both of which may be mediated by the central nervous system. In addition, myocardial damage and vulnerability can result from a chronic condition such as ischemia, inflammation or a variety of forms of necrosis contributed to by the behavior and life-style of an individual. Furthermore, electrical instability of the heart is mediated predominantly by central nervous system influences both chronically and acutely. Underlying myocardial and coronary arterial disease states may also contribute to electrical instability.

In the presence of these chronic factors, there may be subacute development of depression or sustained vigilance activity leading to exhaustion and the consequences of pituitary adrenal cortical stimulation referred to earlier. Thus, the myocardium is under chronic bombardment leading to a 'softening up' process. Similar factors accelerate coronary atherosclerotic obstructive processes as well. High BP, for example, may not only accelerate atherosclerosis but may also increase myocardial oxygen requirements.

When all of these factors and others operate on a chronic and subacute basis, a vulnerable myocardial state exists. Biobehavioral factors are often important triggering mechanisms which bring about the convergence of each of the spheres of weakness into a state of synergy at a single point in time.

The common denominator in the final common pathway leading to SCD could be the impatience and hostility of type A behavior, a life crisis, inappropriate neuroticism, depression, or restricted coping options and the like.

In each of the major contributing spheres, the role of the central nervous system is evident. In short, understanding the response to life-style, behavior, and stress is integral to understanding SCD. Vulnerability to SCD may be a product of the chronic, subacute, and acute factors that are largely biobehavioral and powerfully mediated through the central nervous system. When understood, SCD is neither sudden nor unexpected.

References

1   Ahmed, S.S.; Levinson, G.E.; Regan, T.J.: Depression of myocardial contractility with low doses of ethanol in normal man. Circulation 48: 378–385 (1973).

2   Baroldi, G.; Falzi, G.; Mariani, F.: Significance of morphological changes in sudden coronary death; in Manninen, Halonen, Sudden coronary death. Adv. Cardiol., vol. 25, pp. 82–95 (Karger, Basel 1978).

3   Baroldi, G.; Falzi, G.; Mariani, F.: Sudden coronary death. A postmortem study in 208 selected cases compared to 97 'control' subjects. Am. Heart J. 98: 20–31 (1979).

4   Cobb, L.A.; Baum, R.S.; Alvarez, H.; Schaffer, W.A.: Resuscitation from out-of-hospital ventricular fibrillation: 4-year follow-up. Circulation 51/52: suppl. III, pp. 223–228 (1975).

5   Cobb, L.A.; Hallstrom, A.P.; Weaver, W.D.; Copass, M.K.; Haynes, R.E.: Clinical predictors and characteristics of the sudden cardiac death syndrome. Proc. USA/USSR 1st Joint Symp. on Sudden Death. DHEW Publ. No. (NIH) 78–1470, pp. 99–116.

6   Cobb, L.A.; Werner, J.A.; Trobaugh, G.B.: Sudden cardiac death. I. A decade's experience with out-of-hospital resuscitation. Modern Concepts cardiovasc. Dis. 49: 31–36 (1980).

7   Dembroski, T.M.; Weiss, S.; Shields, J.; Haynes, S.; Feinleib, M.: Coronary-prone behavior (Springer, New York 1978).

8   Dusting, G.J.; Moncada, S.; Vane, J.R.: Prostaglandins, their intermediates and precursors. Cardiovascular actions and regulatory roles in normal and abnormal circulatory systems. Prog. cardiovasc. Dis. 21: 405–430 (1979).

9   Eliot, R.S.: Twentieth century stress and the heart; in Eliot, Stress and the heart, pp. 7–12 (Futura, New York 1974).

10 Eliot, R.S.; Clayton, F.C.; Pieper, G.M.; Todd, G.L.: Influence of environmental stress on the pathogenesis of sudden cardiac death. Fed. Proc. 36: 1719–1724 (1977).

11 Eliot, R.S.; Todd, G.L.; Clayton, F.C.; Pieper, G.M.: Experimental catecholamine-induced acute myocardial necrosis; in Manninen, Halonen, Sudden coronary death. Adv. Cardiol., vol. 25, pp. 107–118 (Karger, Basel 1978).

12 Engel, G.L.: Psychologic factors in instantaneous cardiac death. New Engl. J. Med. 294: 664–665 (1976).

13 Engel, G.L.: Psychologic stress, vasodepressor (vasovagal) syncope, and sudden death. Ann. intern. Med. 89: 403–412 (1978).

14 Fleischman, A.I.; Bierenbaum, M.L.; Stier, A.: Effect of stress due to anticipated minor surgery upon in vivo platelet aggregation in humans. J. hum. Stress 2: 33–37 (1976).

15 Friedman, M.; Byers, S.O.: Effect of environmental influences on alimentary lipemia of the rat. Am. J. Physiol. *213:* 1359–1364 (1967).

16 Friedman, M.; Byers, S.O.; Brown, A.E.: Plasma lipid responses of rats and rabbits to an auditory stimulus. Am. J. Physiol. *212:* 1174–1178 (1967).

17 Friedman, M.; Byers, S.O.; Elek, S.R.: Neurogenic hypercholesterolemia. II. Relationship to endocrine function. Am. J. Physiol. *223:* 473–479 (1972).

18 Friedman, M.; Manwaring, J.H.; Rosenman, R.H.; et al.: Instantaneous and sudden deaths. Clinical and pathological differentiation in coronary artery disease. J. Am. med. Ass. *225:* 1319–1328 (1973).

19 Friedman, M.; Rosenman, R.H.; Carroll, V.: Changes in the serum cholesterol and blood clotting time in men subjected to cyclic variation of occupational stress. Circulation *17:* 852–861 (1958).

20 Gunn, C.G.; Friedman, M.; Byers, S.O.: Effect of chronic hypothalamic stimulation upon cholesterol-induced atherosclerosis in the rabbit. J. clin. Invest. *39:* 1963–1972 (1960).

21 Haft, J.I.: Role of blood platelets in coronary artery disease. Am. J. Cardiol. *43:* 1197–1206 (1979).

22 Haft, J.I.; Arkel, Y.S.: Effect of emotional stress on platelet aggregation in humans. Chest *70:* 501–505 (1976).

23 Hennekens, C.H.; Rosner, B.; Cole, D.S.: Daily alcohol consumption and fatal coronary heart disease. Am. J. Epidem. *107:* 196 (1978).

24 Hinkle, L.E.; Thaler, H.T.: The clinical classification of cardiac deaths. Circulation *65:* 457–464 (1982).

25 Hinkle, L.; Carver, S.; Plakum, A.: Slow heart rate and increased risk of cardiac death in middle-aged men. Archs intern. Med. *129:* 732–748 (1972).

26 Buell, J.C.; Eliot, R.S.: The clinical and pathological syndromes of sudden cardiac death: an overview; in Solomon, Parron, Dews, Biobehavioral factors in sudden cardiac death. Health and behavior: a research agenda interim report, No. 3, pp. 13–28 (National Academy Press, Washington 1981).

27 Kerzner, J.; Wolf, M.; Kosowsky, B.D.; Lown, B.: Ventricular ectopic rhythms following vagal stimulation in dogs with acute myocardial infarction. Circulation *47:* 44–50 (1973).

28 Lapin, B.A.; Cherkovich, G.M.: Environmental changes causing the development of neuroses and corticovisceral pathology in monkeys; in Levi, Society, stress and disease: the psychosocial environment and psychosomatic diseases, vol. 1, pp. 266–279 (Oxford University Press, London 1971).

29 Liang, B.; Verrier, R.L.; Lown, B.; Melman, J.: Correlation between circulating catecholamine levels and ventricular vulnerability during psychological stress in conscious dogs. Proc. Soc. exp. Biol. Med. *161:* 266–269 (1979).

30 Lown, B.; Temte, J.V.; Reich, P.; et al.: Basis for recurring ventricular fibrillation in the absence of coronary heart disease and its management. New Engl. J. Med. *294:* 623–629 (1976).

31 Lown, B.; Verrier, R.L.: Neural activity and ventricular fibrillation. New Engl. J. Med. *294:* 1165–1170 (1976).

32 Lown, B.; Verrier, R.L.; Rabinowitz, S.H.: Neural and psychological mechanisms and the problems of sudden cardiac death. Am. J. Cardiol. *39:* 890–902 (1977).

33 Mason, J.W.: A review of psychoendocrine research on the pituitary adrenal cortical system. Psychosom. Med. *30:* 576–607 (1968).

34 Nerem, R.: Social environment as a factor in diet induced aortic atherosclerosis in rabbits. Hugh Lofland Conf. on Arterial Wall Metabolism, Boston 1979.

35 Ostfeld, A.M.; Shekelle, R.B.: Psychological variables and blood pressure; in Stamler, Stamler, Pullman, The epidemiology of hypertension, pp. 321–331 (Grune & Stratton, New York 1967).

36 Pieper, G.M.; Clayton, F.C.; Todd, G.L.; Eliot, R.S.: Transmural distribution of metabolites and blood flow in the canine left ventricle following isoproterenol infusions. J. Pharmac. exp. Ther. 209: 334–341 (1979).

37 Rabinowitz, S.H.; Lown, B.: Central neurochemical factors related to serotonin metabolism and cardiac ventricular vulnerability for repetitive electrical activity. Am. J. Cardiol. 41: 516–522 (1978).

38 Rabkin, S.W.; Mathewson, F.A.L.; Tate, R.B.: Chronobiology of cardiac sudden death in men. J. Am. med. Ass. 244: 1357–1358 (1980).

39 Regan, T.J.; Koroxenidis, G.; Moschos, C.B.; Oldewurtel, H.A.; Luhan, P.H.; Hellems, H.J.: The acute metabolic and hemodynamic responses of the left ventricle to ethanol. J. clin. Invest. 45: 270 (1966).

40 Regan, T.J.; Levinson, G.E.; Oldewurtel, H.A.; Frank, M.J.; Weisse, A.B.; Moschos, C.B.: Ventricular function in noncardiacs with alcoholic fatty liver: role of ethanol in the production of cardiomyopathy. J. clin. Invest. 48: 397 (1969).

41 Reynolds, R.C.: Community and occupational influences in stress at Cape Kennedy. Relationships to heart disease; in Eliot, Stress and the heart, pp. 33–49 (Futura, New York 1974).

42 Romo, M.: Factors related to sudden death in acute ischaemic heart disease. Acta med. scand. suppl. 547: 7–82 (1973).

43 Rosenman, R.H.; Brand, R.J.; Jenkins, C.D.; et al.: Coronary heart disease in the Western Collaborative Group Study. Final follow-up experience of 8½ years. J. Am. med. Ass. 233: 872–877 (1975).

44 Schneider, R.A.: Patterns of autonomic response to startle in subjects with and without coronary artery disease (Abstract). Clin. Res. 15: 59 (1957).

45 Stout, L.C.; Bohorquez, F.: Significance of intimal arterial changes in non-human vertebrates; in Altschule, Symp. on Atherosclerosis. Medical Clinics of North America, vol. 58, pp. 245–255 (Saunders, Philadelphia 1974).

46 Stout, L.C.; Lemmon, W.B.; Bohorquez, F.; et al.: Increased aortic arteriosclerosis with chronic electric shock in miniature pigs (Abstract). Am. J. Path. 70: 55a (1973).

47 Thomas, C.B.; Murphy, E.A.: Further studies on cholesterol levels in the Johns Hopkins medical students: the effect of stress at examinations. J. chron. Dis. 8: 661–668 (1958).

48 Troxler, R.G.; Sprague, E.A.; Albanese, R.A.; Fuchs, R.; Thompson, A.J.: The association of elevated plasma cortisol and early atherosclerosis as demonstrated by coronary angiography. Atherosclerosis 26: 151–162 (1977).

49 Verrier, R.L.; Calvert, A.; Lown, B.: Effect of posterior hypothalamic stimulation on the ventricular fibrillation threshold. Am. J. Physiol. 228: 923–927 (1975).

50 Warheit, G.J.: Occupation, a key factor in stress at the Manned Space Center; in Eliot, Stress and the heart, pp. 51–65 (Futura, New York 1974).

51 Weiss, S.M. (ed.): Coronary-prone behavior and coronary heart disease: a critical review panel sponsored by NHLBI. Circulation 63: 1199–1215 (1981).

52 Yano, K.; Rhoads, G.G.; Kagan, A.: Coffee, alcohol and risk of coronary heart disease among Japanese living in Hawaii. New Engl. J. Med. 297: 405 (1977).

17 Behavior and Hypertension

Stevo Julius, Christopher Cottier

This selective review is from the vantage point of two investigators who, based on their research on the pathophysiology of hypertension, became convinced that behavior must play an important role in hypertension. The review will also reflect our dissatisfaction with the slow progress in documenting the relationship of behavior and hypertension. The historical reasons for the present state of knowledge will be discussed and after a selective review of the literature, suggestions for future research will be given.

Background

It is common knowledge that emotional stimuli can raise the blood pressure (BP). Short emotional elevations of the BP under designed experimental stressful conditions have been reported frequently [12, 42, 55]. From such experiments evolved the notion that repeated emotional increases of the BP may eventually lead to the disease of sustained human hypertension. Since emotional elevations of the BP also occur in healthy humans, those destined for development of future hypertension must have some distinct characteristics that predispose them for the disease. In essence they must be either (a) hyperreactors to stress so that an excessive *magnitude* or *duration* of BP response leads to hypertension or (b) exposed to more stress either through their stress-prone personality or through more stressful socioeconomic conditions. Much of the research was done to find these predisposing factors to hypertension and some of the work will be reviewed.

It is fair to say that at present behavioral factors in hypertension are of interest only to few investigators. It may be useful to briefly trace the reasons for the contemporary predominance of 'organic' as opposed to behavioral research in order to develop future research agenda and avoid future pitfalls. Why, 75 years after *Geisböck* [30] reported that hypertensive patients 'had a great deal of responsibility, and after long periods of psychic overwork became nervous', is there still a lack of good evidence causally connecting behavior and hypertension?

The root or the problem may well be in the direction of the experimental research. Whereas it is relatively easy to create hypertension by Doca-salt, renal artery stenosis, renal wrapping and by genetic inbreeding, the principle that repeated neurogenic pressor episodes lead to sustained hypertension has not been adequately demonstrated. *Folkow and Rubinstein* [25] failed to elicit sustained hypertension with prolonged electrical stimulation of the defense area. Operant conditioning in monkeys also causes only transient hypertension; the BP between schedules returns to normal levels [9, 41]. Experiments with removing various negative baroreceptor feedback loops either peripherally [15] or centrally [57] have failed to produce sustained hypertension. In a very complete review of four different inbred strains of genetically hypertensive rats, *Hallbäck and Folkow* [35] found various degrees of involvement of an autonomic component in the development of hypertension, but could not build a convincing case that any of these 'spontaneous' hypertensions is purely neurogenic. At best one can find evidence for increased reactivity to stress in the Okamoto strain and in the New Zealand strain. Probably closest to a 'stress'-induced hypertension are the mice of *Henry* et al. [40], where a complex social stress induces longstanding hypertension and increased cardiovascular morbidity, but the nature of stress is so complex that the behavioral component in the process of hypertension can hardly be defined.

The second problem in gaining acceptance for the importance of behavioral aspects in the development of human hypertension stems from studies on the personality patterns in patients with hypertension. Research into personality is dominated by conceptual thinking, which influences both the method of assessment and the interpretation of results. Even when the first psychoanalytical and highly subjective descriptions were replaced by predefined instruments of measurement, the differences in nomenclature precluded comparison. How can one compare reports using such terms as 'kinesthetic perception' and 'structural versus unstructured neurosis' [65] with those that deal with 'anger in' and 'anger out' [38]? Similarly, where behavioral paradigms have been employed, the techniques varied from viewing erotic movies [55], applying mental arithmetics [24], investigating the degree of yielding [37], giving Raven's Progressive Matrices [43] to psychodrama [39]. In some of these the behavior, in others the physiologic responses, were the observed variables. This variety of approaches is not conducive to the development of a uniform body of knowledge about personality, behavior and hypertension.

A third source of disbelief into the important role of behavior in human hypertension is the questionable success of behavioral approaches to the treatment of hypertension. In our opinion, the potential of behavioral approaches to the treatment of hypertension has been overestimated, and it is likely that in the future these forms of hypertensive treatment will continue to be less effective than the pharmacotherapy of hypertension. Further refinements in modalities of behavioral treatment may lead to improvement, but unwarranted popularization of these methods may in the ultimate line do much harm. Effectiveness of behavioral treatment and the question of involvement of behavior in the etiology of hypertension are not necessarily connected. Nevertheless, if expectations in the medical community and in the general public are too high, the relative ineffectiveness of behavioral treatment will be misconstrued to mean that behavior is not causally involved in hypertension. In Ann Arbor, we have witnessed the inauguration of two 'life-style and stress management centers' to treat hypertension. The process of polarization into 'organic-minded' physicians and those who believe only in behavioral approaches has already started. The unwarranted promotion of behavioral aspects may alineate the organic-minded majority and could, at least in the USA, eventually seriously influence the funding for behavioral research.

Evidence

Involvement of the Autonomic Nervous System in Human Hypertension
If behavior is a causal factor in the development of hypertension, then the physiologic consequence must be a shift of balance between centrally originating inhibitory and excitatory influences towards a state of 'net' increase in the cardiovascular drive. It is therefore of interest to review the evidence (a) for an increased autonomic drive in hypertension, and (b) that this increased drive has a central nervous origin as opposed to a peripheral hyperresponsiveness to a normal autonomic tone [68, 71].

The best evidence for involvement of the autonomic nervous system in human essential hypertension is in the so-called 'hyperkinetic' mild to moderate hypertension. Such patients have a borderline or mild BP elevation, a fast heart rate (HR) and an elevated cardiac output [19, 28, 48, 56, 63, 66, 75]. Not all patients with borderline hypertension will develop later sustained hypertension [46]. However, there is some evidence in the literature that patients with hyperkinetic borderline hypertension may be at the highest risk for hypertension [59]. Tachycardia at youth without a BP elevation carries an excessive risk for future hypertension, and when tachycardia and 'transient hypertension' at youth are combined, the risk of later hypertension is particularly high [54].

Tachycardia in the 'hyperkinetic' hypertensive is frequently associated with a higher cardiac output [48]. This elevation of cardiac output is entirely neurogenic and can be abolished by a blockade of autonomic influences on the heart [50]. Interestingly, however, when the excessive cardiac output is removed, the vascular resistance increases and the BP remains elevated [51]. We have, therefore, utilized α-adrenergic blockade to determine whether this elevation of vascular resistance is also neurogenic [21]. In borderline hypertension [21] as well as in mild established hypertension [22], a neurogenic elevation of the vascular resistance was characteristically present only in high-renin patients. Such patients also had elevated plasma norepinephrine values [22]. Literature on plasma catecholamines in hypertension is somewhat controversial, but a recent thorough review by *Goldstein* [32] suggests that the norepinephrine may be elevated in young subjects with mild forms of hypertension. Our own findings show a correlation between the HR and plasma norepinephrine in young patients with borderline hypertension [23], indicating that the 'hyperkinetic' patients may be those with a higher sympathetic tone.

Similar conclusions about the importance of the neurogenic component in hyperkinetic borderline hypertension have been found by *Safar* et al. [64] and *Weiss* et al. [74]. After analyzing the hemodynamic findings in such patients, they conclude that in comparison to patients with established hypertension, the borderlines show more evidence for sympathetic overactivity.

Sympathetic overactivity, however, is not the only autonomic abnormality found in borderline hypertension. β-Adrenergic blockade with large intravenous doses of propranolol was not sufficient to bring the cardiac output into the normal range; it was also necessary to abolish the parasympathetic inhibition of the heart by intravenous atropine [50]. This pointed toward a dysregulation in the sympathetic-stimulatory and in the parasympathetic-inhibitory control of the HR. Abnormality in two components of the autonomic cardiac control pointed toward a central nervous rather than a peripheral receptor abnormality. Futher analysis of the magnitude of the response showed that these patients had an increased sympathetic stimulation and decreased parasympathetic inhibition of the heart. Such a reciprocal change in the sympathetic and parasympathetic tone is characteristic for the function of the higher integrative centers in the medulla oblongata. We therefore concluded that hyperkinetic borderline hypertension is mediated by an abnormal central integration of the autonomic control [49]. This led to investigations of the afferent and descending inputs into the integrative centers of cardiovascular control. In contradistinction to other investigators [11, 72], who studied more severe patients, we could not find an abnormal sensitivity of arterial baroreceptors in hyperkinetic borderline hypertension [45]. Therefore, a primary abnormality in baroreceptor function did not appear to be responsible for the abnormal integration of the central autonomic discharge in borderline hypertension.

A number of descending pathways from the paleocortex can alter the function of integrative centers in the medulla oblongata as well as directly change the overall autonomic discharge from the central nervous system. It was first suggested by *Brod* et al. [12] that patients with hypertension exhibit a hemodynamic pattern much akin to the acute 'defense reaction'. Consequently it is of interest to review whether patients with borderline hypertension have a personality prone to increased alertness, e.g. to a more permanent activation of the defense mechanism, with the resultant increase of central nervous autonomic discharge.

Personality and Hypertension

In this section we will review only those studies of personality in hypertension that lend themselves to comparison. As a rule, attention will be paid to works using clearly understandable terms, even if the conceptual framework is different. We will avoid papers that describe patients in terms of absence or presence of psychiatric abnormalities for two reasons: (a) lack of agreement as to what a psychiatric diagnosis means (for example, 'neurosis', 'schizoid traits':) and (b) the unproven assumption that mental normalcy can be assessed by absence of abnormal traits. A number of differences within the scope of normally present personality traits may be much more relevant. Given these constraints, there emerges a reasonably consistent picture. (a) Generally, the most consistent personality aberrations in hypertension are in the area of assertiveness, expression of anger and ability to socially interact. (b) Personality differences are more frequently found in young patients and patients with mild hypertension. (c) Patients with hypertension are not characterized by a type A personality.

One of the first attempts to assess personality traits in hypertension by an objective instrument appeared in 1933, when *Ayman* [1] found his patients to be 'sensitive', 'given to inner excitement', 'shy', and 'easy to offend'. In 1942, *Hamilton* [36] described his patients with mild hypertension as 'submissive', 'less assertive', 'less self-confident', and somewhat 'introverted'. *Harris* et al. [39] and *Kalis* et al. [52] studied a group of female subjects with borderline hypertension. In the first report, observations were made while subjects acted in a psychodrama; in the second report the patients were recalled for an interview. Subject's performance was rated by independent observers using prepared scales for assessment of various traits. Compared to normotensive subject, patients with borderline hypertension were judged to 'derive less pleasure from life', 'showed motoric unrest, but made obvious attempts to control themselves and hide their emotional feelings'.

We used the same personality inventory on three separate occasions. In the first study on Michigan students [37] with borderline hypertension, we found them to be 'sociable', 'sensitive' but also 'submissive' and 'suspecting'. The Cattell 16-PF Test was later translated into Serbo-Croatian and standardized on 386 male students at the University of Zagreb, Yugoslavia [47]. The test was then given to 75 students whose BP was measured during 5 consecutive days; 24 subjects had borderline hypertension. As in the Ann Arbor study, the borderline hypertensives showed a higher 'sociability' and 'submissiveness'. Additionally, in Yugoslavia, patients with borderline hypertension were also described as 'adventurous' and 'talkative'. The 16-PF Test was again used in Ann Arbor [22], but now in patients with mild, established high-renin hypertension. High-renin patients were more 'submissive'. They were also shown to have a more controlled personality having a higher 'super ego'. Thus, these three studies describe the patient as being submissive but at the same time outward oriented. The trait of submissiveness, which patients reported in questionnaires was confirmed in a test of actual behavior [37]. *Harburg* devised a test of experimental yielding where partners engaged in a discussion on topics on which they held opposing views. They stated their initial position on a scale, were instructed to discuss and arrive at a compromise, and were to mark on the scale how much they yielded. Patients with borderline hypertension anticipated that they would not yield, but during the actual experiments changed their private opinion and moved closer to the position of their normotensive counterparts. In addition to these findings with the 16-PF questionnaire, the patients with high-renin mild hypertension were tested with the 'anger in'-'anger out' scale developed by *Harburg* for the Detroit area study of psychosocial and familiar factors in hypertension [38]. Patients with mild hypertension showed a significantly higher proportion of 'anger in' behavior than control subjects [21]. These findings are much like the results of the large-scale Detroit study where hypertension was associated with 'keeping in anger when attacked' and 'feeling guilty when expressing anger' [38]. The majority of patients with hypertension in the Detroit study had mild BP elevations.

As can be seen from this selective review, various investigators have used different approaches and different descriptive nomenclature. Nevertheless, a reasonably consistent broad picture emerges. The personality of patients with borderline and mild hypertension is characterized by submissiveness to other people's views, by a motivation for contact with other people, by an attempt to control behavior as to be socially acceptable and by difficulties in expressing hostile feelings.

The studies quoted deal with 'prehypertension', borderline hypertension, and mild hypertension as these populations were mostly utilized for research. It is not clear whether such characteristics also prevail in patients with established hypertension. However, it is interesting to note that in two studies where personality traits were assessed in mild and more severe hypertension the personality deviations were more characteristic of milder forms of hypertension [62, 65]. Unfortunately, due to the nature of the measuring instruments or the purpose of the study, personality traits described in these two studies cannot be compared with the results of other studies.

A word of caution with all personality studies in subjects with mild hypertension is in order. The association between behavioral traits and hypertension does not prove that the personality plays a role in the development of hypertension. In that regard, a recent study by *Baer* et al. [2] is of particular interest. These investigators found that *all* family members of a hypertensive propositus, including the wife, show more negative nonverbal behavior. Thus, a certain behavioral pattern is fostered by a hypertensive head of household. However, the pathogenic significance of this is obscure; wives of hypertensive husbands are not shown to have more hypertension.

Some important negative results on the relationship between personality and hypertension also deserve analysis. Hypertension is one of the strongest risk factors for coronary heart disease (CHD). Type A personality is another well-recognized risk factor for coronary morbidity. It would therefore be reasonable to expect some association between the coronary-prone and the hypertensive personality. However, type A behavior does not seem to be characteristic for patients with essential hypertension [69]. This may well point toward different mechanisms by which two different personality patterns lead to a higher coronary riks.

Blood Pressure Reactivity to Stress in Patients with Hypertension
Conceptually a characteristic personality predisposes a subject to future hypertension through an excessive vulnerability or responsiveness to stress. By virtue of his personality, a subject is more prone to increased alertness

leading to a more frequent, larger, and longer lasting central nervous activation of pressor responses. How good is the evidence that patients with hypertension and those destined to hypertension are 'pressor hyperresponders' to
mental stress? The first well-designed report was provided by *Brod* et al. [12].
Mild and severe patients in their study were equally hyperresponsive to the
stress of mental arithmetics. Results in severe patients are difficult to interpret
as peripheral arteriolar hypertrophy may render the patients hyperresponsive to a normal sympathetic tone. In milder and borderline hypertensives,
the vasculature is not hypertrophic and they tend to have a normal pressure
responsiveness to various pressor maneuvers such as cold pressor stress [16],
static exercise [67], dynamic exercise [48], and infusion of dextran [51]. Thus,
if such patients are hyperresponsive to mental stress, this is a specific feature
and not a general characteristic due either to structural changes in the vessels
or due to an overall defect in the reflex control of the circulation. Indeed,
patients with mild hypertension show a specific pattern of hyperresponsiveness to mental stress. *Nestel* [58] found that the BP and urinary catecholamine
response to mental arithmetics are excessive in patients with mild and borderline hypertension. These observations have been taken one step further
by important observations of *Falkner* et al. [24]. They compared normotensive children without a genetic background of hypertension with normotensive children who had a positive parental history for hypertension and with
borderline hypertensive children. During and after mental arithmetics, subjects with borderline hypertension had a higher and longer increase of the
BP and HR. Normotensive offspring of hypertensive parents had an intermediary response: less than the borderline hypertensives and more than normotensives without a genetic background. Similar results with somewhat
different experimentation were obtained by *Light and Obrist* [55]. BP
response to elicited stress and spontaneous BP variability were analyzed.
Stress hyperreactors, that is those whose HR and BP responded most, were
then compared with lesser reactors. Again in this study, the hyperresponders
had a more prevalent family history of hypertension. In view of the previous
discussion about the hyperkinetic state and the prognostic value of elevated
HR for future hypertension, it is interesting to note that in both these studies
[24, 55] the BP increase was associated with a simultaneous increase of the
HR. *Hollenberg* et al. [43] recently added new interesting data on BP responsiveness to mental stress. In addition to the HR and BP response to a nonverbal IQ test and Raven's Progressive Matrices, they also studied the response
of the renal vasculature by the Xenon washout technique. Although they
claim that they compared 'hypertensive' to normotensive subjects, the hyper-

tension in their study was mild indeed. The mean intraarterial BP of 98 ± 3.8 mm Hg in their study is rather similar to the average BP of patients with borderline hypertension [48, 50]. As in two previous studies, when challenged with a mental stress, these patients responded with a faster HR and higher BP but in addition also exhibited a substantially larger decrease in the renal blood flow. In this study, normotensive subjects with a positive family history reacted to mental stress with a response intermediary between normotensive subjects without family history and patients with hypertension.

Behavioral Treatment of Hypertension

Three major categories of behavioral treatment of hypertension will be reviewed: biofeedback, relaxation, and meditation. As the material is large, we decided to highlight our comparison of various studies in a tabular fashion. Papers on biofeedback are reviewed in table I. *Blanchard* et al. [8], *Goldmann* et al. [31] and *Kristt and Engel* [53] reported significant decrements in BP. In contrast, *Elder and Eustis* [20], *Hager and Surwit* [34], and *Green* et al. [33] were unable to find a meaningful decrease of BP in their studies. The methods used range from a comparatively simple noncontinuous BP feedback to a portable continuous BP feedback apparatus that enables the subjects to train at home. Many of the studies are subject to serious methodological problems. Only *Goldmann* et al. [31] and *Hager and Surwit* [34] used appropriate control groups. In many studies a variable part of the study population concomitantly received antihypertensive drugs and biofeedback training. Several studies have no initial baseline period and all but *Elder and Eustis* [20] reported only within-session BP determinations. The longest follow-up lasted 3 months. The overall impression is that none of the biofeedback techniques reported successful long-term effective BP lowering.

Table II presents the studies on meditation. Most authors sent their subjects to a standard course in transcendental meditation and were therefore unable to evaluate the compliance. The comparison of results is beclouded by a lack of information about the intensity of training programs. With the exception of *Pollak* et al. [61], all authors found significant reductions in BP. Only *Stone and DeLeo* [70] used a control group; unfortunately, in this study, the patients were not randomized. The patients had mild essential hypertension and received no antihypertensive medication. BP fell over 6 months from 146/95 to 131/85 mm Hg. The study of *Stone and DeLeo* [70] illustrates one of the main problems: it is very difficult to introduce an acceptable control group into trials of behavioral modification. The subjects in the control group could not expect their BP to change, if they were seen, as in the study

Table I. Behavioral therapy in hypertension – biofeedback

Author(s), year	Refer-ence	Number of subjects	Age (range)	Etiology of hyperten-sion, severi-ty, initial BP on no drugs	Method	Duration of therapy	Results	Commentary
Elder and Eustis, 1975	20	22	50 (23–80)	ess. hpt. (?)	BP displayed on chart; reinforce-ment by lamps and verbal instruc-tions; 10 sessions in 82 days	82 weeks in spaced, 12 weeks in massed design	meaningful BP decrease only within session; in-between session: overall BP basal 146/85; last session: 139/82	20 patients on drugs; no control group; baseline short; inhomogeneous population; com-pliance unknown; baseline inadequate; simple biofeedback system
Blanchard et al., 1975	8	5	–	unknown	sphygmomano-metric BP display every 30 min on TV	daily sessions for 1–2 weeks; 2 subjects hospitalized	reduction of systolic BP from 154 to 128 mm Hg, but no time frame given	2 patients on drugs; no control group; baseline – none; presentation of data incomplete; small number, subjects in part hospitalized
Goldmann et al., 1975	31	18	54 (35–68)	unknown 167/109	constant pressure systolic BP bio-feedback [68], light and sound feedback, beat to beat; control: rest and relax	9 weeks, 2-hour session each week	comparison session 1 and 9: BP 167/109 and 159/94; no change in control group	no baseline; high drop-out rate (7); no follow-up and in-between session BP measurements
Kristt and Engel, 1975	53	5	59 (46–70)	ess. hpt. (?) mod.–severe	constant pressure systolic BP bio-feedback [68], light signal; home training with constant systolic pressure, Korot-koff sound	3 weeks in hospital, then 3 months at home	decrement office BP pretrial versus 3-month follow-up 163/95 vs 144/87; versus home BP 141/? vs 125/?	no control group; all subjects on drugs; inhomogeneous population, severe concomitant disease; small number, no meaningful statistics possible
Hager and Surwit, 1978	34	30	?	ess. hpt. (?)	constant cuff pressure systolic BP biofeedback, beat to beat, light signal, portable, training at home	twice daily training at home over 4 weeks	decrease of BP after 1 month 4/2 mm Hg; no difference between bio-feedback and relaxation	no baseline; some patients on drugs; biofeedback home training; low basal BP of 130/83; 13 drop-outs, reason not speci-fied; controls (10) practical relaxation response
Green et al., 1980	33	12	44 (27–57)	mild hpt.	finger-thermister biofeedback, elements of auto-genic training; twice daily home practice	5–104 weeks	reduction in BP in patients on no drugs: 6/3 mm Hg; on drugs: 9/6 mm Hg	no controls, variable observation time

Table II. Behavioral therapy in hypertension – meditation

Author(s), year	Reference	Number of subjects	Age (range)	Etiology of hypertension, severity, initial BP on no drugs	Method	Duration of therapy	Results	Commentary
Datey et al., 1969	17	47	46 (22–64)	32 ess. hpt. 12 renal hpt. 3 arterio. hpt.	1 month baseline; 37 on drugs; Shavasan yogic exercise: regular slow breathing, temperature change, nostrils focused on by the subject	unspecified (1 patient shown: 9 months)	reduction of BP in no-drug group (mean 134–107 mm Hg); reduction of drugs in other groups of 30% and more in half of the patients	no controls; moderate to severe hypertension; duration of training in Shavasan not mentioned; success expressed only in % reduction of antihypertensive drugs in most patients
Benson et al., 1974	5	14	53 (?)	unknown mild–moderate	6 weeks baseline; all on drugs; transcendental meditation, taught at TM Center, not by authors	duration training period unclear; follow-up 20 weeks	premeditational period, mean BP 146/92; post-meditational period (20 weeks), mean BP 135/87 (significant for systolic and diastolic BP)	no controls; etiology of BP unknown; random-0-sphygmomanometer used; very high drop-out rate (50 of initial 64); all subjects on drugs
Blackwell et al., 1976	7	7	46 (39–59)	unknown	4 weeks baseline; all on drugs; transcendental meditation (Maharashi Yogi), instructions in decreasing frequeny over up to 5 months at TM Center; home training	12 weeks; follow-up after 6 months	reduction in BP at home 13/7, at clinic 3/4 mm Hg at 6 months; no statistical significance calculated	no controls; small number; all on medication
Stone and De Leo, 1976	70	19	28 (21–36)	ess. hpt. 143/90	10–14 days baseline; meditation by breath-counting in 14; 5 subjects in control group; no intervention, only same BP determinations, as treatment group; home training	5 training sessions; home training; follow-up of 6 months	treatment group: BP baseline versus BP at 6 months: 146/95 vs 131/85; control group: no change	5 controls, not randomized; well-classified essential hypertension
Pollak et al., 1977	61	20	40 (22–69)	ess. hpt.	3 months baseline; 9 on drugs; transcendental meditation, instruction in decreasing frequency at TM Center over 6 months; home training	4 months; follow-up of 6 months	no significant BP reduction after 6 months	no controls; compliance unknown; PRA unchanged

Table III. Behavioral therapy in hypertension – relaxation

Author(s), year	Refer-ence	Number of subjects	Age (range)	Etiology of hypertension, severity, initial BP on no drugs	Method	Duration of therapy	Results	Commentary
Patel, 1975	60	40	57	ess. hpt. (?)	relaxation (not specified); control: simple bed rest	each group 6 sessions in 12 days	decrement of BP (7/8 mm Hg) only in relaxation group; no change in biofeedback and control group	37 on drugs; no baseline; 5 controls; simple biofeedback technique; no in-between session BP measurements; initial systolic BP not equal in the 3 groups
Beimann et al., 1978	4	2	27, 35	ess. hpt. (?) 137/98 150/90	baseline 12, 20 days; progressive muscle relaxation (Berstein, Berkovic), home training; identification of anxiety-related stimuli	40, 70 days	after 6-month follow-up, home BP: decrease from 137/97 to 122/81; 149/88 to 132/79	no controls; patients selected for anxiety; small number; patients on low salt diet
Bali, 1979	3	18	37 (30–44)	ess. hpt. (?) 158/105	baseline 2 months; matched pairs; progressive muscle relaxation (Jacobson), modified; home training	2 months instruction, 6–10 sessions; follow-up 12 months	significant BP decrease by 12/9 mm Hg in treatment, no change in control group; 12-month follow-up: decrease 14/11 mm Hg; significant decrease in anxiety levels	control = bed rest; homogeneous group; good design but control only for 2 months, not for 12-month follow-up; intervention in control group sessions unclear
Brauer et al., 1979	10	31	57	ess. hpt. (?) mild–moderate	all on drugs; short baseline; 3 groups: (a) muscle relaxation (Marquis) by therapist; (b) MR by tape only; (c) nonspecific psychotherapy	weekly session over 10 weeks, daily home training until 6 months	change of BP from baseline to 6-month follow-up in groups: (a) 153/93 to 136/83; (b) 150/95 to 145/93; (c) 145/93 to 144/94	drugs changed throughout study; best and significant reductions in group treated by therapist; interesting placebo effect most profound after 10 weeks
Cottier et al., 1981	14	26	35 (20–50)	mild hpt.	6 weeks baseline; progressive muscle relaxation (Berkovic); 9 sessions within 4 months; all subjects on placebo tablets	4 months	no significant BP reduction in office, home and 24-hour BP in whole group; some subjects responded with important BP decreases	9 controls, randomized; attempt to improve control with placebo

of those authors, only for frequent BP determination. Expectation of a positive outcome may be very important and must be taken into consideration before one can accept the specificity of effect of a treatment modality.

An overview of studies on relaxation is given in table III. *Bali* [3] and *Brauer* et al. [10] reported decreases in BP over 12 and 6 months, respectively. The range of the decrease was between 9–20 mm Hg systolic and 6–14 mm Hg diastolic pressure. *Taylor* et al. [73] and *Cottier* et al. [14] did not find significant decrements in BP over 6 and 4 months. Subjects in the reviewed studies had mild to moderate hypertension.

The, patients of *Brauer* et al. [10] were on antihypertensive drugs and changes in treatment were allowed during the study. Most of the authors used a relaxation technique based on *Jacobson's* [44] progressive muscle relaxation but all regimens differed in some aspects.

All authors asked their subjects to train regularly at home, but we know little about compliance. Only *Cottier* et al. [14] obtained repeated BP measurements outside the office at the patient's home. The intervention in the control groups varied widely from simple bed rest to specific psychotherapy and placebo. *Bali's* [3] control was limited to only 2 months. Similarly as in meditation studies, in relaxation studies the control subjects did not expect their BP to decrease.

The overall review of the literature in behavioral treatment of BP allows the following generalizations: (1) On the whole, relaxation and meditation approaches appear to be more effective, and certainly are much more practical than biofeedback treatment. (2) The majority of investigations are essentially pilot studies. The populations were highly selected, the number of subjects small and a control group was often not available. (3) A majority of the studies investigated patients on antihypertensive drugs. In these studies the success was expressed as the decrease in number of drugs required. Such results are difficult to evaluate. (4) Rarely was the effect of treatment on BP evaluated outside the office or laboratory. (5) Compliance, especially when patients were expected to train at home, was generally not reported. (6) Designing a study with appropriate controls is very difficult. If control subjects are simply asked to come to the laboratory and have their BP checked, they will not expect their BP to decrease. This may well explain why many of the control groups did not show the expected hypotensive effect of placebo. In pharmacologic studies, where an effect is anticipated, placebo tablets invariably lower the BP. (7) In the majority of studies, some subjects responded particularly well to behavioral treatment, even if the overall group results were disappointing. No attempt has been made to identify physiologic or personality characteristics of these responders. In this new area of research the effectiveness of single behavioral methods should be established first. We have therefore not reviewed trials, where a combination of methods have been used. Conflicting results have been reported by *Patel* [60], *Frankel* et al. [26], *Bertilson* [6], and *Datey* [18], but especially the work of *Patel* [60] shows, that an intensive program of combined behavioral treatment may lead to sustained lowering of BP.

Implications for Research

One of the most pressing needs is to establish a viable animal model of hypertension by repeated stress-induced pressor episodes. Utilization of various stressors with genetic tendency for hypertension, or with such environmental tendencies for hypertension as high salt intake and overweight, may be a particularly useful approach. An interesting lead in this regard has already been established in Dahl-salt sensitive rats [27]. The model of neurogenic hypertension need not mimic the pathophysiology of human hypertension. What is needed is a demonstration of the basic fact that sustained hypertension can be initiated by frequent neurogenic pressor episodes. A successful model of sustained neurogenic hypertension would greatly enhance the plausibility of human research on behavior and hypertension.

Genetic work in humans has seldom been combined with behavioral research. Particularly useful may be an analysis of genetic distance from the hypertensive propositi as it relates to behavioral styles and to physiologic responses to stress. New promising markers of hypertension have been reported [13, 29]. Although these have not yet been established as predictors of hypertension, behavioral investigation of normotensive groups with and without the marker may be of particular interest.

What happens to the sympathetic tone in the course of hypertension? Why is it relatively easy to find sympathetic overactivity in early phases of human and some animal hypertension, whereas later these factors are difficult to demonstrate [32]?

If some forms of hypertension are neurogenic, behavioral treatment should have a good chance for success. In this context, it would be useful to initially characterize patients's autonomic status and their behavioral characteristics in order to relate them prospectively to the success of behavioral treatment. Differences in responsiveness to behavioral treatment in primary and secondary hypertension may be useful to determine the specific versus nonspecific effect of behavioral treatment of hypertension.

In the area of behavioral treatment, relaxation and meditation methods offer a more effective and a more practical approach than biofeedback. Studies measuring out of office BP, preferably with a 24-hour monitoring device, are highly desirable.

The fact that both hypertension and type A behavior predict CHD, but that the type A behavior is not characteristic of hypertension, offers an interesting field for research about the specificity of personality patterns and the physiologic responses. Are the pathologic substrate, the mode of provocation of infarction and the character of the acute lesion different? What neurohumoral differences underlie the different personality patterns – the hypertensive and the coronary-prone?

If real progress is to be made in future behavioral research on human hypertension, the investigators must attempt to agree on some preferred instrument of measurement. Whereas it is not advisable to limit an investigator's choice, it would be a tremendous adavantage if new specific instruments or paradigms could be cross-validated against some standardized methods. The present day lack of comparability across numerous studies is bewildering and precludes a meaningful integration of the knowledge.

References

1 Ayman, D.: Personality type of patients with arteriolar essential hypertension. Am. J. med. Sci. *186:* 213–233 (1933).

2 Baer, P.E.; Vincent, J.P.; Williams, B.J.; Bourianoff, G.G.; Bartlett, P.C.: Behavioral response to induced conflict in families with a hypertensive father. Hypertension *2:* suppl. I, pp. I-70–I-77 (1980).

3 Bali, L.R.: Long-term effect of relaxation on blood pressure and anxiety levels of essential hypertensive males: a controlled study. Psychosom. Med. *41:* 637–646 (1979).

4 Beimann, I.; Graham, L.E.; Ciminero, A.R.: Self-control progressive relaxation training as an alternative nonpharmacological treatment of essential hypertension: therapeutic effects in the natural environment. Behav. Res. Therapy *16:* 371–375 (1978).

5 Benson, H.; Rosner, B.A.; Marzetta, B.R.; Klemchuck, H.M.: Decreased blood pressure in pharmacologically treated hypertensive patients who regularly elicited the relaxation response. Lancet *i:* 289–291 (1974).

6 Bertilson, H.S.: Treatment program for borderline hypertension among college students: relaxation, finger temperature biofeedback, and generalization. Psychol. Rep. *44:* 107–114 (1979).

7 Blackwell, B.; Bloomfield, S.; Gartside, P.; Robinson, A.; Hanenson, I.; Magenheim, H.; Nidich, S.; Zigler, R.: Transcendental meditation in hypertension: individual response patterns. Lancet *i:* 223–226 (1976).

8 Blanchard, E.B.; et al.: A simple feedback system for the treatment of elevated blood pressure. Behav. Ther. *1975:* 729.

9   Brady, J.V.; Anderson, D.E.; Harris, A.H.: Behavior and the cardiovascular system in experimental animals; in Zanchetti, Neurological and psychological mechanisms in cardiovascular disease (Il Ponte, Milan 1972).

10 Brauer, A.P.; Horlick, L.; Nelson, E.; Farquhar, J.W.; Agras, W.S.: Relaxation therapy for essential hypertension: a veterans administration outpatient study. J. behav. Med. 2: 21–29 (1979).

11 Bristow, J.D.; Honour, A.J.; Pickering, G.W.; Sleight, P.; Smyth, H.S.: Diminished baroreflex sensitivity in high blood pressure. Circulation 39: 48–53 (1969).

12 Brod, J.; Fencl, V.; Hejl, Z.; Jirka, J.: Circulatory changes underlying blood pressure elevation during acute emotional stress (mental arithmetic) in normotensive and hypertensive subjects. Clin. Sci. 18: 269–279 (1959).

13 Canessa, M.; Adragna, N.; Solomon, H.S.; Connolly, T.M.; Tosteson, D.G.: Increased sodium-lithium countertransport in red cells of patients with essential hypertension. New Engl. J. Med. 302: 772–776 (1980).

14 Cottier, C.; Shapiro, K.; Julius, S.: Progressive muscle relaxation in mild hypertension (in press, 1981).

15 Cowley, A.W., Jr.; Liard, J.F.; Guyton, A.C.: Role of the baroreceptor reflex in daily control of arterial blood pressure and other variables in dogs. Circulation Res. 32: 564–576 (1973).

16 Cuddy, R.P.; Smulyan, H.; Keighley, J.F.; Markason, C.R.; Eich, R.H.: Hemodynamics and catecholamine changes during a standard cold pressor test. Am. Heart J. 71: 446–454 (1966).

17 Datey, K.K.; Desmukh, S.N.; Dalvi, C.P.; Vinekar, S.L.: 'Shavasen': a yogic exercise in the management of hypertension. Angiology 20: 325–333 (1969).

18 Datey, K.K.: Role of biofeedback training in hypertension and stress. J. postgrad. Med. 26: 68–73 (1980).

19 Eich, R.H.; Peters, R.J.; Cuddy, R.P.; Smulyan, H.; Lyons, R.H.: The hemodynamics in labile hypertension. Am. Heart J. 63: 188–195 (1962).

20 Elder, S.T.; Eustis, N.K.: Instrumental blood pressure conditioning in outpatient hypertensives. Behav. Res. Therapy 13: 185–188 (1975).

21 Esler, M.D.; Julius, S.; Randall, O.S.; Ellis, C.N.; Kashima, T.: Relation of renin status to neurogenic vascular resistance in borderline hypertension. Am. J. Cardiol. 36: 708–715 (1975).

22 Esler, M.; Julius, S.; Zweifler, A.; Randall, O.; Harburg, E.: Gardiner, H.; DeQuattro, V.: Mild high-renin essential hypertension. Neurogenic human hypertension? New Engl. J. Med. 296: 405–411 (1977).

23 Esler, M.; Zweifler, A.; Randall, O.; Julius, S.; DeQuattro, V.: Agreement among three different indices of sympathetic nervous system activity in essential hypertension. Mayo Clin. Proc. 52: 379–382 (1977).

24 Falkner, B.; Onesti, G.; Angelakos, E.T.; Fernandes, M.; Langman, C.: Cardiovascular response to mental stress in normal adolescents with hypertensive parents. Hemodynamics and mental stress in adolescents. Hypertension 1: 23–30 (1979).

25 Folkow, B.; Rubinstein, E.H.: Cardiovascular effects of acute and chronic stimulation of the hypothalamic defense area in the rat. Acta physiol. Scand. 68: 48–57 (1966).

26 Frankel, B.L.; Patel, D.J.; Horwitz, D.; Friedewald, D.T.; Gaardner, K.R.: Treatment of hypertension with biofeedback and relaxation techniques. Psychosom. Med. 40: 276–293 (1979).

27   Friedman, R.; Dahl, L.K.: The effect of chronic conflict on the blood pressure of rats with a genetic susceptibility to experimental hypertension. Psychosom. Med. *37:* 402–416 (1975).

28   Frohlich, E.D.; Tarazi, R.C.; Dustan, H.P.: Hyperdynamic beta-adrenergic circulatory state: increased beta-receptor responsiveness. Archs intern. Med. *123:* 1–7 (1969).

29   Garay, R.P.; Meyer, P.: A new test showing abnormal net Na$^+$ and K-fluxes in erythrocytes of essential hypertensive patients. Lancet *i:* 349–353 (1979).

30   Geisböck, W.: Die Bedeutung der Blutdruckmessung für die Praxis. Dt. Arch. klin. Med. *83:* 363–374 (1905).

31   Goldmann, H.; Kleinmann, K.; Snow, M.; Bidus, D.; Korol, B.: Relationship between essential hypertension and cognitive functioning: effect of biofeedback. Psychophysiology *12:* 569–573 (1975).

32   Goldstein, D.S.: Plasma norepinephrine in hypertension. A study of the studies. Hypertension *3:* 48–52 (1981).

33   Green, E.E.; Green, A.M.; Norris, P.A.: Self-regulation training for control of hypertension. Prim. Cardiol. *6:* 126–137 (1980).

34   Hager, J.L.; Surwit, R.S.: Hypertension self-control with a portable feedback unit or meditation-relaxation. Biofeedback Selfregulation *3:* 269–276 (1978).

35   Hallbäck, M.; Folkow, B.: Cardiovascular responses to acute mental 'stress' in spontaneously hypertensive rats. Acta physiol. scand. *90:* 684 (1974).

36   Hamilton, J.A.: Psychophysiology of blood pressure. I. Personality and behavior ratings. Psychosom. Med. *4:* 125–133 (1942).

37   Harburg, E.; Julius, S.; McGinn, N.F.; McLeod, J.; Hoobler, S.W.: Personality traits and behavioral patterns associated with systolic blood pressure levels in college males. J. chron. Dis. *17:* 405–414 (1964).

38   Harburg, E.; Erfurt, J.C.; Hauenstein, L.S.; Chape, C.; Schull, W.J.; Schork, M.A.: Socioecological stress, suppressed hostility, skin color, and black-white male blood pressure: Detroit. Psychosom. Med. *35:* 276–296 (1973).

39   Harris, R.E.; Sokolow, M.; Carpenter, L.G.; Friedman, M.; Hunt, S.: Response to psychologic stress in persons who are potentially hypertensive. Circulation *7:* 874–879 (1953).

40   Henry, J.P.; Ely, D.L.; Stephens, P.M.: The role of psychosocial stimulation in the pathogenesis of hypertension. Verh. dt. Ges. inn. Med. *80:* 1724–1740 (1974).

41   Herd, J.A.; Morse, W.H.; Kelleher, R.T.; Jones, L.G.: Arterial hypertension in the squirrel monkey during behavioral experiments. Am. J. Physiol. *217:* 24–29 (1969).

42   Hokanson, J.E.; Burgess, M.; Cohen, M.F.: Effects of displaced aggression on systolic blood pressure. J. abnorm. Soc. Psychol. *67:* 214 (1963).

43   Hollenberg, N.K.; Williams, G.H.; Adams, D.F.: Essential hypertension: abnormal renal vascular and endocrine responses to a mild psychological stimulus. Hypertension *3:* 11–17 (1981).

44   Jacobson, E.: Variation of blood pressure with skeletal muscle tension and relaxation. Annls intern. Med. *12:* 1194–1212 (1939).

45   Julius, S.: Neurogenic component in borderline hypertension; in Julius, Esler, The nervous system in arterial hypertension, pp. 301–330 (Thomas, Springfield 1976).

46   Julius, S.: Borderline hypertension: epidemiological and clinical implications; in Genest, Koiw, Kuchel, Hypertension, pp. 630–640 (McGraw Hill, New York 1977).

47   Julius, S.: The psychophysiology of borderline hypertension; in Weiner, Hofer, Stunkard, Brain, behavior, and bodily disease, pp. 293–303 (Raven Press, New York 1981).

48   Julius, S.; Conway, J.: Hemodynamic studies in patients with borderline blood pressure elevation. Circulation *38:* 282–288 (1968).

49   Julius, S.; Esler, M.: Autonomic nervous cardiovascular regulations in borderline hypertension. Am. J. Cardiol *36:* 685–696 (1975).

50   Julius, S.; Pascual, A.V.; London, R.: Role of parasympathetic inhibition in the hyperkinetic type of borderline hypertension. Circulation *44:* 413–418 (1971).

51   Julius, S.; Pascual, A.V.; Sannerstedt, R.; Mitchell, C.: Relationship between cardiac output and peripheral resistance in borderline hypertension. Circulation *43:* 382–390 (1971).

52   Kalis, B.L.; Harris, R.E.; Sokolow, M.; Carpenter, L.G., Jr.: Response to psychological stress in patients with essential hypertension. Am. Heart J. *53:* 572–578 (1957).

53   Kristt, D.A.; Engel, B.T.: Learned control of blood pressure in patients with high blood pressure. Circulation *51:* 370–378 (1975).

54   Levy, R.L.; White, P.D.; Stroud, W.D.; Hillman, C.C.: Transient tachycardia: prognostic significance alone and in association with transient hypertension. J. Am. med. Ass. *129:* 585–588 (1945).

55   Light, K.C.; Obrist, P.A.: Cardiovascular reactivity to behavioral stress in young males with and without marginally elevated casual systolic pressures. Comparison of clinic, home, and laboratory measures. Hypertension *2:* 802–808 (1980).

56   Lund-Johansen, P.: Hemodynamics in early essential hypertension. Acata med. scand. suppl. *482,* pp. 1–105 (1967).

57   Nathan, M.A.; Reis, D.J.: Chronic labile hypertension produced by lesions of the nucleus tractus solitarii in the cat. Circulation Res. *40:* 72–81 (1977).

58   Nestel, P.J.: Blood pressure and catecholamine excretion after mental stress in labile hypertension. Lancet *i:* 692–694 (1969).

59   Paffenbarger, R.S., Jr.; Thorne, M.C.; Wing, A.L.: Chronic disease in former college students. VIII. Characteristics in youth predisposing to hypertension in later years. Am. J. Epidemiol. *88:* 25–32 (1968).

60   Patel, C.H.: Twelve-month follow-up of yoga and biofeedback in the management of hypertension. Lancet *i:* 62–65 (1975).

61   Pollak, A.D.; Weber, M.A.; Case, D.B.; Laragh, J.H.: Limitations of transcendental meditation in the treatment of essential hypertension. Lancet *i:* 71–73 (1977).

62   Richter-Heinrich, E.: Psychophysiological personality patterns of hypertensive and normotensive subjects. Psychother. Psychosom. *18:* 332–340 (1970).

63   Safar, M.E.; Weiss, Y.A.; Levenson, J.A.; London, G.M.; Milliez, P.L.: Hemodynamic study of 85 patients with borderline hypertension. Am. J. Cardiol. *31:* 315–319 (1973).

64   Safar, M.E.; Weiss, Y.A.; London, G.M.; Frackowiak, R.F.; Milliez, P.L.: Cardiopulmonary blood volume in borderline hypertension. Clin. Sci. mol. Med. *47:* 153–164 (1974).

65   Safar, M.E.; Kamieniecka, H.A.; Levenson, J.A.; Dimitriu, V.M.; Pauleau, N.F.: Hemodynamic factors and Rorschach testing in borderline and sustained hypertension. Psychosom. Med. *40:* 620–630 (1978).

66   Sannerstedt, R.: Hemodynamic response to exercise in patients with arterial hypertension. Acta med. scand. suppl. 458, pp. 1–83 (1966).

67   Sannerstedt, R.; Julius, S.: Systemic haemodynamics in borderline arterial hypertension: resposne to static exercise before and under the influence of propranolol. Cardiovasc. Res. *6:* 398–403 (1972).

68   Shapiro, A.P.: An experimental study of comparative responses of blood pressure to different noxious stimuli. J. chron. Dis. *13:* 293–311 (1961).

69   Shekelle, R.B.; Schoenberger, J.A.; Stamler, J.: Correlates of the JAS type A behavior pattern score. J. chron. Dis. *29:* 381–394 (1976).

70   Stone, R.A.; DeLeo, J.: Psychotherapeutic control of hypertension. New Engl. J. Med. *294:* 80–84 (1976).

71   Suck, A.F.; Mendlowitz, M.; Wolf, R.L.; Gitlow, S.E.; Naftchi, N.E.: Identification of essential hypertension in patients with labile blood pressure. Chest *59:* 402–406 (1971).

72   Takeshita, A.; Tanaka, S.; Kuroiwa, A.; Nakamura, M.: Reduced baroreceptor sensitivity in borderline hypertension. Circulation *51:* 738–742 (1975).

73   Taylor, C.B.; Farquhar, J.W.; Nelson, E.; Agras, S.: Relaxation therapy and high blood pressure. Archs gen. Psychiat. *34:* 339–342 (1977).

74   Weiss, Y.A.; Safar, M.E.; London, G.M.; Simon, A.C.; Levenson, J.A.; Milliez, P.L.: Repeat hemodynamic determinations in borderline hypertension. Am. J. Med. *64:* 382–387 (1978).

75   Widimsky, J.; Fejfarová, M.H.; Fejfar, Z.: Changes of cardiac output in hypertensive disease. Cardiologia *31:* 381–389 (1957).

18 A Cardiac-Behavioral Approach in the Study of Hypertension[1]

Paul A. Obrist, Alan W. Langer, Kathleen C. Light, John P. Koepke

Our research concerns the significance of the organism-environment interaction (stress, if you like) in the etiology of essential hypertension. This presentation will overview our research strategy, some working hypotheses, and then some recent data from our laboratory [28, 31].

Research Strategy

Our strategy can be most simply labeled as mechanistic and prospective. Mechanistic because our first concern is with the control of the blood pressure (BP) and how these control mechanisms are influenced by life's events. Prospective because we do not study established hypertension but rather possible etiological routes using young adult normotensive humans and in some cases conscious dogs.

This strategy has evolved from the following considerations. The vascular and myocardial events whose interaction controls the BP are subject to numerous extrinsic (neurohumoral) and intrinsic (local) influences [9]. The complexity led *Page and McCubbin* [35] to propose a mosaic model which, among other things, views hypertension as evolving from a number of etiological pathways and events. Thus, hypertension likely is not a condition reflecting a homogenous etiology, anymore than is an elevated body temperature. It is a symptom indicative of some derangement in bodily processes which in time can have serious consequences. But an elevated BP is uninformative of how this symptom evolved and thus of rational ways to prevent or treat it. As a consequence, significant insight into the etiology of hypertension is dependent on deciphering the mechanisms by which the BP is controlled.

[1] Research cited in this paper performed by the authors was supported by Research Grants HL18976, HL23718 and HL24643, National Heart, Lung and Blood Institute.

A prospective strategy is deemed necessary by two considerations. First, hypertension is a progressive condition [35], with its origins likely early in life [23]. In this regard, effective prevention requires early identification. Second, the events that initiate the process may be quite different from those that sustain it [2]. Furthermore, it is conceivable that the significance of behavioral influences may vary as the process progresses, or even may vary among different etiological routes. This implies that efforts to decipher the etiological process retrospectively in cases of established hypertension could prove misleading.

While these considerations argue for a mechanistic prospective strategy, they create problems in light of the complexity of control and the long time span involved in the etiology. These concern questions like, what mechanisms one should focus on, and in what age group and subpopulation should the effort be initiated? It is beyond anyone's grasp to deal with the many potentially relevant etiological routes and it is not practical to deal with too young a population, e.g. children. Also, since only a minority (though still a large number) of individuals will become hypertensive, we need some way to identify subgroups on whom to invest our energies. Guidelines do exist. For example, there is epidemiological evidence that offspring of hypertensive parents are more apt to become hypertensive than offspring of normotensives [14], but this observation has not yet illuminated the etiological process, nor is it a particularly powerful predictor.

In order to provide a focus to facilitate our efforts we have developed some hypotheses, derived from a variety of data, which suggest one etiological route that may be important, while also implicating behavioral events. Furthermore, the hypotheses suggest a subpopulation which may be at risk. These hypotheses shall be discussed next, but first, the following points should be underscored: (1) we are dealing with working hypotheses not articles of faith, and they are thus subject to experimental evaluation. (2) Even if these hypotheses prove relevant in one form or another, they would likely depict only part of the etiological process. (3) These hypotheses deal first with ways in which the BP is controlled. Even if they prove irrelevant to the disease state, their evaluation should shed light on control mechanisms in the behaving organism. (4) Finally, our hypotheses do not deal with the relationship between a disease state and some behavioral dimension like type A-B behavior and coronary heart disease (CHD). Rather, they focus on the interaction of behavior and BP control with the hope that this will ultimately link both to the disease state.

Hypotheses

There are two interrelated hypotheses, both concerned with BP control, which serve as the basis for formulating when elevations of the BP may have pathophysiological significance.

β-Adrenergic Mechanisms. β-Adrenergic refers to the sympathetic receptor sites on the myocardium and in some vascular beds, which upon excitation result in increased heart rate (HR) and cardiac contractility, but vascular dilation. This is in contrast to other sympathetic receptor sites specific to the vasculature which upon excitation result in constriction and are labeled α-adrenergic [44]. This proposes that increased β-adrenergic (sympathetic) excitation of the myocardium can be one of the early stages in the hypertensive process. We are also considering the possibility that such β-adrenergic influences extend to the kidney, and in particular to the renal handling of sodium. Thus, neurogenic influences enter into the control of the BP through their influence on the cardiac output, which can reflect either a direct myocardial effect, or an expansion of plasma volume in the case of sodium retention, or a summation of the two.

Evidence suggesting a direct myocardial mechanism is derived primarily from individuals with marginally elevated BP (borderline hypertension in some parlance), where a certain percentage evidence an elevated cardiac output mediated by increased sympathetic drive [20]. Renal involvement is suggested by the evidence that renin, a kidney hormone involved in the control of sodium balance, is subject to influence by β-adrenergic mechanisms [45]. Renin has also been found to be elevated in individuals with borderline hypertension who evidenced increased β-adrenergic myocardial effects [7], and in siblings of hypertensives who had an impaired excretion of a sodium load (i.e. blunted natriuresis) [14].

Admittedly, such evidence is suggestive at best. For example, marginally elevated BP values only weakly predict a later hypertension [18]. Furthermore, in established hypertension, vascular, not myocardial, influences on the BP are primary [35]. Nonetheless, this evidence serves the purpose of pointing to a potential mechanism which is evident early in adulthood and thus could be a precursor to established hypertension.

Concept of Metabolic Appropriateness. This hypothesis addresses the question of why β-adrenergic mechanisms might serve in this etiological capacity. We propose that this is because they involve cardiovascular and renal adjustments which are excessive relative to metabolic functions and needs [see ref. 43 on disorders of regulation]. For example, an elevated cardiac output in the absence of any appreciable increase in tissue oxygen and nutrient requirements results in tissue overperfusion [37]. This has no immediate life-threatening consequences as would underperfusion, but there is evidence suggesting that the vasculature will eventually autoregulate [15] so as to reduce the excessive blood flow to a more efficient level [5]. Vascular resistance is elevated to accomplish this. In turn, the BP now comes under greater vascular control. There are also other possible vascular complications like structural changes [8] or a decrease in β-adrenergic vasodilatory tone (β-adrenergic blunting) [3] all of which act to increase the resistance to flow.

In the case of the kidney, any retention of sodium which is not metabolically necessitated is an obviously inefficient adjustment in light of the constancy of plasma sodium concentration. A consequence can be plasma volume expansion which, as *Guyton* [15] has proposed, triggers a chain of events ending in an elevated vascular resistance and hence an elevated BP. The elevated pressure in this instance has even been viewed as a means of restoring balance between sodium intake and output (i.e. pressure natriuresis). Furthermore, sodium retention could act directly on the vasculature, either through structural changes or by increasing vascular responsivity to adrenergic excitation [2, 6]. In the words of *Page and McCubbin* [35], we can see the 'mosaic' forming.

With either the myocardium or the kidney, we have a vital organ subject to control by β-adrenergic mechanisms which can modify their response to metabolic requirements in a manner which indicates an exaggerated (in contrast to deficient) adjustment, a consequence of which is an alteration in the control of the BP.

The potential significance of this hypothesis can be seen in another way; this addresses a problem created by the variability (reactivity) of the BP. Available evidence indicates that the BP is quite variable, reaching hypertensive levels at one time or another (i.e. episodically) in most adult humans. This is illustrated best by the large increases in systolic blood pressure (SBP) observed during exercise [4]. But even under less metabolically demanding conditions, appreciable elevations of the BP are encountered in normotensive individuals engaged in their everyday activities [1]. This suggests that the reactivity of the BP per se does not carry unequivocal meaning in regard to the hypertensive process; since, as we have previously indicated, not everyone becomes hypertensive. Also, this ambiguous quality of the BP reactivity to various 'stressful' stimuli has not consistently differentiated normotensives from hypertensives nor has it proven to have much predictive value with regard to the development of hypertension [6, 21, 42, 43]. This situation suggests that there must be individuals for whom a reactivity of the BP is of no consequence, but others where it may be of consequence. No doubt, an understanding of a number of variables would act to clarify matters, such as *Weiner* [43] has suggested with regard to the nature of personal interactions and the experimental climate. One such variable we propose is that the BP reactivity is of significance to the hypertensive process when it involves mechanisms which are indicative of metabolically inappropriate adjustments of the myocardium and kidney. On the other hand, this means that there will be circumstances where a reactivity of the BP and the underlying myocardial and vascular mechanisms are in large part appropriate to the metabolic requirements of a situation. Thus, an elucidation of BP control mechanisms and the metabolic appropriateness of cardiovascular and renal adjustments becomes a requisite for our understanding of the significance of the BP reactivity.

With these hypotheses in mind, we would like to review some data which illustrate our research strategy and bear on this conceptual framework. Keep in mind that this work is concerned not only with these hypotheses but with the question of the significance of behavioral processes, a problem which has not produced uniform agreement or as *Paul* [36, p. 624] has aptly concluded – 'It is not established that repetitive or continuous psychological stress leads to sustained elevations of BP in anyone.'

Data

Our first task has been to demonstrate that behavioral tasks can evoke β-adrenergic influences on the myocardium and kidney as evaluated by pharmacological intervention with neurogenic mechanisms. Our work with myocardial effects, particularly HR, has been the most extensive so far undertaken. Also, this work relates to still other issues; thus we shall discuss this research first.

With the myocardium, an evaluation of neurogenic mechanisms may appear to be proving the obvious, but efforts by behavioral scientists to evaluate neurogenic influences have not been at the forefront of our efforts (much was apparently assumed). Also, when we first began to decipher neurogenic mechanisms, vagal or parasympathetic influences on the myocardium were found to dominate, even mask, sympathetic effects. This was observed with the classical aversive conditioning paradigm [34]. A reasonably conclusive demonstration of β-adrenergic influences was not achieved until we resorted to active coping tasks, like shock avoidance, where β-adrenergic effects were seen both in regard to phasic and tonic myocardial changes (phasic refers to short-term changes, usually encompassing a matter of seconds, in association with discrete stimuli or events such as the anticipatory HR changes seen between conditioned and unconditioned stimuli; tonic refers to more long-term effects, usually encompassing minutes, such as the average HR in each minute of baseline or during some task). The tonic changes proved to be the most robust. Not only were these myocardial effects seen with HR, but also with several different indirect measures of cardiac contractility [13, 29, 30, 32, 33].

The significance of active coping as a behavioral variable is indicated further by contrasting neurogenic influences during shock avoidance to those during passive stressors like the cold pressor. Here, shock avoidance evokes a more appreciable tonic β-adrenergic myocardial effect. But beware – the picture is more complex than this simple active-passive dichotomy implies, as a later discussion of individual differences will indicate.

Our next step was to evaluate tonic BP control under these conditions. We find rather consistent evidence of β-adrenergic myocardial influences on the SBP, an effect consistent with our one hypothesis concerning β-adrenergic influences. However, the picture is more complicated when we consider the diastolic blood pressure (DBP).

Comparing conditions where β-adrenergic influences are maximal (i.e. shock avoidance) to those where they are less pronounced (i.e. cold pressor), the SBP parallels the myocardial effects, while the DBP tends to reverse this relationship. For example, shock avoidance evokes the largest SBP changes, but the smallest DBP effect. β-Adrenergic blockade attenuates the SBP increase but results in a larger DBP effect. In contrast, the cold pressor evokes a smaller SBP but a larger DBP change, while pharmacological β-adrenergic blockade has little effect on either aspect of the BP. In other words, the two aspects of the BP are influenced differentially as a function of the degree of β-adrenergic excitation, which in turn is influenced by certain qualitative differences among conditions.

These results suggest that under conditions of maximal β-adrenergic activation, myocardial control of the BP, particularly the SBP, is more evident. When β-adrenergic influences are less obvious, vascular control of the BP is the most evident. Such an interpretation is consistent with the vasodilatory effects of β-adrenergic excitation. It is also supported by a recent pilot study [25]. Subjects demonstrating the greatest myocardial effects during an active coping task, evidenced after β-adrenergic blockade, the greatest attenuation of both HR and SBP, but the greatest increase in DBP. This latter result also indicates that such subjects have a propensity for greater α-adrenergic mediated vasoconstriction but which is attenuated by increased β-adrenergic vasodilation.

The importance of these observations is that they provide evidence for a behavioral influence on β-adrenergic control of the BP. While the lesser DBP effects might be considered to weaken the relevance of these observations to the hypertensive process, it should be kept in mind that it is not uncommon to find an elevated SBP (i.e. > 140 mm Hg), but a normotensive DBP (< 90 mm Hg) in some young adults considered borderline hypertensive [38]. Also consider that in the hypothesized progression of the hypertensive process, an initial β-adrenergic contribution would be anticipated to have a lesser effect on the DBP, to the extent that it evokes active vasodilatory mechanisms. In time, this influence could weaken for any number of reasons, e.g. intrinsic increases in vascular smooth muscle tone or β-adrenergic blunting.

The evidence cited so far represent only the first steps toward implicating behaviorally evoked β-adrenergic mechanisms in the etiological process. Two other lines of evidence strengthen the significance of myocardial events in this proposed etiological route. First, we find appreciable individual differences in β-adrenergic reactivity. Second, these individual differences are directly related to the incidence of hypertension in the parents of our study subjects.

The establishment of reliable individual differences is a necessary condition for initiating efforts to identify the individual at risk. It is intuitively reasonable to expect that the more reactive individual should be the individual singled out (at least initially) as our future hypertensive. If all subjects reacted in a similar quantitative manner, it would weaken our case that we are dealing with a significant component of the etiological process with our focus on β-adrenergic mechanisms.

There are two aspects of the individual difference data to note [25, 26, 28]. First, they are most appreciable when using a resting baseline obtained after subjects are acclimated to the laboratory environment (this baseline is, in contrast to a resting baseline, obtained when the individual first comes to the laboratory, and just prior to exposure to the stressors; this initial baseline is usually more elevated but to varying degrees among subjects, ranging from no difference to an appreciable difference [28]). The magnitude of the individual differences is illustrated in one study of 56 subjects. Here HR reactivity to shock avoidance averaged 57 bpm in the 14 most reactive subjects (upper quartile) but 9 bpm in the 14 least reactive subjects (lower quartile). As with HR, large individual differences in SBP are observed and they are directly related to the HR effects, i.e. the HR reactor is the SBP reactor. Second, these individual differences extend across a variety of active coping tasks and to a lesser extent to more passive tasks. They are even apparent in the resting state obtained before the individual is acclimated to our procedures. Thus, individual differences appear to be a reasonably stable characteristic of the individual. Subjects characterized as hyperreactors generalize their reactivity to most any novel, challenging or threatening situation. However, the vitality of this phenomenon awaits field studies using more naturalistic conditions.

The relationship between β-adrenergic reactivity and the incidence of hypertension in the parents of our study subjects was evaluated because it would serve in the most direct possible way as a means to ascertain the significance of β-adrenergic mechanisms in the etiological process, short of expensive and time consuming longitudinal studies (this does not deny the significance nor necessity for longitudinal studies; it is premature to launch such efforts until more evidence is available relevant to the working hypotheses; for example, evidence that β-adrenergic hyperreactivity extends to conditions found in every day life, and also involves renal processes would further encourage such an effort). Since hypertension evidences familial trends between parents and offspring (although the basis or mechanisms of such trends are hardly known), it was reasoned that if β-adrenergic reactivity was an early event in the process, then subjects who are characterized as β-adrenergic reactors should more commonly have hypertensive parents.

This anticipated relationship has now been found in five studies. The first and most exhaustive effort [16] demonstrated that subjects having the greatest HR response to a shock avoidance task had a much greater incidence of hypertension among their parents. Follow-up studies using active coping tasks with appetitive incentives (e.g. money) or more realistic life stressors (e.g. preparing a speech), found a similar but usually less pronounced relationship. SBP was also found to relate to parental hypertension but in a less robust manner.

Two other observations derived from these data reinforce the significance of β-adrenergic mechanisms: (1) No relationship has been found between HR and parental history with conditions which evoke a lesser β-adrenergic effect such as the painful cold pressor. (2) Elevations of the casual SBP (i.e. measurements taken under conditions more comparable to clinical assessment procedures such as a BP screening clinic) were found to relate to parental hypertension, primarily in subjects who evidenced greater β-adrenergic reactivity to laboratory procedures like shock avoidance [26]. Note that such casual episodic elevations of the SBP were also found in the laboratory non-reactor, thus, they are not unique to the hyperreactor. The point here is that an episodic elevation of the BP appears to have significance only in those individuals who evidence some propensity to β-adrenergic reactivity. This suggests, as previously discussed, that a reactivity of the BP takes on greater predictability once we begin to obtain insight into control mechanisms. However, a word of caution is necessary. These latter two observations were derived from relatively small samples of subjects, thus replication is essential. Nonetheless, the various aspects of our data involving parental hypertension encourage us to pursue a further evaluation of β-adrenergic mechanisms.

Coincident with these studies using a young adult human population have been experiments with conscious dogs where we have initiated efforts towards evaluating the question of metabolic appropriateness. In the process, we have obtained our first evidence demonstrating stress evoked β-adrenergic influences on the renal handling of sodium. All studies have used as the stressor a shock avoidance task, with treadmill exercise serving as the reference to make a judgment of metabolic appropriateness.

The first study [24] demonstrated that shock avoidance evokes a disproportionate increase in the cardiac output relative to any increase in O_2 consumption (measured by the arteriovenous blood oxygen content difference). This effect is best illustrated by data from one dog where comparable levels of cardiac output were reached during shock avoidance and exercising at 3 mph on a treadmill. Yet the O_2 consumption is noticeably less during shock avoidance and is more like that seen during rest, when the cardiac output is appreciably less. This study did not evaluate β-adrenergic influences on the cardiac output-O_2 relationship. However, under similar conditions in another study they were observed to influence myocardial performance, as evaluated by intraventricular dP/dt and HR [13]. Unfortunately, O_2 consumption was not evaluated. Thus, this piece of the puzzle remains missing.

Two other studies have focused on the kidney. One [12] demonstrated that shock avoidance results in the renal retention of sodium likely through tubular mechanisms. In this study, dogs were first volume loaded with saline, hence increasing their excretion rates. While exercise tended to increase excretion rates further, shock avoidance tended to decrease them. The most pronounced effect was seen in a dog who evidenced similar large HR changes during both conditions (i.e. > 60 bpm), yet exercise *increased* sodium and water excretion while shock avoidance *decreased* it by comparable amounts, i.e. 50%. What is striking in this example is that excretion rates were appreciably increased by the volume loading and still further by exercising, yet a behavioral event like avoidance evokes mechanisms that can overpower this fundamental homeostatic control of plasma volume. The second study [22] has demonstrated the involvement of β-adrenergic mechanisms in the shock avoidance evoked sodium retention, thus suggesting that both the myocardium and kidney are engaged by adrenergic mechanisms undert these conditions.

Studies like these with dogs are now being extended to our young adult human population so that we can evaluate the operation of similar mechanisms. We do have one encouraging lead. In our most recent study using an active coping task, plasma renin was found to be higher in our myocardial reactors. This suggests that humans, like dogs, could be retaining sodium under these conditions. In any case, our results underscore the possibility that β-adrenergic mechanisms can simultaneously disrupt two fundamental metabolic processes, involving the myocardium on one hand, and the kidney on the other. We believe this disruption could prove to be an essential condition in the evolution of cardiovascular pathophysiology.

Postscript

A point was made in the discussion of this paper which questions the validity of one of the mechanisms proposed to be involved in the transition from borderline to established hypertension, namely the role of tissue overperfusion in triggering vascular autoregulation. The evidence cited [19, 27] indicates that borderline hypertensives with an elevated cardiac output also have an elevated O_2 consumption, which would indicate that the elevated cardiac output is metabolically appropriate and thus not a reflection of tissue overperfusion. However, there are other data and considerations which point to the possible significance of this mechanism.

The data stem from observations of a reduction in the arteriovenous oxygen content difference in the presence of an elevated cardiac output. The former is the most direct way we have for assessing overperfusion since when it is reduced it indicates that less O_2 is being extracted. When such a reduction occurs even in the presence of an increase in oxygen consumption, this is suggestive of overperfusion. One should be mindful of the observation that during exercise, the increases in oxygen consumption and cardiac output are accompanied by increases in the arteriovenous oxygen difference [4]. Our work with conscious dogs [24] illustrates the point. While shock avoidance increased both the cardiac output and O_2 consumption, the arteriovenous oxygen difference was more comparable to the resting state. A similar effect has also been reported in humans when comparing individuals with normal to those with an elevated resting state cardiac output. For example, *Stead* et al. [41] observed in the subgroup with an elevated cardiac output, a 23% higher O_2 consumption but a 33% smaller arteriovenous O_2 content difference. An even more dramatic effect was reported by *Gorlin* et al. [11] who observed in the presence of an elevated cardiac output a 17% increase in O_2 consumption but a 60% reduction in the arteriovenous O_2 content difference. While the focus of these studies was not on borderline hypertension, an elevated SBP (i.e. > 140 mm Hg) was commonly reported. Also considering that these were resting state values obtained in individuals usually less than 30 years of age, there seems reason to believe that in principle, we are dealing with 'borderline' hypertension and no differently than in the studies purporting to demonstrate a metabolically appropriate cardiac output [27]. Also even in these latter efforts there is evidence that the arteriovenous O_2 content difference is slightly less than in normotensive controls [39, 40]. Thus, even these data suggest a mildly metabolically inappropriate adjustment in these populations of borderline hypertensives although not one of sufficient magnitude to suggest any significant degree of overperfusion. It is even possible that some resting state conditions fail to provide a situation where overperfusion would be particularly evident since the elevation of cardiac output when encountered are usually rather small, i.e. $< 10\%$ [17]. A more appropriate condition would be one where appreciable increases in β-adrenergic excitation are encountered such as we have observed in our hyperresponders. Remember in this case that during shock avoidance the average increase in HR in the more responsive subjects approaches 100% of the resting value. Of course, not having as yet measured the cardiac output or the O_2 consumption, we cannot claim to have demonstrated overperfusion. However, this likelihood is suggested by a report of *Gliner* et al. [10] that stress-induced increases in cardiac output parallel increased HR under conditions where there is likely minimal increases in oxygen consumption.

Finally, it should be kept in mind that studies such as those of *Julius* [17] which evaluate hemodynamics in borderline hypertension use a strategy which differs from ours in at least one significant way. This is that they select subjects on the basis of their BP regardless of the hemodynamic process and find for example that only a certain percentage (commonly less than half) evidence an elevated cardiac output. It is not surprising, therefore, that evidence for a disruption of the cardiac output, O_2 consumption relationship is not a particularly robust effect.

In summary, this issue is subject to experimental evaluation and there is sufficient evidence to warrant at least an exploration of the problem. Even then, should we fail to demonstrate what appears to be tissue overperfusion, it does not close the books on the significance of β-adrenergic mechanisms since their influence could be manifested with still other transition processes like sodium retention.

References

1   Bevan, A.T.; Honour, A.J.; Stott, F.H.: Direct arterial pressure recording in unrestricted man. Clin. Sci. *36:* 329–344 (1969).
2   Brown, J.J.; Fraser, R.; Lever, A.F.; Morton, J.J.; Robertson, J.I.S.; Schalekamp, M.A.D.H.: Mechanisms in hypertension: a personal view; in Genest, Koiw, Kuchel, Hypertension: physiopathology and treatment, pp. 529–548 (McGraw-Hill, New York 1977).
3   Buhler, F.R.; Kiowski, W.; Brummelen, P. van; Amann, F.W.; Bertel, O.; Landmann, R.: Plasma catecholamines and cardiac renal and peripheral vascular adrenoceptor-mediated responses in different age groups of normal and hypertensive subjects. Clin. exp. Hypertens. *2:* 409–426 (1980).
4   Carlsten, A.; Grimby, G.: The circulatory response to muscular exercise in man (Thomas, Springfield 1966).
5   Coleman, T.G.; Samar, R.C.; Murphy, W.R.: Autoregulation versus other vasoconstrictors in hypertension: a critical review. Hypertension *1:* 324–330 (1979).
6   Doyle, A.E.; Mendelsohn, F.A.O.; Morgan, T.O.: Pharmacological and therapeutic aspects of hypertension, vol. 2 (CRC Press, Boca Raton 1980).
7   Esler, M.; Julius, S.; Zweifler, A.; Randall, O.; Gardiner, H.; DeQuattro, V.: Mild high-renin essential hypertension – neurogenic hypertension. New Engl. J. Med. *296:* 405–411 (1977).
8   Folkow, B.U.B.; Hallback, M.I.L.; Lundgren, Y.; Sivertsson, R.; Weiss, L.: Importance of adaptive changes in vascular design for establishment of primary hypertension, studies in man and in spontaneously hypertensive rat. Circulation Res. *32/33:* suppl., pp. I-2–I-16 (1973).
9   Frohlich, E.D.: Hemodynamics of hypertension; in Genest, Koiw, Kuchel, Hypertension: physiopathology and treatment, pp. 15–49 (McGraw-Hill, New York 1977).
10 Gliner, J.A.; Bedi, J.F.; Horvath, S.M.: Somatic and non-somatic influences on the heart: hemodynamic changes. Psychophysiology *16:* 358–362 (1979).
11 Gorlin, R.; Brachfeld, N.; Turner, J.D.; Messer, J.V.; Salazar, E.: The idiopathic high cardiac output state. J. clin. Invest. *38:* 2144–2153 (1959).

12   Grignolo, A.; Koepke, J.P.; Obrist, P.A.: Renal function, heart rate and blood pressure during exercise and shock avoidance in dogs. Am. J. Physiol. R. *242:* R482–R490 (1982).

13   Grignolo, A.; Light, K.C.; Obrist, P.A.: Beta-adrenergic influences on cardiac dynamics during shock-avoidance in dogs. Pharmacol. Biochem. Behav. *14:* 313–319 (1981).

14   Grim, C.E.; Luft, F.C.; Miller, J.Z.; Rose, R.J.; Christian, J.C.; Weinberger, M.H.: An approach to the evaluation of genetic influences on factors that regulate arterial blood pressure in man. Hypertension *2:* I-34–I-42 (1980).

15   Guyton, A.C.: Arterial blood pressure and hypertension (Saunders, Philadelphia 1980).

16   Hastrup, J.L.; Light, K.C.; Obrist, P.A.: Parental hypertension and cardiovascular response to stress in healthy young adults. Psychophysiology *19:* 615–622 (1982).

17   Julius, S.: Neurogenic component in borderline hypertension; in Julius, Esler, The nervous system in arterial hypertension, pp. 301–330 (Thomas, Springfield 1976).

18   Julius, S.: Borderline hypertension: epidemiologic and clinical implications; in Genest, Koiw, Kuchel, Hypertension: physiopathology and treatment, pp. 630–640 (McGraw-Hill, New York 1977).

19   Julius, S.; Conway, J.: Hemodynamic studies in patients with borderline blood pressure elevation. Circulation *38:* 282–288 (1968).

20   Julius, S.; Esler, M.D.: Autonomic nervous cardiovascular regulation in borderline hypertension. Am. J. Cardiol. *36:* 685–696 (1975).

21   Julius, S.; Schork, M.A.: Borderline hypertension: a critical review. J. chron. Dis. *23:* 723–754 (1971).

22   Koepke, J.P.; Grignolo, A.; Obrist, P.A.: Decreased urine and sodium excretion rates during signaled shock avoidance in dogs: role of beta-adrenergic receptors (Abstract). Fed. Proc. *40:* 553 (1981).

23   Kuller, L.H.; Crook, M.; Almes, M.J.; Detre, K.; Reese, G.; Rutan, R.: Dormont High School (Pittsburg, Pennsylvania) Blood Pressure Study. Hypertension *2:* I-109–I-116 (1980).

24   Langer, A.W.; Obrist, P.A.; McCubbin, J.A.: Hemodynamic and metabolic adjustments during exercise and shock avoidance in dogs. Am. J. Physiol. Heart circulat. Physiol. *5:* H225–H230 (1979).

25   Light, K.C.: Cardiovascular responses to effortful active coping: implications for the role of stress in hypertension development. Psychophysiology *18:* 216–225 (1981).

26   Light, K.C.; Obrist, P.A.: Cardiovascular reactivity to behavioral stress in young males with and without marginally elevated systolic pressure: a comparison of clinic, home and laboratory measures. Hypertension *2:* 802–808 (1980).

27   Lund-Johansen, P.: Hemodynamic alterations in essential hypertension; in Onesti, Kim, Moyer, Hypertension: mechanisms and management, pp. 43–50 (Grune & Stratton, New York 1973).

28   Obrist, P.A.: Cardiovascular psychophysiology – a perspective, pp. 237 (Plenum Publishing, New York 1981).

29   Obrist, P.A.; Gaebelein, C.J.; Teller, E.; Langer, A.W.; Grignolo, A.; Light, K.C.; McCubbin, J.A.: The relationship between heart rate, carotid dP/dt, and blood pressure in humans as a function of the type of stress. Psychophysiology *15:* 102–115 (1978).

30   Obrist, P.A.; Howard, J.L.; Lawler, J.E.; Sutterer, J.R.; Smithson, K.W.; Martin, P.L.: Alterations in cardiac contractility during classical aversive conditioning in dogs: methodological and theoretical implications. Psychophysiology *9:* 246–261 (1972).

31   Obrist, P.A.; Light, K.C.; Langer, A.W.; Koepke, J.P.: Psychosomatics; in Coles, Donchin,

Porges, Psychophysiology: systems, processes and applications (Guilford, New York, in press, 1983).

32 Obrist, P.A.; Lawler, J.E.; Howard, J.L.; Smithson, K.W.; Martin, P.L.; Manning, J.: Sympathetic influences on the heart in humans: effects on contractility and heart rate of acute stress. Psychophysiology *11:* 405–427 (1974).

33 Obrist, P.A.; Light, K.C.; McCubbin, J.A.; Hoffer, J.L.: Pulse transit time: relationship to blood pressure and myocardial performance. Psychophysiology *16:* 292–301 (1979).

34 Obrist, P.A.; Wood, D.M.; Perez-Reyes, M.: Heart rate during conditioning in humans: effects of UCS intensity, vagal blockade, and adrenergic block of vasomotor activity. J. exp. Psychol. *70:* 32–42 (1965).

35 Page, I.H.; McCubbin, J.W.: The physiology of arterial hypertension; in Hamilton, Dow, Handbook of physiology: circulation, vol. I, sect. 2, pp. 2163–2208 (Am. Physiological Society, Washington 1966).

36 Paul, O.: Epidemiology of hypertension; in Genest, Koiw, Kuchel, Hypertension: physiopathology and treatment, pp. 613–629 (McGraw-Hill, New York 1977).

37 Peart, W.S.: Personal views on mechanisms of hypertension; in Genest, Koiw, Kuchel, Hypertension: physiopathology and treatment, pp. 588–597 (McGraw-Hill, New York 1977).

38 Safar, M.E.; Weiss, Y.A.; Levenson, J.A.; London, G.M.; Milliez, P.L.: Hemodynamic study of 85 patients with borderline hypertension. Am. J. Cardiol. *31:* 315–319 (1973).

39 Sannerstedt, R.: Hemodynamic response to exercise in patients with arterial hypertension. Acta med. scand., suppl. 458, pp. 1–83 (1966).

40 Sannerstedt, R.: Hemodynamic findings at rest and during exercise in mild arterial hypertension. Am. J. med. Sci. *258:* 70–79 (1969).

41 Stead, E.A.; Warren, J.V.; Merrill, A.J.; Brannon, E.S.: The cardiac output in male subjects as measured by the technique of arterial catherization. Normal values with observations on the effects of anxiety and tilting. J. clin. Invest. *24:* 326–331 (1945).

42 Weiner, H.: Psychosomatic research in essential hypertension; in Koster, Musaph, Viser, Psychosomatics in essential hypertension. Biblthca psychiat., No. 144, pp. 58–115 (Karger, Basel 1970).

43 Weiner, H.: Psychobiology and human disease (Elsevier, New York 1977).

44 Weiner, N.: Norepinephrine, epinephrine and the sympathomimetic amines; in Goodman, Goodman, Gilman, The pharmacological basis of therapeutics, pp. 138–175 (McMillan, New York 1980).

45 Zanchetti, A.; Bartorelli, C.: Central nervous mechanisms in arterial hypertension: experimental and clinical evidence; in Genest, Koiw, Kuchel, Hypertension: physiopathology and treatment, pp. 59–75 (McGraw-Hill, New York 1977).

19 Behavior, Autonomic Function and Animal Models of Cardiovascular Pathology

Neil Schneiderman

Emotional behavior and environmental stress as well as hereditary and constitutional factors have been implicated in the pathogenesis of essential hypertension and coronary heart disease (CHD) in humans. Personality variables such as chronically suppressed anger, resentment and fear have been related to the development of essential hypertension [4, 58, 226] as have situational variables such as occupational stress [32] and living in a stressful residential neighborhood [111]. Similarly, personality variables such as aggressiveness, impatient irritability, and potential for hostility appear to be characteristic of the type A coronary-prone behavior pattern, which has been established as a potential risk factor for CHD [220]. CHD has also been related to behaviorally stressful life events [209].

Although both essential hypertension and CHD generally appear to have a multicausal basis, the psychosocial factors associated with each seem to involve the type of struggles that are likely to mobilize the sympathetic nervous system (SNS) chronically or at least more often than in less stressed individuals. Moreover, experimental evidence indicates that under controlled laboratory conditions type A coronary-prone individuals respond with greater cardiovascular and/or catecholamine changes to behavioral challenges than do type B persons [44, 89]. Although more controversial, there is also at least some evidence that hypertensives may respond with greater blood pressure (BP) elevations to environmental stressors such as the cold pressor test than do normotensives [57, 129].

While it is important to examine physiologic reactivity and autonomic nervous system functioning in experiments conducted upon human subjects, and it is valuable to correlate psychologic functioning with hypertension and CHD in retrospective and prospective studies, it would be unethical deliberately to induce such pathology by experimental means in humans. Cause-effect relationships, however, can be established between emotional behavior and cardiovascular pathology by resorting to animal experimentation. Such experimentation can also provide a vehicle for studying how presumed pathophysiological mechanisms might mediate relationships between behavior and cardiovascular pathology. Animal research has indicated that behavioral variables can induce hypertension and cause cardiovascular pathology. It has provided evidence that behavioral factors can accelerate the development of atherosclerosis, and under appropriate circumstances can lead to fatal arrhythmias. Animal research has also provided important clues concerning possible pathophysiologic mechanisms that may mediate relationships between behavior and cardiovascular pathology. Particularly salient in these studies has been the role of the autonomic nervous system as a putative mediator. In this chapter we shall first describe some aspects of the neural and hormonal control of the circulation. This will be followed by a brief discussion of cardiovascular functioning during aversive situations. We shall then describe the presumed role of the sympathoadrenomedullary axis in the development of hypertension and CHD before specifically describing animal experiments relating animal behavior to hypertension, arteriosclerosis, stress-induced cardiomyopathy and lethal arrhythmias. The chapter concludes with a discussion of possible relationships that may exist among psychologic processes, physiologic reactions, and the specificity of cardiovascular pathology.

Neural and Hormonal Control of the Circulation

The heart and vasculature are innervated by the secretions of the autonomic nervous system (ANS), which in turn are under the control of the central nervous system (CNS). Autonomic control of the circulation involves: (a) intrinsic detector (afferent) neurons that provide information to the CNS concerning the state of the heart, blood, and vasculature; (b) the CNS, which processes this information and integrates it with other relevant information derived from both the internal milieu and from the external environment, and (c) effector neurons of the parasympathetic nervous system and the effectors of the sympathoadrenomedullary axis that innervate the heart and vasculature.

Peripheral Autonomic Regulation. Intrinsic cardiovascular adjustments originate in the responses of chemoreceptors and mechanoreceptors located within the circulatory system. Information about respiratory performance is provided by arterial chemoreceptors located in the aortic and carotid bodies. Information about mean pressure and about changes in pressure occurring in different parts of the cardiovascular system are provided by arterial, pulmonary, atrial, and ventricular mechanoreceptors. Mechanoreceptors sensitive to arterial pressure are known as baroreceptors. Major groups of these stretch receptors lie within the walls of the carotid sinus and aortic arch, although some receptors are located along the thoracic aorta as well as along the subclavian, common carotid, and mesenteric arteries [96].

An increase in baroreceptor stimulation leads to a pronounced reflexive decrease in heart rate (HR) and a diminution in BP unless the reflex is gated within the CNS. The reflexive bradycardia or slowing of HR is mediated by the cardiac branches of the vagus nerves. Systemic injections of atropine methylnitrate that blockade the cholinergic innervation of the vagus nerves at the heart, and thereby abolish the bradycardia, do not eliminate the reflexive, systemic hypotension. This suggests that the diminution in pressure is largely due to an inhibition of vasoconstrictor activity. Although a considerable amount of research has focused upon the role of the systemic arterial baroreceptors in neural control of the circulation, mechanoreceptors in the heart and pulmonary circulation are also important, participating in the control of HR, arterial pressure, renin release, plasma volume, and vascular resistance.

At one time the arterial baroreceptor reflex was conceptualized as a simple pressure regulator that minimized generallized disturbances of the circulation [145]. More recent formulations have emphasized that it is the interaction of the intrinsic baroreceptor and chemoreceptor inputs with those of extrinsic influences impacting upon the CNS that determine the neural control of the systemic circulation [146].

The efferent pathways involved in the neural control of the circulation include ANS ganglionic transmission as well as sympathetic and parasympathetic effector activity. Although cholinergic nicotinic receptors predominate in ganglionic transmission, autonomic ganglia also contain muscarinic (cholinergic), α- and β-adrenergic, and histaminergic receptors capable of modulating ganglionic transmission. Sympathetic (β-adrenergic) and parasympathetic influences upon the heart play an important role in regulating HR and cardiac output, whereas sympathetic influences upon the blood vessels are reflected in vasomotor tone. Although α-adrenergic mediation of vasoconstrictor tone plays a preeminent role in regulating vasomotor tone, neurogenic vasodilator mechanisms including sympathetic cholinergic [254], dopaminergic [194], histaminergic [204], β-adrenergic [258], and sustained dilator [13] influences are also important.

The cells of origin of the sympathetic (thoracolumbar) division of the ANS are situated in the intermediolateral cell column in the lateral horns of the thoracic and upper lumbar segments of the spinal cord. First-order neurons synapse at sympathetic ganglia; second-order neurons innervate target organs. The cells of the adrenal medulla are actually specialized postganglionic sympathetic neurons. Whereas the other secondary neurons of the sympathetic division release their transmitter, usually norepinephrine, at neuromuscular junctions, the adrenal chromaffin cells release both norepinephrine and epinephrine into the circulatory system, which distributes these neurosecretions throughout the body.

The concept of α- and β-adrenergic receptors was originally proposed by *Ahlquist* [3]. Although subclassifications have been added, the basic formulation has remained useful. Vasoconstrictor effects of catecholamines are mediated via α-adrenergic receptors at the arterioles. α-adrenergic receptors are selectively blocked by drugs such as phentolamine, and are powerfully activated by norepinephrine. In contrast, the chronotropic (ventricular rate) effects of catecholamines at the heart are mediated by β-adrenergic receptors and are blocked by drugs such as propranolol. Epinephrine has a more powerful effect in activating the β-receptors of the heart than does norepinephrine.

The heart is sympathetically innervated by the cardiac accelerator nerves, which liberate norepinephrine. This neuronal innervation occurs primarily at the S-A node and the A-V node with some additional innervation also occurring at the ventricles. Recent work [9] has determined, however, that the β-adrenoceptors are not distributed in the same manner as the noradrenergic innervation of the heart by the cardiac accelerator nerves. Thus, the ratio of receptors of endogenous norepinephrine in the dog and rat heart was found to be almost 6 times higher in the left ventricle, which is only minimally innervated neuronally than in the maximally innervated right atrium. *Baker and Potter* [9] therefore concluded that most cardiac adrenoceptors are not at nerve endings, but are localized where they can respond optimally to circulating epinephrine, the distribution of adrenoceptors being similar to that of the coronary blood flow. They also found that circulating levels of norepinephrine rarely appraoch concentrations likely to influence most cardiac adrenoceptors.

Most experimental evidence is consistent with the view that adrenoreceptors at nerve endings in the heart are preferentially activated by neurally released norepinephrine during tasks such as exercise [47], and that the increases in plasma norepinephrine during exercise also reflect the release of norepinephrine at nerve endings innervating vasoconstrictors. In contrast, during life-threatening situations (e.g. hemorrhage, severe acidosis, hypogly-cemia, hypoxia, and the discharge of pheochromocytomas) circulating plasma levels of epinephrine reach concentrations that are adequate for this catecholamine to activate β-adrenoceptors throughout the heart. Some forms of psychological stress involving harassment [89] as well as smoking [259] also result in the preferential release of epinephrine.

Thus far, we have seen that the sympathetic division of the ANS exerts important effects upon the functioning of the heart and blood vessels. By influencing cardiac output and peripheral resistance, the sympathetic division exerts important effects upon BP and upon the overall state of the circulation. A third important variable influencing BP is plasma volume, and this, too, is importantly influenced by sympathetic activity.

Decrease in effective circulating blood volume, in part detected as a decrease in arterial pressure by vascular baroreceptors in the renal arteriolar wall, leads to a decrease in sodium excretion, which is in part mediated through direct effects of renal adrenergic nerves on proximal reabsorption of sodium [88]. Diminished renal perfusion also leads to the secretion of renin from the juxtaglomerular cells. Renin secretion is increased when endogenous sympathetic activity increases, and decreased when sympathetic activity decreases. Direct catecholamine effect upon the juxtaglomerular cells is mediated via stimulation of β-adrenergic receptors and involves the formation of cyclic AMP [216].

The enzyme, renin, acts on angiotensinogen, a plasma protein, to form angiotensin. Angiotensin, in turn, accelerates the release of aldosterone from the adrenal cortex, which then stimulates sodium reabsorption by the renal tubules. The sodium that is actively reabsorbed is accompanied by water. Increases in water retention increase effective blood volume thereby serving as negative feedback, turning off the renin-angiotensin-aldosterone system.

The efferent fibres of the cranial portion of the parasympathetic (craniosacral) division of the ANS supply the head and viscera as well as the heart. In contrast, fibres of the sacral division supply the genitalia, bladder and large bowel. The vascular beds of skin and skeletal muscle are not innervated by the parasympathetic division. The parasympathetic innervation of the heart occurs via the cardiac branch of the vagus nerves. Most of the cardiac ganglion cells are located near the S-A node and A-V conduction tissue. The influence of vagus nerve activity on the heart can be quite powerful. Even during strong sympathetic activation, concomitant activation of the parasympathetic outflow to the heart results in bradycardia [205].

Central Autonomic Regulation. The involvement of the CNS in cardio-vascular regulation has been under scrutiny since *Bernard* [16] transected the spinal cord and observed a marked fall in BP. Subsequently, *Owsjannikow* [195] and *Dittmar* [48] implicated the brain stem in BP regulation. Research since then has suggested that central regulation of the cardiovascular system involves neuronal integration at virtually every level of the CNS from the neocortex to the spinal cord.

In recent years the recognition that several antihypertensive drugs, including clonidine [229], α-methyldopa [117], and propranolol [159] may act principally through their actions on the CNS, and that the benzodiazepines can dampen the circulatory as well as behavioral effects of stressful emotional stimuli [31], has provided one focus for research interest into CNS control of the circulation. Several investigators, for example, have argued that the hypotensive effect of propranolol may be due to central β-adrenergic blockade [41, 159]. A major rationale for this view is that while the major peripheral action of propranolol is β-adrenergic blockade of the heart result-ing in a decrease in pulse rate and cardiac output, the reduction in BP requires days to weeks of chronic drug administration [247]. In support of the CNS mediation hypothesis, *Lewis* [159] showed that intracerebroventricular administration of propranolol in conscious rabbits resulted in decreased sym-pathetic splanchic nerve activity and hypotension.

Clonidine is another antihypertensive drug that has both central and peripheral effects. In both cat and rat, for instance, clonidine stimulates cen-tral and peripheral α-adrenergic receptors [144]. The peripheral effects of clonidine, however, cannot account for its potent antihypertensive effects. *Chan and Koo* [29b] and *Chen and Chan* [30] claim to have localized an area in the medial medullary reticular formation of rats and cats, which appears to be necessary for the effects of clonidine to occur. In addition to this region, the nucleus tract of solitarius in the medulla, the ventral surface of the lower brain stem, and the anterior hypothalamus have also been implicated in the hypotensive effects of clonidine.

Microinjection of clonidine or norepinephrine into the anterior hypo-thalamus produces a depressor response and bradycardia. The effects are mediated by α-receptors since localized prior injection of phentolamine abolishes the depressor and bradycardia effects induced by norepinephrine or clonidine [256]. Transection experiments, however, have localized the site of clonidine's action upon tonic levels of BP to the medulla [230]. Present evidence suggests that the α-adrenergic action of clonidine upon the anterior hypothalamus, and perhaps also the nucleus tract of solitarius, is to facilitate phasic depressor and bradycardia adjustments including the baroreceptor reflex.

In addition to the search for CNS sites involved in the action of antihypertensive drugs, research interest has long focused upon the role of the CNS in circulatory adjustments that occur during behavior. One important pathway, originating in the frontal cortex, is responsible for the sympathetically mediated vasodilation occurring in skeletal muscle during exercise [71, 128]. Another pathway, linked to the amygdala and hypothalamus, is involved in the increases in HR, cardiac output, vasodilation in skeletal muscle, and vasocontriction in the viscera during fight-or-flight reactions [1]. Still a third pathway, which also has been linked to the hypothalamus, is involved in the elaboration of depressor and bradycardia responses [136].

The functional organization of the hypothalamus with regard to cardiovascular responses and behaviors elicited by intracranial stimulation show important differences among species. *Hess* [125], for instance, provided evidence that the autonomic and behavioral mechanisms involving the feline hypothalamus are organized into an anterior 'trophotropic' zone concerned with parasympathetic related functions and a posterior 'ergotropic' zone concerned with emergency functions such as defensive threat and escape behavior, which involve the mobilization of the SNS. In contrast, *Ban* [10] provided evidence that the rabbit hypothalamus reveals a mediolateral functional organization with regard to circulatory and behavioral responses to intracranial stimulation. Thus, the medial hypothalamus mediates sympathetic and the lateral hypothalamus mediates parasympathetic activity.

Recent experiments in my laboratory have confirmed and expanded *Ban's* [10] formulation of a mediolateral functional organization of the rabbit hypothalamus with regard to cardiovascular responses and behavior. In one study, for example, we found that microstimulation of the medial hypothalamus, particularly the ventromedial hypothalamic nucleus elicited tachycardia and a pressor response associated with circling movements, hind-limb thumping and other responses usually associated with aggressive behavior [86]. In contrast, stimulation of an intermediate zone, including the anterior and posterior hypothalamus, elicited pronounced primary bradycardia (nonreflexive) and a pressor response as well as other manifestations of sympathetic arousal (e.g. pupil dilation). The animals tended to show behavioral immobility except for rather slow, orienting-like movements of the head. A third pattern of responses, identified by microstimulation of the lateral hypo-thalamus elicited profound bradycardia, a small depressor response and quiet inactivity.

Several experiments in my laboratory using intracranial stimulation, coagulative lesions, horseradish peroxidase histochemistry and extracellular single unit recording techniques have indicated that the bradycardia elicited by stimulation of the lateral hypothalamus involves a pathway originating at least as far rostrally as the central nucleus of the amygdala [86]. This path-way descends polysynaptically through the lateral hypothalamus, lateral zona incerta of the caudal diencephalon [141], parabrachial nucleus [106], and cardioinhibitory vagal preganglionic motoneurons in the medulla [161, 233].

Of considerable importance in our research has been the finding that stimulation of the ventromedial hypothalamus in rabbits produces a pressor response and tachycardia, whereas stimulation of the anterior and posterior hypothalamus produces a pressor response and bradycardia. In both instances the animals are clearly aroused sympathetically. In the former case stimulation of the ventromedial hypothalamus inhibits vagal cardioinhibi-tory motoneurons [134]; whereas in the latter case stimulation of the anterior hypothalamus activates vagal cardioinhibitory motoneurons [262].

In preliminary work we have also observed that stimulation of the ven-tromedial hypothalamus in the rabbit leads to increases in serum catechol-amines, and damage to the endothelium of the aorta, which is observable via the electron microscope. These findings are consistent with results reported by Soviet investigators. *Sudakov and Yumatov* [245], for example, found that stimulation of the ventromedial hypothalamus of rabbits produced a pressor response and an increase in plasma epinephrine that was abolished by adrenalectomy. In another study *Ulyaninsky* et al. [253] found that intermit-tent electrical stimulation of the ventromedial hypothalamus in rabbits for up to 2 weeks elicited cardiac arrhythmias (atrial fibrillation, ventricular extrasystoles, and ventricular fibrillation) associated with increased catechol-amine content in the blood and myocardium. On the initial day of stimula-tion 5 of 43 experimental animals went into ventricular fibrillation and died. Fibrillation was preceded by ventricular extrasystoles in 4 of 5 rabbits. The fifth animal did not have a prodromal arrhythmia prior to ventricular fibrilla-tion. In rabbits in which stimulation of the hypothalamus resulted in pro-nounced rhythm disorders, the ultrastructure of the myocardial cells exhibited foci of hypercontraction. There was also obvious swelling and destruction of the mitochondria as well as the presence of lipid droplets.

Cardiovascular Functioning during Aversive Situations

Just as the experiments in my laboratory have indicated that two separate patterns of autonomically mediated cardiovascular responses are associated with sympathetic activation, the same division of cardiovascular responses can be shown to occur during aversive animal behavior experiments, a finding which holds both across species and across experimental situations. This finding is consistent with *Hilton's* [127] observations that (a) the CNS is organized to produce integrated patterns of response rather than changes in single, isolated variables, and (b) the repertoire of patterned cardiovascular responses is very small, thus facilitating the job of examining the neuraxis for pathways mediating these patterns.

The animal behavior literature indicates that mammals confronted with an aversive situation generally tend to reveal one pattern of autonomic activity if fight, flight or other appropriate active coping responses are being attempted, but another pattern if active coping responses seem unavailable. The former pattern, sometimes referred to as the defense reaction was described in the previous section [1, 27, 49, 125]. It is characterized by increased movement, HR, cardiac output, and vasodilation in skeletal muscle. The second pattern, which occurs in aversive situations in which an active coping response does not seem available, is characterized by extreme vigilance, an inhibition of movement, an increase in SNS activity, but also a vagally mediated decrease in HR [260]. Examples of the two patterns of response, one associated with active coping and the other with anticipation of an aversive situation, have both been described within individual experiments [2, 7, 8, 155].

Anderson and Tosheff [7], for instance, examined the cardiovascular responses of dogs during daily 1-hour sessions of unsignaled shock-avoidance as well as during the 1 h preceding the avoidance task when the animals were kept in a restraint harness within the experimental chamber. In terms of the coping versus noncoping distinction, the avoidance situation is one in which the performance of the avoidance response can be conceptualized as the utilization of a coping mechanism. Briefly, *Anderson and Tosheff* [7] found that placing their dogs in a restraint harness for a 1-hour period immediately preceding the avoidance contingency was associated with a preparatory cardiovascular response pattern consisting of a progressive increase in total peripheral resistance and arterial pressure accompanied by progressive decreases in HR and cardiac output. In contrast, once the avoidance contingency was initiated, HR, and cardiac output increased substantially accompanied by a further increase in BP.

In similar fashion differences in cardiovascular response patterns have been described in cats before and during confrontation with other animals [2, 8]. In general, preparation for fighting was associated with bradycardia, decreased cardiac output, hind-limb vasoconstriction and increased peripheral resistance. Conversely, during actual fighting, HR, cardiac output and hind-limb blood flow increased, whereas total peripheral resistance decreased.

Although the basic distinction between the two patterns of cardiovascular responses associated with two classes of behavioral contingency seems fairly robust, it should be kept in mind that the responses may change somewhat over time as a function of autoregulation, neuronal and hormonal processes.

At the outset of avoidance conditioning, uncertainty is greatest, the animal is shocked most often, and cardiovascular responsiveness is usually greatest. Forsyth [72], for example, exposed rhesus monkeys to different variations of an unsignaled avoidance procedure for 15 daily sessions. All of the groups initially showed increases in HR and BP, but over the course of the experiment, BP and HR declined in all groups except the one placed on the longest (16 h/day), most stringent (5-second shock-shock interval) schedule. Similarly, during signal avoidance conditioning in the dog, *Lawler* et al. [154] measured the effective refractory period of the dog heart at different stages of conditioning. They found that the effective refractory period was decreased significantly at avoidance onset during the first 5 avoidance sessions, but was unaltered during the next 5 sessions. Decreases in effective refractory period were most pronounced during the first session; the decrease was similar to that reported during stellate ganglion stimulation of catecholamine infusion [109].

During the early stages of unsignaled conditioning dogs or monkeys engaged in an unsignaled avoidance task typically reveal an increase in systemic arterial pressure that is associated with an increase in HR and cardiac output but a decrease in total peripheral resistance [7, 74]. *Forsyth* [74], however, found that if his monkeys were subjected to a prolonged avoidance session (24–72 h), the increase in BP became associated with an increase in total peripheral resistance. Besides examining the determinants of BP, he examined regional blood flow using a radioactive microsphere injection technique. Injections made 20 min after the onset of training revealed a large increase in blood flow to the heart, liver, and skeletal muscle, but a decrease in flow to the kidney. In contrast, an injection of microspheres made after 72 successive hours of avoidance conditioning revealed increased blood flow to the heart, spleen, pancreas, and liver at the expense of the kidneys, skeletal muscle, and gastrointestinal organs. The increased resistance in skeletal muscle was the predominant contributor to the increase in total peripheral resistance. Interestingly, when rhesus monkeys in an earlier experiment were subjected to a 72-hour unsignaled avoidance session, marked elevations in urinary epinephrine occurred during the first 24 h, then progressively declined; norepinephrine levels increased modestly during the avoidance session [169].

In summary, the behavioral data suggest that during aversive situations in which fight, flight or coping takes place, mammals are likely to show increases in HR, cardiac output, BP, and vasodilation in skeletal muscle, which closely resemble the defensive reaction. In contrast, during aversive situations in which fight, flight, or active coping does not occur, animals are likely to show a decrease in HR and cardiac output associated with an increase in peripheral resistance and in BP. Although the cardiovascular changes have been linked to autonomic activity, and to the liberation of peripheral catecholamines, fine grain analyses relating neuronal and hormonal activities to intensity, duration, and kind of behavioral situation are clearly needed.

Sympathoadrenomedullary Hypotheses of Cardiovascular Pathology

The sympathoadrenomedullary axis plays an important role in increasing metabolic and cardiovascular activity during emotional behavior. During fight, flight, or active coping in situations perceived as threatening, for example, the SNS releases norepinephrine from nerve terminals and epinephrine and norepinephrine from the adrenal medulla. This stimulates the heart to increase its rate and force of contraction and the veins to increase the return of venous blood. As a result, cardiac output is increased. The arterioles in the skin and splanchnic beds constrict, causing an increase in total peripheral resistance, which is at least partially offset by vasodilation in skeletal muscle. Activation of the SNS also stimulates: (a) the liver, to release glucose, (b) adipose tissue, to mobilize free fatty acids, and (c) the kidney, to release renin and to decrease the excretion of sodium and water.

Although the SNS plays an important role in mediating relationships between emotional behavior and cardiovascular reactivity, it should not be thought of as the sole factor. Its actions are coordinated with parasympathetic nervous system activity, intrinsic metabolic adjustments and endocrine changes [157, 168, 237]. The last includes activation of the adrenal cortex.

Before turning to a consideration of sympathoadrenomedullary hypotheses of cardiovascular pathology, it should be emphasized that sympathetic activation can be highly adaptive in challenging situations. However, if the challenge is too severe, too prolonged or perhaps too often repeated, or if the individual already has pronounced organ or tissue damage, activation of the SNS can aggravate existing disorders or initiate new pathology. It would therefore appear that *Selye's* [235] general adaptation syndrome may be conceptually useful not only in terms of pituitary-adrenocortical activity but also in terms of SNS function.

Emotional behavior, presumably related to SNS activation, has been related to angina pectoris [190], arrhythmias [164], atherosclerosis [12, 149], hypertension [95], myocardial ischemia and infarction [206, 225], sudden death [162], and thrombosis [100]. Also, injections of even modest concentrations of catecholamines have been shown to produce atherosclerosis [81], arrhythmias [98], and myocardial ischemia and necrosis [55, 219].

There are many ways in which SNS activity might mediate relationships between emotional behavior and cardiovascular pathology. These include (a) precipitation of life-threatening arrhythmias, (b) alterations in the metabolism of myocardial cells, (c) induction of cardiac ischemia due to an increased need for myocardial oxygenation in conjunction with atherosclerotic stenosis of the coronary arteries, (d) decreased excretion of sodium and water, (e) increased cardiac work in pumping blood at a higher arterial pressure, (f) increased resistance to blood flow through the arterioles, (g) deposition and incorporation into coronary artery plaques of thromboembolitic components of the blood, and (h) facilitation of necrosis, calcification and rupture of plaques, which in turn could produce thrombosis and myocardial infarction.

Essential Hypertension. The exact mechanisms by which catecholamines may mediate relationships between emotional behavior and hypertension have not yet been documented. However, several important clues, and a few plausible hypotheses are available. The pathophysiological mechanisms associated with sustained hypertension include increased arteriolar resistance and increased retention of sodium and water. Renal, endocrine and neurogenic mechanisms have been implicated in different subgroups of patients and show varying degrees of interrelationship among the subgroups.

This led *Page* [16] to propose that a mosaic of factors contributes to the development of essential hypertension, and most contemporary students of primary hypertension to believe that the pathogenesis of the disorder is far less homogeneous than was once suspected. Nevertheless, a fairly large percentage of borderline hypertensive individuals reveal considerable SNS activity characterized by elevated levels of plasma catecholamines and renin, and a high cardiac output [58].

According to *Julius* and his collaborators, behavioral factors may in part lead to increased sympathoadrenomedullary activity, which in turn causes the kidney to secrete renin, the heart to increase its output and the arterioles to increase their resistance, with all three factors contributing towards the hypertension [58]. *Folkow* and his collaborators have also contended that neurogenic factors play a role in the development of hypertension by inducing vessel constriction, but these investigators emphasize that it is the increased pressure caused by the vasoconstriction, which produces the vascular thickening and mechanically increased resistance resulting in sustained hypertension [67, 68, 70]. Another influential hypothesis has been offered by *Guyton* [99]. According to this suggestion sustained hypertension results from the malfunction of renal mechanisms involved in fluid volume control. Whereas *Guyton* [99] has been concerned primarily with long-term influences sustaining the hypertension, *Brown* et al. [23] have suggested that in the initial stages of essential hypertension, nonrenal neurogenic factors are important, but that over time a renal abnormality develops due to the neurogenic rises in pressure. The means by which emotional stress can lead to increases in arterial pressure is shown in figure 1. Note that according to this schema a failure in homeostasis could result from dysfunction of the kidney, adrenal cortex, precapillary vessels or heart.

It would thus appear that the various hypotheses proposed to explain hypertension are not incompatible with one another, but merely emphasize different aspects of the same problem. One aspect is in assessing how neurogenic mechanisms can serve as intermediaries between behavior and the development of hypertension. The hypotheses of *Julius* and of *Folkow* provide a suitable framework for studying this issue. A second aspect of the problem is how neurogenic events underlying hypertensive responses ultimately can lead to a sustained hypertension. The issue here is that sustained hypertension represents a disordered regulation of homeostasis since (a) the baroreceptor reflex ordinarily should help to restore systemic arterial pressure to normotensive levels after hypertensive episodes, and (b) healthy kidneys usually counteract increased arterial pressure, perfusing them by

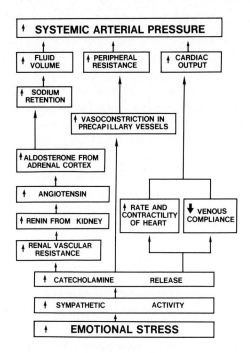

Fig. 1. The intermediate steps by which sympathetic nervous system activity could mediate relationships between emotional stress and increases in systemic arterial pressure.

increasing urine output, thereby decreasing fluid volume [238]. *Folkow's* hypothesis provides a partial framework for understanding how neurogenic mechanisms can lead to structural changes underlying sustained hypertension; whereas, *Guyton's* hypothesis provides a framework for understanding how the hypertension is maintained.

Another suggestion as to how emotional stress can be related to sustained hypertension as well as to CHD is encompassed in a hypothesis proposed by *Carruthers* [29a]. Briefly, he has proposed that emotional stress causes the release of catecholamines from the SNS, which mobilizes free fatty acids in considerable excess of metabolic requirements. This in turn contributes to morphological changes of the arterial wall in two ways. First, the free fatty acids in the plasma increase the intensity of platelet aggregation [26], leading to smooth muscle proliferation and vessel thickening (i.e. arteriosclerosis). Second, the excess free fatty acids are taken up directly by arterial walls or are converted to triglycerides, which are later deposited in arterial walls as atheromas (i.e. atherosclerosis). Thus, the narrowing of arterial lumina and increases in vessel wall resistance could contribute to the development of sustained hypertension.

Atherosclerosis. An approximate sequence of events by which the release of catecholamines from the SNS might mediate the relationship between emotional behavior and the development of atherosclerotic plaques may be conceptualized in the following manner [see *Herd*, this volume]. The initiating event in the atherosclerotic process appears to involve damage to the arterial endothelium [221]. This single layer of cells provides an interface between the blood and the rest of the vascular structure. Activation of the SNS during emotional stress can produce an increase in arterial pressure, which might result in damage to the endothelial lining of arterial vessels due to turbulence and shear stress. Catecholamines released during such emotionally stressful situations could also insult the endothelium directly [85, 207, 227].

Ordinarily the intact endothelium is nonreactive to platelets. Injury to the endothelium, however, disrupts at least two factors involved in the prevention of platelet adhesion. The first of these is the production of prostaglandin I_2 [126]; the second is the functioning of the glycocalyx, which is a carbohydrate-rich cell-coat covering the lumen side of the endothelium [40, 249]. When disruption of the endothelium is small, functional platelets seal the gaps [261]. When more pronounced injury occurs, however, the platelets adhere to exposed subendothelial tissue structures. These adherent platelets recruit additional platelet constituents. The platelets also contain a growth factor that promotes smooth muscle proliferation [138].

Catecholamines released during exertion or emotional stress can also mobilize lipid stores from adipose tissues [115]. The mobilized lipids are hydrolyzed to free fatty acids for energy production in muscular activity [269]. In this manner SNS activation evoked by physical exertion including fight-or-flight reactions can lead to the effective utilization and rapid clearance of free fatty acids from the circulation. In contrast, when lipid mobilization induced by strong emotion is not accompanied by vigorous physical activity, the free fatty acids are not cleared as rapidly, and some of them become converted to triglycerides by the liver. These are then circulated in the blood as a component of very low density lipoproteins [232]. Eventually some remnants of these very low-density lipoproteins (VLDL) are converted into low-density lipoproteins (LDL) and again released into the circulation. The major source of LDL in humans are the VLDL [240]. This is important

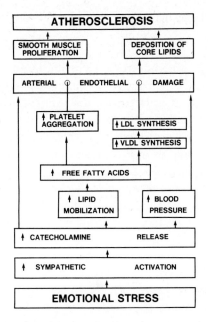

Fig. 2. Summary diagram showing some of the key steps by which increased sympathetic nervous system activity and the release of peripheral catecholamines are hypothesized to mediate the relationship between emotional stress and the development of atherosclerosis.

for the study of atherogenesis, because it is the LDL that are the source of most lipid in atheroma [174].

The exact mechanisms by which lipoproteins produce atherosclerosis are presently unknown. It is clear, however, that complex interactions among lipoproteins, blood platelets, arterial endothelium, arterial smooth muscle cells, and macrophages are involved [24]. Figure 2 provides a simplified summary diagram of the manner by which catecholamines may mediate relationships between emotional stress and atherosclerosis. Although the focus of this chapter is upon the role of catecholamines in the development of CHD, it is important to note that other hormones which become elevated during stress may be linked to the pathogenesis of atherosclerosis. The pituitary-adrenocortical system can also become activated during psychosocial stress leading to prolonged elevations of plasma corticosterone [21; *Henry* and *Herd,* this volume]. This is particularly important as a putative atherogenic mechanism because, cortisol has been shown to potentiate diet-induced atherosclerosis in cynomolgus monkeys [243], and an association between elevated plasma cortisol and early atherosclerosis has been demonstrated by coronary angiography [251].

   Coronary Heart Disease. Coronary atherosclerosis is a major predisposing factor for myocardial ischemia, which in turn is responsible for a variety of clinical states, including angina pectoris, acute myocardial infarction and sudden cardiac death. Angina pectoris refers to a relatively brief (less than 20 min) episode of chest pain due to myocardial ischemia. This is caused by an imbalance between oxygen supply and oxygen demand. Stimulation of the sympathetic nerves to the heart or infusion of norepinephrine have been shown to produce transient coronary vasoconstriction of the coronary arteries [17, 63, 257], which is apparently mediated by α-adrenergic receptors. Usually, the direct vasoconstrictive effect is soon overcome by vasodilation. However, in individuals with pronounced coronary atherosclerosis, it is possible that myocardial ischemic pain sometimes results from a failure of the initial sympathetic vasoconstriction produced by strong emotion or exertion to be overcome by normal vasodilator mechanisms [228]. In any event it is clear that the increased myocardial oxygen requirements associated with sympathetic arousal during the elicitation of strong emotions (e.g. increased HR, myocardial contractility, myocardial systolic wall stress) can initiate an attack of angina pectoris in some individuals, particularly if they already have severe coronary atherosclerosis. Episodes of angina pectoris are usually accompanied by evidence of increased blood and urinary concentrations of catecholamines [190].
   Acute myocardial infarction refers to the ischemic necrosis of myocardial tissue due to an acute decrease in coronary flow and/or by an abrupt increase in myocardial oxygen demand that cannot be met by adequate blood flow through the coronary arteries. One scenario for acute myocardial infarction, then, could have an individual with marked coronary atherosclerosis responding to a psychosocial situation with strong emotion and a pronounced sympathoadrenomedullary response. Although the release of catecholamines during sympathetic activation should ordinarily increase myocardial oxygenation, it also may drastically increase myocardial oxygen requirements. If the need for myocardial oxygen is not adequately met in this situation, because of severe narrowing or obstruction of coronary arteries, persistent ischemia with resultant myocardial infarction may result.
   The most vulnerable part of the heart to acute myocardial infarction is the subendocardium (inner third) of the left ventricle [53]. Although this region has the lowest partial pressure of oxygen of any part of the heart, its

oxygen demands are the greatest. Increased sympathetic activity producing enhanced ventricular contractility and rate also increases myocardial oxygen demand. So too does the increased afterload brought about by a sympathetically induced increase in arterial pressure. At the same time, the blood flow to the ventricle is dependent upon diastole, which becomes shortened.

It would therefore appear that to the extent that myocardial necrosis is observed in the inner third of the left ventricular myocardium following behavioral stress, sympathetic arousal and the release of catecholamines would appear to be implicated. But one difficulty that can occur in assessing the role of emotional behavior and of SNS activation in producing myocardial infarction is that infarction itself is accompanied by an immediate increase in blood catecholamines due to neurogenic reflexes elicited from within the infarcted and contiguous areas [166]. In addition, following onset of an acute myocardial infarction, patients may respond to the emotional stress and pain of the event with an intense sympathoadrenomedullary response.

Sudden cardiac death refers to natural death, due to cardiac causes that occurs between a few seconds and several hours after the onset of symptoms [178, 250]. According to *Moss* [178] most investigators in the field use a 1-hour period after onset to define sudden death. *Friedman* et al. [80], however, have further subdivided sudden cardiac death into instantaneous (less than 30 s after onset of symptoms) and noninstantaneous (minutes to hours) categories. In any event, the major aspects of sudden cardiac death are that: (a) natural death due to cardiac causes occurs soon after onset of terminal symptoms; (b) time and mode of death are unexpected, and (c) the patient may or may not have had known preexisting CHD.

In the vast majority of cases severe, occlusive coronary atherosclerosis appears to be the major predisposing cause of sudden cardiac death. The terminal pathophysiological event is ventricular fibrillation. Although the precipitating causes of the ventricular fibrillation are not completely known, observations that victims of sudden cardiac death are more likely to have been subjected to an acute psychological stressor than were victims of a non-fatal infarct [180] are consistent with results of animal studies, which have suggested that activation of the SNS and the neurogenic release of catecholamines are important factors in precipitating ventricular fibrillation [253].

In summary, current evidence suggests that SNS activity and the release of catecholamines associated with emotional behavior can interact with predisposing factors (e.g. atherosclerosis; left ventricular hypertrophy; the effects of prior infarcts) to result in ventricular fibrillation and sudden cardiac death. The state of the coronary vessels, condition of the heart and its conduction system and the ability of the heart to extract oxygen as well as the duration and severity of psychological stress, appear to be important variables.

Hypertension

Page's [196, 197] widely accepted mosaic theory contends that hypertension can begin and also develop in multiple ways. Although some cases of essential hypertension may arise from a single regulatory defect, the extensive interrelationships that exist among the multiple, dynamic, regulatory mechanisms controlling BP, suggest that in many instances the origin and development of hypertension are multifactorally determined. Hereditary, environmental, and psychological factors have all been implicated. In recent years animal models have begun to be useful in establishing how organism-environment interactions can influence genetic predispositions, and how one aspect of regulatory functioning can influence another.

At present there is scant evidence to suggest that behavioral factors alone can produce chronic hypertension. Organism-environment interactions, however, have been shown to produce short-term hypertension that outlasts immediate stimulus contingencies. More important, evidence is beginning to accumulate, which indicates that behavioral variables can interact with other variables to produce or exacerbate chronic hypertension. In this respect, the animal models that have already been developed (e.g. behavioral, genetic, organic lesion) are likely to be useful in documenting interactive factors that can produce hypertension, and in providing important clues concerning the physiological mechanisms involved. It also appears likely that neurogenic factors, including SNS activity associated with emotional behavior, may contribute significantly to the development of essential hypertension.

Noncontingent Environmental Stimulation. Several reports emanating from World War II suggest that individuals subjected to battlefield conditions may show increased BP levels [95, 224]. *Graham* [95], for example, found that 187 of 695 men from an armored brigade that had spent at least a year engaged in desert warfare against Rommel's forces had diastolic BP (DBP) greater than 100 mm Hg. When 33 of these hypertensives were retested after 2 months away from the front, 28 showed normal pressures. Similar reports of increased pressure levels associated with the events of World War II were reported for soldiers at the Finnish front [52] and for the besieged civilian population of Leningrad [179]. Blast victims of the Texas City disaster in the USA also showed transient but pronounced elevations in BP following the explosion of a ship and several nearby Monsanto chemical plants [224].

In the animal laboratory several experiments have produced hypertension in rats using aversive auditory [62, 171, 223, 242] and multimodal sensory stimuli such as motion, noxious sounds and flashing lights [25, 200, 242].

The results of these experiments are provocative, but not convincing, with regard to the development of pronounced, chronic hypertension. Although some of the animals were exposed to the aversive stimulation for as long as 10 months, maximum systolic pressures tended to peak between 150 and 160 mm Hg. Only the experiment conducted by *Perhach* et al. [200], which showed elevated BP readings persisting for 20 weeks after cessation of exposure to the noxious stimuli, provided evidence that the elevated pressures might have some permanence. Even here, however, the procedures used to record BP did not rule out the possibility that the observed elevations observed after the termination of aversive stimulation were BP-conditioned responses formed by an association between the indirect tail-cuff recording procedure and aversive stimulation. Previously *Dykman and Gantt* [51] reported that a stimulus, which produced an elevation of BP in dogs after being paired with electric shocks could still do so 13 months following conditioning.

A recent experiment conducted on rhesus monkeys also showed higher levels of BP in 2 chair-restrained rhesus monkeys exposed continuously to realistic patterns of industrial noise for 9 months than in a control monkey not exposed to the noise [201]. Moreover, the BP, which was recorded chronically from indwelling arterial catheters, remained elevated in the noise exposed animals for 27 days of monitoring following noise termination. Although these results are of interest, it should be pointed out that the average daily systolic pressure for the noise exposed animals was only about 105 mm Hg and that the average peak hourly systolic BP (SBP, recorded at about 9 a.m.) was only about 130 mm Hg.

The experiments just described provide a few insights into the physiological and morphological changes associated with the effects of noncontingent environmental stimulation upon elevations in BP. *Perhach* et al. [200] reported significant decreases in SBP following administration of guanethidine, catapres, chlorisondamine, hydralazine, hydrochlorothiazide, phentolamine, propranolol, or sotalol. Although the statistics are not reported, these investigators also claim that there was an increase in the ratio of heart weight-body weight in the animals that developed hypertension. This finding agrees with the results of *Buckley and Smookler* [25], who found that their hypertensive rats exhibited left ventricular hypertrophy and vacuolization of all three zones of the adrenal cortex. Unfortunately, *Buckley and Smookler* [25] did not evaluate the persistence of the BP elevations after the multimodal sensory stimulation was discontinued.

The results reported by *Smookler* et al. [242] suggests that the peripheral SNS plays a crucial role in noxious stimulation-induced hypertension since administration of 6-hydroxydopamine as a chemical sympathectomy prevented the hypertension from developing. This role of the peripheral SNS, however, seems to be a passive one that is secondary to some other mechanism, since in nonsympathectomized animals the responses to sympathetic nerve stimulation, or administration of norepinephrine, or isoproterenol were virtually identical between the hypertensive and normotensive rats.

Contingent Environmental Stimulation. Behavioral experiments designed to examine the effects of operant or instrumental conditioning upon the development of hypertension have basically been of two kinds. In one, changes in BP are observed as concomitants of the performance of an instrumental response such as lever-pressing to avoid shock [73, 124]. This, in a rough sort of way, is analogous to the situation of the air traffic controller, who must respond appropriately to the blips moving across the screen, with the thought lurking in the background that failure to act appropriately will have aversive consequences. In the second kind of experiment, rewards and/or punishments are made contingent upon prespecified increases in BP [14, 114]. Such experiments are appropriate for asking questions about whether repeatedly increasing BP during training sessions can lead to physiologic and/or morphologic changes that might contribute to the development of sustained hypertension.

Several experiments conducted upon nonhuman primates have examined BP changes as a function of key or lever-press performance on a shock avoidance task. In one experiment *Herd* et al. [124] trained 6 squirrel monkeys to press a key that turned off a light associated with delivery of electric shock. As training progressed, each monkey learned to press the key and the number of shocks decreased while mean arterial pressure increased. Eventually, over a period of 4–11 months, arterial pressure for 4 of the 6 monkeys was elevated before, during and after each session, even if noxious stimuli were not delivered. However, the persistence of the elevated pressure beyond training was not reported. In a similar experiment in which α- and/or β-adrenergic blocking agents were administered, the results suggested that both cardiac and vasomotor factors were responsible for the elevations in BP, and that compensation by one mechanism took place when the other was compromised by pharmacologic blockade [142].

BP responses to long-term avoidance schedules have also been examined in the rhesus monkey [73]. In this experiment 6 chair-restrained rhesus monkeys with indwelling arterial catheters were subjected to unsignaled (Sidman) avoidance schedules for 12–16 h/day for 7–14 months after a pretraining baseline period. Control animals showed little change from baseline, but after several months the pressures of 5 of 6 experimental animals gradually increased from approximately 130/80 to about 160/100 mm Hg; pulse rate tended to diminish as arterial pressure increased. No consistent pathologic findings were found except for atheromatous plaques surrounding the catheter tip in the abdominal aorta.

In the experiments by *Herd* et al. [124] and by *Forsyth* [73] shock avoidance was made contingent upon the performance of a key or lever press response while BP was monitored concurrently. *Benson* et al. [14] further observed that if the manipulandum was removed and the schedule was altered so that increases in BP per se turned off the signal light and prevented the delivery of shock, squirrel monkeys continued to avoid the shock by increasing BP. Moreover, when the contingencies were changed so that the lowering of BP terminated the signal light and avoided shock, BP returned to normotensive levels.

A programmatic series of experiments at Johns Hopkins University has investigated in considerable detail the direct conditioning of BP increases in restrained baboons. In an initial experiment in which food delivery and shock avoidance were made contingent upon specified increases in DBP for 12 h/day, sustained increases in both SBP and DBP were maintained throughout the 12-hour conditioning sessions; HR became elevated at the start of each session and then gradually declined [114]. During the ensuing 12-hour conditioning-off recovery period, HR continued to fall and BP returned to basal level within 6–8 h. In instances in which cardiac output has been measured, it has paralleled HR [112].

During similar experiments in which reinforcement was made contingent upon increases in BP, selective α- and β-adrenergic blockade attenuated but did not eliminate the operantly conditioned BP elevations [113]. Plasma norepinephrine increased significantly during sessions, and increases in epinephrine approached significance [93]. The experimental findings of this last study were consistent with the hypothesis that early in a session adrenomedullary secretion of epinephrine accounts for increased HR and cardiac output; whereas, later in a session the relative contribution of peripheral vasoconstriction mediated by norepinephrine increases. Although plasma renin activity correlated well with baseline HR and BP, no evidence of acute changes in plasma renin activity were associated with the observed cardiovascular changes during training. Morphological changes do not appear to have been examined in any of these studies.

Psychosocial Stimulation. Studies in which occupational stress [32] or living in a stressful residential neighborhood [111] have been related to hypertension suggest that psychosocial variables may contribute to the development of hypertension. In the animal literature the comprehensive series of studies conducted by *Henry* [this volume] and his collaborators upon Agouti CBA (brown) mice provides the most convincing evidence that psychosocial variables can lead to sustained hypertension.

In an early study attempts were made to induce hypertension in mice by: (a) mixing of animals previously maintained in different boxes; (b) crowding; (c) subjecting groups to threat from a predatory cat, and (d) inducing conflict for territory by placing equal numbers of males and females in an interconnecting box system [120]. Although elevations in BP induced by some of these manipulations were maintained for several months, pressures often returned towards normal values when the stimulation was discontinued.

In subsequent experiments mice were typically isolated from the time of weaning at 12–14 days of age until they were 4 months old [118, 119, 123]. Then, groups of approximately 30 experimental animals of both sexes were placed in the complex population environment consisting of boxes joined by narrow interconnecting tubes to a single central feeding and watering area. The tubes were sufficiently narrow so that only one mouse could pass through at a time. In contrast to control animals raised in social environments, the previously isolated, experimental animals experienced repeated confrontations leading to vigorous fighting that produced epilation and scarring.

After several months in the complex environmental cage the previously isolated mice developed evidence of sustained hypertension accompanied by interstitial nephritis, increased heart weight, myocardial fibrosis and arteriosclerosis of the intramural coronary vessels and aorta [118, 119, 123]. It appears likely that the sustained hypertension and degenerative effects observed as a function of psychosocial stress were related to SNS activation and to the release of catecholamines into the circulation. Thus, for example, increases were seen in the adrenal medullary enzymes, tyrosine hydroxydase and phenylethanolamine *N*-methyltransferase [122]. In a subsequent study, it was also shown that plasma renin activity was greater in experimental than in control mice [255]. Observation of BP reduction by the angiotensin enzyme inhibitor SQ14225 indicated that renin was involved in maintaining BP during later but not the initial stages of an experiment [unpublished observations]. It would therefore appear that the experiments conducted by *Henry* and his collaborators have not only been able to demonstrate an association between psychosocial stress and sustained hypertension, but have provided important clues concerning the manner in which the SNS helps mediate the relationship.

Genetic-Behavioral Interactions. Page's [196] mosaic theory implies that the hereditary factors underlying hypertension consist of a spectrum of variants more or less randomly mixed in the genetic coding of human reproduction. The development of selectively bred rat strains has provided an important tool for (a) isolating putative genetic variants that might contribute to human hypertension, and (b) examining the manner in which these genetic variants are influenced by environmental factors.

The spontaneously hypertensive rat (SHR) developed by *Okamoto and Aoki* [193] is the most widely used experimental model for the study of genetic factors in hypertension. Hypertension in the SHR appears to be due to a relatively few major genetic components acting in concert [110]. Pronounced increases in tonic BP begin at about 5 or 6 weeks of age. Hypertension then develops rapidly over the next couple of months, with an established phase being reached before 6 months of age. SBP in the mature SHR is approximately 190–200 mm Hg.

During the early accelerating phase of their hypertension, young SHR, like borderline hypertensive humans, display a 'hyperkinetic' circulation with increased cardiac output related to enhanced sympathetic discharge reminiscent of the defense reaction [69, 135]. In contrast, older SHR, like chronic hypertensive humans, have a normal or subnormal cardiac output, but a high peripheral resistance. At this stage sympathetic tone appears to be reduced, but secondary structural changes including left ventricular hypertrophy and arteriosclerotic changes in the large arteries and precapillary resistance vessels are apparent.

A large number of experiments have shown that young SHR show greater increases in SNS activity, plasma catecholamines, and cardiovascular reactivity than normotensive control rats when subjected to flashing lights footshock, loud noises, vibrations, physical restraint or cold temperatures [104, 181–185, 268]. In order to test the hypothesis that the ultimate development of hypertension in SHR is due to the hyperreactivity to environmental stimulation, *Hallbäck* [103] socially isolated SHR at weaning until they were 7 months of age. She found that the social isolates exhibited significantly lower baseline BP than group-reared SHR although both groups revealed similar cardiovascular responses to acute aversive stimulation. Subsequently, *Hallbäck-Norlander and Lundin* [105] found that HR and cardiac output showed greater increases to loud noises in SHR than in control rats, whereas anesthesia lowered HR and cardiac output more in SHR than in controls. The cardiovascular findings are consistent with reports that if blood is sampled from chronic indwelling catheters in undisturbed SHR and age-matched controls while in their home cages, no strain differences in plasma norepinephrine or epinephrine are observed. In contrast, SHR exhibit excessive and prolonged discharges of both catecholamines during immobilization [181, 182] or anticipation of footshock [183].

In summary, the experimental findings suggest that exposure to aversive stimulation facilitates the development of hypertension in SHR whereas removal of environmental stimulation can impede its development. The cardiovascular and catecholaminergic hyperreactivity to environmental stimulation shown by SHR appear to be central in origin, and the hyperreactivity may play a role in the pathogenesis of hypertension.

One limitation of the SHR as a model is that unlike humans, SHR invariably develop severe hypertension unless they are socially isolated. In order to get a better understanding of the pathogenic significance of aversive stimulation in animals with a genetic susceptibility for hypertension, *Lawler* et al. [152] mated SHR with Wistar-Kyoto normotensive rats and used the offspring in an experiment. The offspring had SBP of about 150 mm Hg when they were 14 weeks old. Beginning at week 15 an experimental group and a mild restraint control group were placed in conditioning cages for 2 h daily, 5 days per week. The experimental group was trained on a conflict-avoidance task in which failure to respond to a signal led to 5 inescapable shocks, whereas responding led to a single inescapable shock. The mild restraint group did not receive this training. Animals in a maturational control group remained in their home cages throughtout the study.

Lawler et al. [152] found that by the time the animals were 29 weeks old, the experimental rats had tonic systolic levels of about 185 mm Hg. In contrast, the SBP of the restraint and maturational controls were 165 and 150 mm Hg, respectively. In a subsequent report, *Lawler* et al. [153] found that experimental animals studied for a 10-week follow-up period without conflict maintained the elevated pressure. When sacrificed these animals showed evidence of myofibrillar degeneration and an elevation in heart weight/body weight ratios.

The borderline hypertensive rat is a potentially interesting experimental model. This is especially true in the light of recent human research indicating that subjects having at least one hypertensive parent show greater HR and BP reactivity on experimental tasks involving mental arithmetic or shock avoidance than do the offspring of normotensive parents [61, 192]. However, in view of previous findings that socially isolated SHR have significantly lower BP than group-raised SHR [103], and the findings of *Lawler* et al. [152, 153] that even minimally handled and restrained offspring of matings between SHR and normotensive rats show higher BP than maturational controls, the utility of the 'borderline' hypertensive model must still be established by direct comparisons with the SHR model.

Another important genetic animal model for hypertension research was developed by *Dahl* et al. [37–39]. This model consists of 2 lines of rats having opposite, genetically determined predispositions toward hypertension. One of these, the Dahl hypertension-sensitive line or S strain, shows increasing levels of hypertension as a function of the amount of sodium chloride in the diet; a diet of 8% NaCl results in SBP exceeding 200 mm Hg. The other line, or R strain, is relatively insensitive to sodium chloride intake. Both strains remain normotensive at relatively low dietary sodium levels.

Although the differences between the R and S strains in their propensity for hypertension is most pronounced with regard to salt load, the S strain is also more prone to become hypertensive in response to deoxycorticosterone-NaCl treatment, cortisone, renal artery clamping, and severe aversive stimulation [38, 39, 77–79]. In one behavioral experiment *Friedman and Dahl* [77] exposed S rats that were maintained on a low salt diet to 13 weeks of experimentation. The major experimental manipulation was a conflict situation in which lever pressing sometimes produced food and sometimes produced shock. Other groups of S rats were either food-deprived, shocked, both food-deprived and shocked but without conflict, or not manipulated experimentally (controls). Throughout the 13 weeks of experimentation the conflict group had higher BP than the other groups. Mean BP of the conflict group was 166 mm Hg and of the unstimulated control group 140 mm Hg. The elevated level in the conflict group decreased gradually to control levels during a 13-week recovery period.

In a subsequent experiment, a modest amount of NaCl was added to the diet of conflict exposed S rats [78]. Although the absolute magnitudes of BP obtained were only slightly higher than in the previous study, BP did not return to baseline when the rats were placed on a low salt diet during the recovery period. Interestingly, the conflict procedure is completely ineffective in producing BP increases in R rats [78]. The results of the behavioral experiments on Dahl strain rats therefore suggest that genetic predisposition, diet and emotional behavior can interact systematically either to produce or not produce sustained increases in BP. Moreover, genetic predispositions may not manifest themselves unless environmental factors challenge the organism.

Experiments examining the genetic predispositions leading to hypertension susceptibility in the S strain point to a polygenetic mode of inheritance. The kidneys, adrenal cortex and SNS all appear to be implicated. In terms of the SNS, S as opposed to R rats exhibit an exaggerated vascular reactivity to vasopressor agents such as norepinephrine and angiotensin, even before the onset of hypertension [131, 246]. Moreover, destruction of peripheral sympathetic nerves with 6-hydroxydopamine (6-OHDA) [246] or guanethidine [84] prevents the onset of NaCl hypertension in S rats.

Other Models of Hypertension. The earliest animal model of hypertension was developed by *Goldblatt* et al. [90], who found that by impeding flow through a renal artery with an adjustable clip they could produce hypertension. Hypertension becomes even more severe if the contralateral kidney is removed. In 1942, *Selye* demonstrated that administration of the mineral corticoid, deoxycorticosterone acetate (DOCA) in baby chicks produces hypertension with associated cardiovascular disease. Mammals, however, tend to be resistant to DOCA unless first 'sensitized' by unilateral nephrectomy and by the addition of 1% NaCl in their drinking water [28].

Hall and Hall [101, 102] found that subjecting rats to electric shock potentiated the incidence and severity of hypertension induced by unilateral nephrectomy, NaCl maintenance and treatment with either DOCA or growth hormone. Furthermore, they found that DOCA plus shock causes more kidney damage than DOCA without shock stress, and that growth hormone plus shock stress potentiated both cardiac and kidney pathology relative to administration of growth hormone alone.

Rats tend to consume a large draught of water following the ingestion of individual food pellets (polydipsia) when they are only permitted to eat pellets intermittently during a few hours/day [59]. Mononephrectomized rats given saline to drink on such a schedule develop hypertension [60]. This hypertension is maintained even after water replaces saline as the drinking fluid. The hypertension is associated with increased heart weight and at least minor kidney damage.

Experiments conducted by *DeChamplain* [42] and *DeChamplain and Van Ameringen* [43] have clearly established that sodium balance influences the activity of the SNS. Moreover, the effects of DOCA and saline appear to be synergistic with one another as well as with their effects mediated by both SNS fibers and the adrenal medulla. Elevated levels of plasma norepinephrine and epinephrine are also seen in rats subjected to DOCA-salt or a high sodium diet when compared with control rats after all 3 groups have been mononephrectomized [75].

Another model of hypertension that clearly involves SNS activity includes the making of bilateral lesions in the nucleus tract of solitarius (NTS) or in the anterior hypothalamus. The hypothalamic effects can be blocked by adrenalectomy [186], whereas the NTS effects require both chemical sympathectomy and adrenalectomy [50]. Both of these experiments were conducted upon rats. In cats, lesions of NTS abolish the baroreceptor reflex and produce labile hypertension [187]. Based upon these findings cats were given Pavlovian classical conditioning after being subjected to bilateral NTS lesions [188]. The conditioned increases in arterial pressure were more than 5 times greater in lesioned that in nonlesioned animals. These findings suggest that the baroreceptor reflexes normally are able to dampen conditioned increases in pressure, and that when these are rendered inoperative, large increases in pressure can occur.

Comment. Animal behavior models have provided unequivocal evidence that aversive situations can elicit dramatic elevations in arterial BP. These increases in pressure are mediated by the sympathoadrenomedullary system. Although such increases in BP can under appropriate circumstances outlast the precipitating stimuli, there is little evidence to support the hypothesis that behavioral variables alone can produce sustained hypertension.

The most convincing evidence to date supporting the notion that emotional behavior alone can produce sustained hypertension has been provided by *Henry* and his collaborators. Therefore, it would seem worthwhile to compare some of the differences between *Henry's* experimental situation with the situations that failed to obtain sustained hypertension. One possibility to consider is the choice of experimental animal. In humans the natural history of hypertension is usually about 35 years or roughly half the life span. In mice, 9 months of behavioral stress would approximate half of these animals' life time, whereas in rhesus monkeys or baboons it is possible for the animals to live 20 years or longer. Therefore, if susceptibility to behaviorally induced hypertension interacts with variables influenced by the aging process, the fairly young animals used in most primate experiments might well not show evidence of sustained hypertension after only 9 months of behavioral manipulation.

Another variable that may account for the differences between *Henry's* results and those of other investigators is genetic susceptibility. It is conceivable that CBA mice have an underlying susceptibility to behaviorally induced hypertension, whereas other mice may not. When *Alexander* [5] performed similar experiments on rats to those performed by *Henry's* group on mice, elevated BP were noted in only one third of socially deprived rats after social stimulation, and even the increases in these animals were fairly small. Since the disparity between the *Henry* and *Alexander* experiments included a species difference, it would be useful to determine whether psychosocial stress can produce sustained hypertension in mouse strains other than the CBA.

Still another variable that may account for the mouse studies having produced evidence of sustained hypertension, whereas the primate studies did not, may have to do with the choice of experimental paradigm. It is possible that the operant conditioning paradigms used in much of the primate research do not mobilize the SNS to the same extent on a long-term basis that repeated confrontations do in complex psychosocial situations. Furthermore, the subjects in these primate operant conditioning experiments experienced prolonged safe periods each day in which the avoidance contingency was not present [73, 114, 124]. In contrast, the mice in *Henry's* experiment were vulnerable to attack 24 h/day.

Another issue that deserves comment is whether elevations in BP by themselves, if large enough and if evoked often enough, necessarily lead to hypertension. One of the major findings of the primate operant conditioning research just reviewed, is that intermittent (even 12 h/day) increases in BP by themselves do not necessarily lead to sustained hypertension, and may not even inevitably lead to pronounced arteriosclerosis. Thus, after thousands of hours of BP elevations that often exceeded 30 mm Hg, *Harris* et al. [114] found no evidence of sustained hypertension. Moreover, *Goldstein* et al. [92] found that following extensive training baroreflex sensitivity actually increased during conditioning off periods compared with the preconditioning baseline.

Although intermittent increases in cardiac output frequently precede the development of sustained hypertension, it is worth noting that some patients with increased cardiac output due to thyrotoxicosis or anemia do not develop sustained hypertension. Thus, while increases in SNS activity and increases in BP are correlated, it may be some aspects of SNS activity rather than the increases in BP per se that are responsible for the development of sustained hypertension. Thickening of the intima of resistance vessels, for example, may require damage of the precapillary vessel endothelium by circulating catecholamines, particularly epinephrine, before smooth muscle proliferation can occur. Also, *Genest* [87] has hypothesized that at least in the early stages of hypertension, the increase in peripheral resistance may be secondary to inappropriate SNS activity in the presence of arteriolar hypersensitivity of hyperresponsiveness to pressor agents such as norepinephrine or angiotensin.

A final issue that deserves comment is the role of emotional behavior as a precipitating factor in hypertension. Although the experimental data do not convincingly support the hypothesis that emotional behavior alone can produce sustained hypertension, it is abundantly clear that behaviors associated with pronounced increases in SNS activity can interact with diet (e.g. salt), renal infection [160] or genetic predisposition to produce hypertension. It is likely that future behavioral research into the causes of hypertension will address itself to examining interactions with atherogenic and high salt diets, genetic predispositions, and various organ insults.

Arteriosclerosis

Animal behavior experiments have implicated aversive behavioral factors in the development of both arteriosclerosis [119, 213] and atherosclerosis [11, 12, 149, 198, 252]. The term arteriosclerosis literally means hardening of the arteries, and includes a variety of conditions that cause the artery walls to become thick and hard. Atherosclerosis may be considered as a subclass of arteriosclerosis in which part of the thickening of the vessel wall is due to deposition of fats or to an irregular intimal lesion referred to as an atheromatous plaque. Usually this plaque has a lipid core made up of free and ester cholesterol covered by a cap of fibrous tissues. The plaque is also associated with necrotic processes; however, the plaque may eventually calcify. The exact mechanisms by which plaques grow and progressively narrow the precapillary vessel lumina are not completely known. However, continued lipid and lipoprotein accumulation in the lesion, hemorrhage into a plaque, and fibrous organization of thrombi forming on the surface of the plaque have all been implicated. Narrowing of a lumen by at least 75% can compromise regional blood flow [130].

Although the specific mechanisms by which emotional stresses induce arteriosclerosis and atherosclerosis remain speculative, there is some evidence that such associations do exist. *Ratcliffe* [211], for instance, found that an increase in the prevalence of arterial lesions found among birds and mammals dying at the Philadelphia Zoo was related to intraspecies social pressures. These lesions, consisting of arteriosclerotic stenosis of small intramural arteries, were not only found in zoo animals, but also in chickens [213] and swine [212] subjected to psychosocial stress. *Henry* et al. [122] also found arteriosclerosis in the intramural coronary vessels of his psychosocially stressed mice as well as in the aorta. In addition, rats [252] and squirrel monkeys [149] subjected to atherogenic diets and to psychological stress have shown elevated levels of serum cholesterol and intramural coronary atherosclerosis relative to control animals. Finally, systematic intraspecies individual differences have been found in serum cholesterol [19, 33, 140] and in coronary artery atherosclerosis among group-housed nonhuman primates [139, 140].

The experiments by *Henry* et al. [118, 119, 122, 123] in which previously isolated mice were placed in a social environment that was conducive to conflict have already been described. In terms of the present discussion, the major points of interest are that (a) the mice developed arteriosclerosis of the intramural coronary arteries and aorta, and (b) the hypertensive and degenerative effects observed were correlated with increases in the adrenal medullary enzymes, tyrosine hydroxylase and phenylethanolamine-N-methyltransferase.

Evidence of morphologic changes occurring in intramural coronary vessels as a function of behavioral stress has also been provided by *Basset and Cairncross* [12]. They observed that daily exposure of rats for up to 2 months to a situation requiring escape from electric shock led to changes in the endothelial linings of the coronary vessels within the heart as well as to the deposit of lipid in arteriole walls. Briefly, *Bassett and Cairncross* [12] found that daily exposure to behavioral stress for 1.5–2 months led to junctional gaps in the endothelial lining of the coronary microcirculation and to increased platelet aggregation.

Normally, the intact endothelium provides a barrier against the free exchange of large lipid molecules such as cholesterol between plasma and the arterial wall. When the endothelium becomes damaged, however, such molecules may equilibrate rapidly [270]. *Bassett and Cairncross* [11, 12] have suggested that due to prolonged stress associated with SNS activity, endogenous inflammatory substances can cause separation of adjacent endothelial cells. One source of these endogenous inflammatory substances could be mast cells, which are found around small blood vessels. *Bassett and Cairncross* [11] found and increase of such mast cells in rats as a function of exposure to irregular, signalled foot shock. Mast cells hold and release histamine [94], which can be triggered by catecholamines [116] in response to SNS arousal.

Thus far, attention has focused upon the singular role of behavioral stress in the development of arteriosclerosis. Prospective epidemiological studies, however, have indicated that the risk factors for atherosclerotic CHD are multicausal in origin [137, 220]. These epidemiological studies in conjunction with animal experiments in which lipid-induced atherosclerosis has been shown to be accelerated by increases, in BP [22, 45, 177] have demonstrated impressive interactions among diet, serum cholesterol values and BP in the development of atherosclerosis. Presumably, catecholamines and/or hemodynamic factors that insult the vascular endothelium can make it vulnerable to chemical factors such as elevated levels of lipids and LDL [221, 222]. Perhaps one reason that nonhuman primates failed to develop sustained hypertension and atherosclerosis in the experiments of *Benson* et al. [14], *Forsyth* [73], *Harris* et al. [114], and *Herd* et al. [124] was that the low fat, low cholesterol laboratory diets fed to the animals may have precluded significant interactions from occurring among serum cholesterol and LDL, catecholamines, and elevated arterial pressure.

The effects of aversive stimulation upon animals given an atherosclerotic diet has received some attention, however, and is likely to receive considerably more in the future. In one experiment rats fed a high lipid diet and exposed to unpredictable grid shocks revealed higher levels of accumulated cholesterol in aorta, kidney, and serum than control rats fed only the high lipid diet [138]. Other experiments have further indicated that behavioral stress superimposed upon an atherogenic diet can accelerate atherogenesis [149, 252].

Lang [149] placed 3 groups of squirrel monkeys on an atherogenic diet for 25 months. One group received transport to a Skinner box, and restraint in the box for 1 h, 5 days/week. The second group received transport, restraint and unsignaled (Sidman) shock avoidance for the same time periods. A third group served as cage controls. Total serum cholesterol, examined immediately prior to termination of the experiment was about equal in the 2 groups exposed to the Skinner box, and both were significantly higher than the cage control group. Coronary atherosclerosis was found postmortem in most of the monkeys that had been transported regularly to the Skinner box, but was not found in the cage control monkeys. The coronary lesions were in the small intramyocardial arteries and consisted of both intracellular and extracellular sudanophilic accumulations in the intima.

In the *Uhley and Friedman* [252] study rats were placed on an atherogenic diet and then served either as cage controls or were placed in a special cage in which one half of the grid floor was charged every 5 min throughout the 6-hour/day experimental session. At the end of 10 months total serum cholesterol and lipid levels were significantly higher in the experimental than in the control group. The experimental animals also revealed significantly more sudanophilic staining in the intima of coronary artery vessels than did control animals. *Uhley and Friedman* [252] contrasted these results with those of an earlier study that used a similar experimental protocol without the atherogenic diet. The experimental animals in the earlier study revealed neither hypercholesteremia nor discernable atherosclerosis.

Although direct linkages among behavioral stress, the release of catecholamines during SNS arousal, hemodynamic changes, diet, lipid mobilization, lipid utilization, and the development of atherosclerosis have not yet been examined in the same experiment, the studies by *Lang* [149], *Paré* et al. [198], and *Uhley and Friedman* [252] indicate that such studies would be feasible and potentially valuable. Such experiments, however, will need to pay more attention to the effects of species, age, sex, psychosocial groupings, and variables associated with behavioral development than has previously been the norm, because such variables are likely to influence the results significantly. One example of the need for specifying behavioral contexts is that in *Lang's* [149] squirrel monkeys handling (and transport to a restraint cage) was associated with increased atherogenesis; whereas, in a study reported by *Nerem* et al. [189], handling and petting of cholesterol-fed rabbits in the laboratory was associated with a decreased number of intimal sudanophilic lesions relative to rabbits that were not handled.

Several studies have recently begun to examine serum cholesterol levels and/or atherogenesis as a function of psychosocial variables in nonhuman primates. In one experiment, for example, *Kaplan* et al. [140] placed male cynomolgus monkeys on a moderately atherogenic diet for 20 months. Half of the monkeys were housed in a socially stable situation, whereas social instability was induced in the other half by frequent reorganization of group membership. Social status in terms of dominance and subordination was evaluated animal's wins and losses during fighting. The major findings of the study were that the dominant animals in the stable condition had less coronary atherosclerosis than the subordinates, whereas the situation was reversed in the unstable situation. One possible interpretation for such findings could be that the dominant animals were able to maintain order while experiencing relatively little SNS arousal in the socially stable situation. In contrast, the increased coronary atherosclerosis seen in the dominant animals housed in an unstable environment might have reflected relatively greater SNS arousal required to retain dominance and/or maintain order.

Another investigation conducted on cynomolgus monkeys by the same group of experimenters examined the relationship between individual differences in HR reactivity to a behavioral challenge and the extent of atherosclerosis [139, 167]. The standardized challenge consisted of having the experimenter display prominently and threateningly before the target animal a large 'monkey glove' usually used in the capture and handling of the animal. The monkeys, who had been fed a moderately atherogenic diet for 20 months, and who had been fitted with ECG telemetry devices, were divided into high and low HR reactors. Soon afterwards, at necropsy, it was found that the high HR reactors revealed significantly more atherosclerosis of the coronary arteries and thoracic aorta than the low HR reactors.

The investigation reported by *Kaplan and Manuck* [139] and by *Manuck and Kaplan* [167] has provided the first direct test of the hypothesis that high HR reactivity to an aversive behavioral challenge is associated with increased atherosclerosis. Their positive outcome is of particular interest with regard to atherosclerotic CHD in humans because, type A relative to type B individuals reveal more: (a) HR reactivity in challenging behavioral situations [44, 89]; (b) coronary atherosclerosis when studied at autopsy [83], and (c) coronary atherosclerosis when studied by coronary angiography [18, 147]. Although the investigation conducted on monkeys has the advantage over the human autopsy and arteriography studies of having been conducted upon relatively healthy individuals, it shares the limitation of having been retrospective. Therefore, what appears to be needed now in order to firmly link SNS reactivity to atherogenesis are prospective studies looking at cardiovascular reactivity, plasma catecholamines, plasma cholesterol and lipoprotein fractions, and atherosclerosis.

The research that has been conducted upon the type A coronary-prone behavior pattern was not only been enriched by the animal behavior literature, but has also provided a useful theoretical framework for animal research. *Coelho and Bramblett* [33], for example, have developed an ethogram of more than 100 separate behaviors in the baboon (e.g. barking, biting, chasing) and dimensionalized them into five major categories reminiscent of coronary-prone behavior in humans. These dimensions are tension, threat, attack, subordination, and affiliation. Interestingly, *Coelho and Bramblett* [33] found that the highest levels of serum cholesterol in their baboons were in animals that were high on threat, attack, and tension, but also on subordination. It would thus appear that these baboons, like their type A human counterparts: (a) are engaged more or less unsuccessfully in a struggle to gain increased control over their environment and (b) have increased levels of serum cholesterol, which may lead to increased atherogenesis [76, 82].

Stress-Induced Cardiomyopathy

Myocardial degeneration has been reported to occur as a function of frightening sensory stimuli in cage restrained wild rats [208], shocks delivered by an animal prod in swine restrained by a muscle relaxant [132, 133], behavioral stress associated with the trapping, handling, and transport of baboons [97], unsignaled, unpredictable foot-shock in domestic rats [176], and avoidance conditioning in squirrel monkeys [35]. It has also been observed as a function of relatively long-term psychosocial stress in mice [119], rabbits [263], and baboons [150].

Captured wild rats developed scattered myocardial lesions after exposure to tape recordings of cats and rats hissing and squealing during fighting, whereas control rats not exposed to the recordings did not suffer myocardial damage [208]. The stress-induced, scattered myocardial lesions, which occurred in the absence of vascular abnormalities, were attributed to 'localized states of anoxia in the ventricular tissue under the metabolic (increased oxygen consumption) and microcirculatory (subendothelial vascular compression, shortened diastone) influence of liberated adreno- and sympathogenic catecholamines'.

Raab et al. [208] observed both coagulation necrosis and coagulative myocytolysis. Coagulation necrosis refers to myocardial cellular death in a state of lost contractility whereas coagulative myocytolysis refers to myocardial cellular death while the cell is hypercontracted. In the case of coagulation necrosis, hypoxia of cardiac muscle related to increased myocardial oxygen demand leads to ischemic necrosis; the myofibrils, seen microscopically as thin wavy fibers, are not damaged except for the stretching of filaments by surrounding viable cells. In contrast, myocardial cellular death during coagulative myocytolysis occurs while the cell is hypercontracted, and this has been attributed to hyperfunctional overdrive rather than to ischemia [55].

Although coagulative necrosis and coagulative myocytolysis may occur differentially as a function of the condition of the heart and vasculature as well as the duration and intensity of sympathetic arousal, experiments such as those conducted by *Raab* et al. [208] indicate that both types of myocardial damage can occur concurrently.

Acute behavioral stress has been clearly shown to produce severe myocardial damage in 6-month-old swine [132, 133]. The behaviorally stressed pigs were initially injected with succinylcholine at a dosage that produced muscular weakness without respiratory distress. They were then shocked on a hind limb with an animal prod 5 or 6 times during the next 15–20 min. Swine that survived the session were shot through the brain and killed instantly 16–48 h later. Control animals, sacrificed in the same way, were neither injected with succinylcholine nor shocked.

Johansson et al. [133] reported that of 23 experimental pigs, 2 died during the experimental session and another died 3 h later. The 3 animals had multiple, intramural, subepicardial, and subendocardial hemorrhages. Myocardial degeneration and necrosis were found in all 23 experimental animals, but in 0 of 9 control animals. Damaged muscle cells were observed throughout the left ventricle, but were most apparent in the subendocardium. Many foci were tiny consisting of only 1 muscle cell or 2; a few measured about 1 mm in diameter and were composed of several damaged cells.

Light and ultrastructural analyses were conducted upon the hearts of many of these same animals by *Johansson* et al. [133]. Experimental pigs revealed evidence of both coagulative necrosis and coagulative myocytolysis. Myofibrils were contracted in cells at the periphery of necrotic foci. Changes within the necrotic areas included the complete lysis of myofilaments. Electron microscopic analyses indicated severe swelling of the tubules of the sarcoplasmic reticulum, damage to myofilaments, mitochondrial damage, loss of glycogen, and increase in the number of lipid droplets. Electron densities, presumably consisting of calcium salts, were also seen. The findings observed in the *Johansson* et al. [133], *Jonsson and Johansson* [132], and *Raab* et al. [208] studies as a function of behavioral stress are similar to the changes seen after infusion of catecholamines [64, 65].

Attempts have been made to determine whether contingent noxious stimulation as well as noncontingent stimulation can lead to pronounced myocardial damage. *Corley* et al. [36], for example, trained squirrel monkeys to press a response lever to postpone tail shock in an unsignaled (Sidman) avoidance situation. Once the animals were trained to press the lever every few seconds to avoid shock, 8-hour avoidance sessions were continually alter-nated with 8 h of rest. The experiments were terminated, and the animals sacrificed, when the animals ceased responding in the avoidance session. All 8 monkeys subjected to the avoidance situation showed microscopic evidence of at least scattered myofibrillar degeneration, whereas caged control animals that were never shocked showed no evidence of myocardial pathology. However, because no controls were instituted for the effects of chair restraint, capture and handling, or shock per se, it is not possible to relate specifically the myocardial damage to the avoidance contingency. These problems were remedied in a subsequent experiment.

Corley et al. [35] subjected 11 pairs of squirrel monkeys to an 'avoid-yoke' procedure in which one member of each pair was able to manipulate a response lever to avoid tail shock. Each time that the 'avoid' animal failed to press the lever in time to postpone shock for 40 s, both this animal and its 'yoked' partner received shock. Thus, both monkeys always received the same number and temporal pattern of shocks, but only the avoid animal had the possibility of exerting control over whether shock would occur. The animals were exposed to a single 24-hour experimental session.

Because the avoidance animals were not chaired or trained to lever press prior to the 24-hour session, both the avoidance animal and its yoked partner received a fairly large number of shocks at the beginning of the session. Consequently, it is hardly surprising that yoked as well as experimental animals showed evidence of myocytolysis and necrosis or that a yoked as well as 3 avoid monkeys died prior to sacrifice. The remaining animals were sacrificed 24–146 h after initiation of the experimental session in order to assess the permanence of the myocardial damage observed.

Cardiac tissue sections were made through the midportion of the left ventricle of all animals, and fuchsin stains (e.g. Masson's trichrome) were used to identify areas of myocardial damage. Although both avoidance and yoked monkeys showed selective staining of myocardial cells, called fuch-sinophilia, the staining was significantly more pronounced in the avoidance monkeys. The fuchsinophilia staining appears to reflect a persistent morpho-logic effect, since it was readily observable in monkeys killed 5 days after the termination of the stress session.

Selye [236] first described fuchsinophilia as an early indicator of myocar-dial damage, and subsequent research specifically related it to myofibrillar degeneration [215]. According to *Fleckenstein* et al. [66], extreme stress causes a release of toxic levels of catecholamines. This, in turn, causes myocardial cells to hypercontract (functional overdrive) and to become overloaded with calcium which, if not reversed, leads to myofibrillar degeneration. In any event, the effects of intense behavioral stress associated with pronounced sympathetic arousal tends to lead to calcium-related changes observable in damaged myocardial fibers. In the experiments just described these were evidenced as (a) fuchsinophilia [35], and (b) changes in electron density that can be visualized using an electron microscope [132].

The next set of experiments to be described also used calcium-related changes in damaged myocardial cells to assess the effects of intense behavioral stress upon the heart, this time using a radiopharmaceutical procedure. This was accomplished by coupling radionuclides to phosphate complexes having a high affinity for tissue-bound calcium, and detecting increased myocardial damage as increased radioactive counts [173, 175, 176]. The radionuclide used in these experiments was ^{99m}Tc. Phosphate complexes that were chosen because they have a high affinity for tissue-bound calcium were methylene diphosphonate (MDP) and stannous pyrophosphate (PP). Validation of the procedure for assessing myocardial damage has been based upon clinical studies with human patients [199] as well as experimental studies with dogs [271], rabbits [46], and rats [156].

In one experiment *Miller* et al. [175] placed rats into one of four treatment conditions: (a) control, (b) epinephrine injection through a cutaneous incision, (c) a 2-hour session in which a 1-mA grid shock was given at variable intervals around a mean of 24 s, or (d) a 12-hour grid shock session. Then, 18 h after epinephrine injection or 8 h after termination of the shock conditions, each animal received an intravenous injection of ^{99m}Tc-PP or ^{99m}Tc-MDP. After 100 or 300 min the animals were sacrificed, Hearts were removed, washed, blotted, weighed, and counted in a scintillation counter. Subsequently, sections were prepared for light microscopy and stained with hematoxylin and eosin.

Neither the catecholamine injection nor grid shock conditions produced mortality prior to the time of sacrifice. The epinephrine injections produced large and relatively uniform, grossly visible foci of damage along the posterior interventricular septum and base of the left ventricle. Intermittent foot shock resulted in myocardial injury that was not macroscopically evident following 2 h of stress. Following 12 h of foot shock, however, widely scattered small foci of grossly visible injury were evident. In terms of whole-heart radionuclide concentrations, higher scintillation counts were obtained 300 than 100 min after injection. ^{99m}Tc-MDP produced higher counts than ^{99m}Tc-PP. Whole heart concentrations of MDP were an order of magnitude greater in the epinephrine injection condition than in the 12-hour foot shock condition. Concentration of MDP was in turn much greater in the 12-hour than in the 2-hour foot shock condition, and the MDP concentration in the 2-hour foot shock condition was significantly greater than in the control condition. The use of ^{99m}Tc-MDP would therefore appear to provide a reasonably sensitive radiobioassay for quantitatively assessing diffuse myocardial damage in behavioral experiments.

In another study Miller and Mallov [176] showed that radionuclide accumulation occurred only in nonanesthetized rats, suggesting that the myocardial damage was CNS-mediated. They also showed that the heightened uptake was not due to increased muscle activity accompanying the stress, since levels of ^{99m}Tc-MDP in the myocardium of restrained rats also given a dose of d-tubocurarine that minimized movement without impairing respiration did not differ significantly from those in nonrestrained, noncurarized rats. In contrast, animals receiving foot shock showed significantly greater uptake than animals not receiving foot shock whether or not they were restrained and curarized. More recently, Miller [173] found that the uptake of ^{99m}Tc-MDP is greatly reduced if foot shocks are preceded by a warning signal than if foot shocks are presented unsignaled. The studies by Miller and his colleagues would therefore appear to provide an important link between psychological aspects of stress (e.g. stimulus predictability) and the extent of myocardial injury.

Arrhythmias

Atherosclerotic CHD is the major cause of death in the Western World. Some 60% of these fatalities occur in nonhospitalized individuals within 2h of the onset of symptoms [6]. In most cases the terminal event is ventricular fibrillation. Although myocardial ischemia associated with atherosclerotic CHD appears to create the biochemical and metabolic conditions that set the stage for ventricular fibrillation, most often acute changes in atherosclerotic lesions or obstructing thrombi are not evident [250]. Instead, it appears that other factors associated with CNS and autonomic functioning may transiently destabilize the heart, thereby setting in motion a chain of events leading to a fatal arrhythmia.

One effect of myocardial ischemia is to alter cardiac mechanics, which in turn can trigger various reflexes. The site of the ischemia can be important in producing different reflex effects. At the onset of clinical myocardial infarction in humans, for example, injury to the posterior wall of the left ventricle is often accompanied by excessive vagal activity, whereas injury to the anterior ventricular muscle tends to be associated with sympathetic over-activity [264].

When the vagal afferent fibers originating in the left ventricle become excited, this can induce pronounced bradycardia and an inhibition of the sympathetic innervation of peripheral vessels [191, 248]. In contrast, activation of sympathetic afferent fibers from the heart have been shown to give rise to cardiocardiac sympathosympathetic reflexes that increase both HR and contractility [165].

Bradycardia has been documented to facilitate the formation of ectopic beats, possibly by increasing temporal dispersion of excitability recovery in the myocardium, and by reducing the threshold for ventricular fibrillation [107, 108]. The sympathosympathetic reflexes have also been shown to contribute to the genesis of cardiac arrhythmias associated with myocardial ischemia, since these arrhythmias are considerably reduced after section of the thoracic dorsal roots that convey the afferent impulses [234].

The interactions among centrally induced efferent activity upon the heart, myocardial ischemia, and the various reflexive adjustments that can be triggered by ischemia have not been studied, but are necessarily complex in a conscious, behaving organism. Thus, for example, the activation of vagal afferents may reflexively induce profound bradycardia and an inhibition of sympathetic activity, which would lead to the unloading of the baroreceptors. This unloading could, in turn, induce a generalized sympathetic activation resulting in increased BP and sympathetic β-adrenergic activity at the heart. If pronounced, simultaneous increases in parasympathetic and sympathetic activity occur in the ischemic heart, this can increase susceptibility to fatal arrhythmias [15].

The very complexity of the interactive central and reflexive cardiovascular adjustments that are likely to be going on during myocardial ischemia in the behaving individual suggests the need for studying these adjustments in the conscious organism. Results of case [56] and retrospective studies [172, 214, 218] showing a close temporal link between acute emotional excitement and lethal or near-lethal ventricular arrhythmias further suggest the need for studying cardiovascular activity in the conscious, behaviorally stressed organism.

Several experiments conducted upon animals have related behavioral stress to sudden death, lethal and near-lethal arrhythmias. In the experiment by *Johansson* et al. [133] previously described, swine were subjected to 'restraint-stress' (i.e. prevention of escape behavior by myorelaxant) in conjunction with electric shock. Cardiomyopathy was observed in all of the experimental animals. Of 3 pigs that died suddenly, death was immediately preceded by ventricular fibrillation in 1 case and by sinus bradycardia terminating in ventricular standstill in 2 others. Major electrocardiographic changes included T wave inversion in all experimental animals and ventricular tachycardia in 14 of 23 animals.

In the experiment by *Corley* et al. [35], also previously described, squirrel monkeys were subjected to 24 h of unsignaled escape/avoidance or to a yoked condition. 4 deaths were associated with the experimental stress. Of these, 2 avoidance monkeys and 1 yoked monkey succumbed during the experimental session; another avoidance monkey seemed to show some recovery from the obvious effects of stress, but died suddenly 48 h later. For the 3 monkeys that succumbed during the session, HR declined from over 200 bpm to ventricular asystole within 5–10 min. The cardiovascular changes and stress-induced deaths did not appear to be related to the extent of cardiomyopathy that was observed in these animals as opposed to those who survived. *Richter* [217] had reported the results of an experiment in which severe behavioral stress led to pronounced bradycardia followed by cardiac arrest.

Skinner et al. [241] have studied the effects of emotional stress on the ECG of conscious pigs in whom the left anterior descending (LAD) coronary artery was occluded. In one group of animals occlusion occurred without prior adaptation to the laboratory situation, whereas in another group as many as 8 daily adaptation sessions were conducted before the animals were brought to the laboratory and the LAD coronary artery was occluded. Each adaptation session consisted of tying the pig's feet together, transporting it from the vivarium to the laboratory, attaching the recording wires and occluder tubes, and then leaving the animal undisturbed for 1 h before returning it to its home cage. The experimental session included the above steps through the attachment of the occluder tubes, which were then used to ligate the coronary artery.

Skinner et al. [241] found that animals not previously adapted to the experimental procedures revealed ventricular fibrillation 9–14 min following occlusion. Usually this fibrillation was preceded by ventricular arrhythmias (e.g. extrasystole, premature ventricular contractions) occurring during the first few minutes of acute coronary occlusion. A period of normal sinus rhythm was reinstated between the initial arrhythmias and the onset of fibrillation. In contrast to the nonadapted pigs, the swine receiving the 8 adaptation sessions did not reveal fibrillation during the next 24 h of monitoring.

The experiment by *Skinner* et al. [241] clearly demonstrated that the behavioral stress of an experimentally naive pig being tied up, transported from the vivarium to the laboratory, and then being prepared for experimentation was sufficient to trigger ventricular fibrillation following occlusion of the LAD coronary artery. Adaptation to these stressful procedures prior to occlusion delayed or prevented the fibrillation.

In order to study cardiac vulnerability to ventricular fibrillation, *Lown* et al. [163] have used nonobtrusive measures to assess electrical instability of the heart and its predisposition for potentially lethal arrhythmias. An assumption made in such experiments is that the nonobtrusive measures of electrical instability of the heart and ventricular fibrillation share a common electrophysiological basis. To the extent that this assumption is correct, and the nonobtrusive measures are derived from measures reflecting normal physiological processes, the nonobtrusive measures can be used as a marker of cardiac vulnerability for ventricular fibrillation. Advantages of the nonobtrusive measures are that they can be used in conscious animals without: (a) ongoing behavior being interrupted, and (b) the heart having to undergo ventricular fibrillation.

In early work, *Han and Moe* [109] found that if three stimuli are presented in close succession during diastole at low current intensities, they will elicit three extrasystoles. If, however, current intensity is progressively increased towards the ventricular fibrillation threshold, there comes a point where the three stimuli will elicit four or more responses (repetitive extrasystoles). The repetitive extrasystole threshold measure: (a) appears not to alter overall cardiac function; (b) does not appear to influence the animal's behavior, and (c) has been reported to be a constant 66% of the current required to reach the ventricular fibrillation threshold [170].

In one experiment using the repetitive extrasystole threshold as an endpoint, 5 dogs were tested in 2 different environments [164]. One environment, designed to minimize behavioral stress, consisted of a cage to which the dogs were acclimatized for 1 h/day for 3 days before testing. The other environment was one in which the animals were individually restrained in a sling during each of 3 daily sessions. During each of these sessions the animals received an electric shock while in the sling. On days 4 and 5 the dogs were examined in each environment, but no cutaneous shocks were presented. The current intensity required to elicit a repetitive extrasystole was found to be 3 times greater in the cage (43 mA) than in the sling (15 mA). *Lown* et al. [164] suggested that the lower repetitive extrasystole threshold obtained in the behaviorally stressful situation was due to increase SNS activity as exemplified by a rapid unpaced HR and somatic tremor. According to *Lown* et al. [163], placing dogs in the behaviorally stressful environment described above also resulted in elevated plasma catecholamines. In another experiment conducted in *Lown's* laboratory, dogs showed decreases in repetitive extrasystole thresholds during a signaled avoidance task [155].

Although *Skinner* et al. [241], *Lawler* [155], *Lown* et al. [163, 164], and *Matta* et al. [170] have provided evidence that is consistent with the view that SNS activation associated with behavioral stress can reduce the threshold for ventricular fibrillation, particularly under conditions of myocardial ischemia, the situation appears to be somewhat more complex. Thus, conditions also exist in which increases in HR and/or myocardial contractility may actually be associated with reductions rather than increases in ventricular arrhythmias. Some individuals with ventricular extrasystoles, for example, show a suppression of these arrhythmias during exercise [148, 202], and patients with premature ventricular contractions during rest can learn to suppress their arrhythmias by means of operantly conditioned (biofeedback training) increases in HR [203]. Finally, in an aversive Pavlovian conditioning experiment conducted upon rhesus monkeys, *Randall and Hasson* [210] have shown that if coronary occlusion takes place after the monkeys have been well-trained to make conditoned responses, the frequency of ventricular arrhythmias is sometimes reduced below basal levels on conditoning trials, even though the conditioned responses include increases in cardiac contractility, HR, and systemic arterial pressure.

Several major differences exist between the *Skinner* et al. [241] experiment in which psychological stimuli facilitated ventricular fibrillation and the *Randall and Hasson* [210] experiment in which the conditioned stimulus sometimes suppressed ventricular arrhythmias. One difference was species; a second was the nature of the psychological stimulus; and a third was the period when the coronary artery was ligated. Although differences in species and in procedures cannot be ruled out, the most important factors appear to be the differences in the stimulus situation and the period in the experiment when the coronary artery was ligated. Interestingly, the changes found with regard to arrhythmias in the studies conducted by *Skinner* et al. [241] and *Randall and Hasson* [210] parallel the changes found in: (a) plasma catecholamines by *Mason* et al. [168] in the rhesus monkey, and (b) effective refractory periods (ERP) of the heart by *Lawler* et al. [154] in dogs.

The pigs in the study by *Skinner* et al. [241] were subjected to the acute, severe, unexpected stress of being bound and transported to an unknown place. In contrast, the monkeys in the study by *Randall and Hasson* [210] were subjected to a predictable, Pavlovian conditioned stimulus in a situation with which the animals were already familiar. Previously, *Mason* et al. [168] had found that during novel, unpredictable, threatening situations, pronounced increases in epinephrine as well as norepinephrine occur, whereas during predictable situations such as those involving Pavlovian conditioning, increases occur in plasma norepinephrine but not epinephrine. Interestingly, *Lawler* et al. [154] found that the ventricular ERP (i.e. time following a paced beat before stimulation elicits an extrasystole) is shortest at the outset of the first session of a signaled avoidance situation when novelty, uncertainty, and perceived threat are likely to be greatest. It would thus appear that while the extensive distribution of β-adrenoceptors in the left ventricle is optimal for having epinephrine facilitate myocardial performance [9], this is accomplished at the risk of making the heart more vulnerable to ventricular arrhythmias during a momentary instability caused by myocardial ischemia.

In contrast to circulating epinephrine, which appears to have its greatest myocardial effects upon the left ventricle, norepinephrine has its greatest effect on the heart at nerve endings innervating the S-A and A-V nodes. It is therefore possible that, in the *Randall and Hasson* [210] experiment, the well-learned, predictable Pavlovian conditioning stimulus elicited the release of norepinephrine from terminals in the vicinity of the S-A and A-V nodes. This may then have produced rapid sinus pacemaker activity that then dominated the cardiac rhythm and in some instances overrode the ischemia-related arrhythmias.

Previous research in the rhesus monkey has established that during aversive Pavlovian conditioning sessions, experienced animals: (a) do not show increases in plasma epinephrine [168]; (b) reveal only moderate arousal in terms of their HR and BP baselines [143], and (c) have HR and BP conditioned and unconditioned responses that are heavily influenced by parasympathetic as well as SNS activity [143]. Interestingly, *Lawler* et al. [175] indicate that once conditioning is well-established (i.e. after five 90-min sessions), ventricular ERP actually increased from the preavoidance baseline during conditioning sessions. It is conceivable that similar sequences of events as those just described may have occurred in pigs that were brought to the experimental laboratory daily in the *Skinner* et al. [241] experiment.

In summary, it appears that in acute, unpredictable, highly fear-arousing situations, epinephrine has an important influence upon myocardial performance, and ERP decreases, whereas in more predictable, less threatening situations myocardial performance is primarily influenced by sympathetic and parasympathetic neuronal innervations, and ERP either remains unchanged or actually increases. When the heart is subjected to acute ischemia in conjunction with the preceding situations, the former is more likely than the latter to lead to ventricular fibrillation.

Conclusions

The results of animal behavior experiments have clearly linked prolonged and/or severe behavioral stress with the development of cardiovascular pathology. These pathologies include hypertension, atherosclerosis, cardiomyopathy, and ventricular arrhythmias. In each case SNS activity and the peripheral release of catecholamines have been implicated as important mediators.

Intense, life-threatening, behavioral stress can directly cause cardiomyopathy and even death [35, 133]. To a limited extent behavioral contingencies such as the predictability or unpredictability of aversive stimulation have been related to the severity of myocardial damage [173]. Physical restraint, which prevents the individual from making a fight, flight or other appropriate coping response, appears to be implicated in stress cardiomyopathy, but this variable requires further study. Although behavioral stress may cause death in an otherwise healthy individual, there is no evidence that behavioral stress alone can lead to a massive infarction.

Unlike cardiomyopathy, which can result solely from behavioral stress, sustained hypertension, atherosclerosis, and most fatal arrhythmias occur in conjunction with other factors. Although behavioral stress alone can induce hypertension that may outlast the immediate, aversive stimulus situation, the development of sustained hypertension appears to depend upon such predisposing factors as diet and genetic background with which psychologic factors may interact. The manner in which these three factors can interact is exemplified by the *Friedman and Iwai* [79] experiment in which genetic predisposition, the consumption of a modest amount of sodium in the diet and behavioral stress together produced sustained hypertension.

Similar interactions among diet, genetic predisposition and long-term behavioral stress, can lead to the development of atherosclerosis, which in turn provides the substrate for atherosclerotic CHD. In this respect, the animal behavior literature has provided convincing evidence that large (20–40 mm Hg), intermittent (12 h/day), fairly long-term (many months) elevations in BP do not necessarily lead to sustained hypertension [114], but the effects of these increases on the development of arteriosclerosis need to be evaluated. It appears likely that it is the SNS arousal, ordinarily associated with large, intermittent, long-term increases in BP rather than the BP increases that lead to sustained hypertension and arterio/atherosclerosis, probably in conjunction with genetic and dietary factors.

Animal behavior experiments have convincingly shown that long-term behavioral stress can interact with diet to enhance atherogenesis. Such an interaction can predispose an individual to ischemic CHD. Acute behavioral stress in such predisposed individuals could precipitate angina pectoris, myocardial infarction or fatal arrhythmias. Thus far, however, the interactions between myocardial ischemia and behavioral stress have only been studied using ligation of a major coronary artery to induce ischemia. The results indicate that severe, unexpected behavioral stress following acute myocardial ischemia can reliably produce ventricular fibrillation.

Although the behavioral changes that are associated with the development of cardiovascular pathology are closely linked to SNS activity and to the peripheral release of catecholamines, investigations of the possible mechanisms that might be mediating pathological processes were until fairly recently hampered by a lack of comprehensive physiological, biochemical and morphological analyses. Recent advances in techniques, and the systematic application of these techniques to the study of relationships between behavior and the development of CHD, are now providing valuable information. Use of tethering procedures in conjunction with computer analysis now allow 24 h/day recordings of BP to be made in the behaving animal. Concurrent use of a remotely controlled, permanently implanted venous catheter permits blood samples to be obtained covertly without the animal being aware of the procedure. This is important when studying behaviorally induced changes in epinephrine, norepinephrine and other humoral agents, whose plasma concentrations change rapidly in the behaving animal.

The development of methods for precisely monitoring plasma catecholamines, lipoprotein fractions, renin, cortisol, and electrolytes now permits close examination of the biochemical mechanisms likely to be mediating behaviorally induced pathology. Similarly, recent advances in technology now allow for detailed examination of the state of the systemic circulation, coronary vessels, condition of the heart and its conduction system, and the ability of the heart to extract oxygen during behavioral experiments.

Although animal behavior experiments have causally related behavioral stress to hypertension, atherogenesis, cardiomyopathy, and lethal ventricular arrhythmias, the exact relationships between specific behavioral variables and CHD have not yet been clearly specified. While improvements in technology will be helpful in establishing these relationships, they are not a panacea. Also needed are improvements in experimental design and in the conceptualization of issues.

One pervasive deficiency in experimental design has been a lack of stimulus control. Consequently, the exact roles of stimulus predictability, availability of coping responses, and the effortfulness of these responses have not yet been related to the development of CHD with adequate precision. Other deficiencies have often included insufficient information about the animals being studied, particularly concerning home cage-living conditions, life history, relative maturity, sex, and psychosocial behavior.

Recently, new experimental designs have been introduced, which permit animals to interact relatively freely in more naturalistic environments while their physiology and behavior are closely monitored. Such designs permit the assessment of individual differences in behavior. Although relatively few animal studies have examined the role of individual differences in the development in CHD, several striking parallels have been found between the behavior of nonhuman and human primates. Thus, for example, *Kaplan and Manuck* [139] found that HR reactivity to an aversive behavioral challenge is positively associated with atherosclerosis. This finding is of particular interest with regard to atherosclerotic CHD in humans, because type A relative to type B individuals have been shown to have greater HR reactivity in challenging behavioral situations [44].

Another example is provided by the work of *Coehlo and Bramblett* [34], who used computer analyses in the development of ethograms, dimensionalized baboon behavior into general categories, and then found that animals scoring relatively low on dominance, but high on tension, threat and attack have relatively high levels of plasma cholesterol. Experiments such as these should provide valuable information about important relationships between psychosocial behavior and the development of atherosclerotic CHD.

The basic thesis of this chapter has been that aversive behavior and the SNS play an important role in the development of cardiovascular pathology. Experiments such as those described by *Coehlo and Bramblett* [34] suggest that the behaviors involved may be quite complex. This implies that the CNS plays a larger role in the development of such pathology than has generally been recognized. Our recent experiments [86] indicate that at least two separate SNS patterns of response are integrated within the brain, and that these are associated with two alternative patterns of behavioral activity. It remains to be demonstrated whether these two SNS patterns, if evoked consistently, can lead to separate forms of pathology.

A third physiological pattern, and one that can be elicited by electrical stimulation of the lateral hypothalamus in the conscious rabbit [86] consists of a bradycardia response, a modest decrease in BP and quiet, behavioral inactivity. It also remains to be seen whether activation of this pathway, which descends from the central nucleus of the amygdala through the lateral hypothalamus and lateral zona incerta, can counteract any of the deleterious effects of prolonged, intense SNS activation, which results in cardiovascular pathology. Interestingly, electrical stimulation of the lateral hypothalamus of the rabbit has been shown to be: (a) rewarding in an instrumental conditioning situation [239], and (b) effective as an unconditioned stimulus leading to a conditioned decrease in BP as the learned response during Pavlovian conditioning [20].

References

1 Abrahams, V.C.; Hilton, S.M.; Zbrozyna, A.: Active muscle vasodilation produced by stimulation of the brain stem: Its significance in the defence reaction. J. Physiol., Lond. *154:* 491–513 (1960).

2 Adams, D.B.; Baccelli, G.; Mancia, G.; Zanchetti, A.: Cardiovascular changes during naturally elicited fighting behavior in the cat. Am. J. Physiol. *216:* 1226–1235 (1968).

3 Ahlquist, R.P.: A study of the adrenotropic receptors. Am. J. Physiol. *153:* 586–600 (1948).

4 Alexander, F.: Psychoanalytic study of a case of essential hypertension. Psychosom. Med. *1:* 139–152 (1939).

5 Alexander, N.: Psychosocial hypertension in members of a Wistar rat colony. Proc. Soc. exp. Biol. Med. *146:* 163–169 (1974).

6 American Heart Association, National Academy of Sciences, & National Research Council: Standards of cardiopulmonary resuscitation (CPR) and emergency cardiac care (ECC). J. Am. med. Ass. *227:* 833–868 (1974).

7 Anderson, C.E.; Tosheff, J.: Cardiac output and total peripheral resistance changes during preavoidance periods in the dog. J. appl. Physiol. *34:* 650–654 (1973).

8 Baccelli, G.; Ellison, G.D.; Mancia, G.; Zanchetti, A.: Opposite responses of muscle circulation to different emotional stimuli. Experientia *27:* 1183–1184 (1971).

9 Baker, S.P.; Potter, L.T.: Biochemical studies of cardiac β-adrenoceptors, and their clinical significance. Circulation Res. *46:* suppl. I, pp. 34–42 (1980).

10 Ban, T.: The septo-preoptico-hypothalamic system and its autonomic function; in Tokizane, Schade, Correlative neurosciences. Prog. Brain Res. (Elsevier, Amsterdam 1966).

11 Bassett, J.R.; Cairncross, K.D.: Morphological changes induced in rats following prolonged exposure to stress. Pharmacol. Biochem. Behav. *3:* 411–429 (1975).

12 Bassett, J.R.; Cairncross, K.D.: Changes in the coronary vascular system following prolonged exposure to stress. Pharmacol. Biochem. Behav. *6:* 311–318 (1977).

13 Beck, L.; Pollard, A.A.; Kayaalp, S.O.; Weiner, L.H.: Sustained dilation elicited by sympathetic nerve stimulation. Fed. Proc. *25:* 1596–1606 (1966).

14 Benson, H.; Herd, J.A.; Morse, W.H.; Kelleher, R.T.: Behavioral induction of arterial hypertension and its reversal. Am. J. Physiol. *217:* 30–34 (1969).

15 Bergamaschi, M.: Role of the sympathetic and parasympathetic innervation in the genesis of ventricular arrhythmias during experimental myocardial ischemia; in Schwartz, Brown, Malliani, Zanchetti, Neural mechanisms in cardiac arrhythmias (Raven Press, New York 1978).

16 Bernard, C.: De l'influence du systeme nerveux grand sympathique sur la chaleur animale. Comptes Rendus *34:* 472–494 (1852).

17 Berne, R.M.; Rubio, R.: Regulation of the coronary blood flow. Adv. Cardiol. *12:* 303–317 (1974).

18 Blumenthal, J.A.; Williams, R.B., Jr.; Kong, Y.; Schanberg, S.M.; Thompson, L.W.: Type A behavior pattern and coronary atherosclerosis. Circulation *58:* 634–639 (1978).

19 Bramblett, C.A.; Coelho, A.M., Jr.; Mott, G.E.: Behavior and serum cholesterol in a social group of cercopithecus aethiops. Primates *22:* 96–102 (1981).

20 Brickman, A.; Schneiderman, N.: Classically conditioned blood pressure decreases induced by electrical stimulation of posterior hypothalamus in rabbits. Psychophysiology *14:* 287–292 (1977).

21 Bronson, F.H.; Eleftherious, B.E.: Adrenal response to fighting in mice: separation of physical and psychological causes. Science *147:* 627–628 (1965).

22 Bronte-Stewart, B.; Heptinstal, R.H.: The relationship between experimental hypertension and cholesterol-induced atheroma in rabbits. J. Path. *68:* 407–414 (1954).

23 Brown, J.J.; Fraser, R.; Lever, A.F.; Morton, J.J.; Robertson, J.I.S.; Schalekamp, M.A.D.H.: Mechanisms in hypertension: a personal view; in Genest, Koiw, Kuchel, Hypertension: physiopathology and treatment (McGraw-Hill, New York 1977).

24 Brown, M.S.; Kovanen, P.T.; Goldstein, J.L.: Regulation of plasma cholesterol by lipoprotein receptors. Science *212:* 628–635 (1981).

25 Buckley, J.P.; Smookler, H.H.: Cardiovascular and biochemical effects of chronic intermittent neurogenic stimulation; in Welch, Welch, Physiological effects of noise (Plenum Publishing, New York 1970).

26 Burstein, Y.; Berns, L.; Heldenberg, D.; Kahn, Y.; Werbin, B.Z.; Tamir, I.: Increase in platelet aggregation following a rise in plasma free fatty acids. Am. J. Hematol. *4:* 17–22 (1978).

27 Cannon, W.R.: Bodily changes in pain, hunger, fear and rage; 2nd ed. (Appleton, New York 1929).

28 Carretero, D.A.; Romero, J.C.: Production and characteristics of experimental hypertension in animals; in Genest, Koiw, Kuchel, Hypertension: physiopathology and treatment (McGraw-Hill, New York 1977).

29a Carruthers, M.E.: Aggression and atheroma. Lancet *ii:* 1170–1171 (1969).

29b Chan, S.H.H.; Koo, A.: The participation of medullary reticular formation in clonidine-induced hypotension in rats. Neuropharmacology *17:* 367–373 (1978).

30 Chen, Y.H.; Chan, S.H.H.: Clonidine-induced hypotension in cats: the role of medial medullary reticular α-adrenoceptors and vagus nerve (Abstr.). Neuroscience *4:* 47 (1978).

31 Chinn, C.: Pharmacological aspects of neural control of the circulation; in Hughes, Barnes, Neural control of the circulation (Academic Press, New York 1980).

32 Cobb, S.; Rose, R.M.: Hypertension, peptic ulcer and diabetes in air traffic controllers. J. Am. med. Ass. *224:* 489–492 (1973).

33 Coelho, A.M.; Bramblett, C.A.: Species specificity in stress modeling in nonhuman primates. Proc. Pre-Meeting Workshop on Stress, Am. Society of Primatologists, Winston-Salem 1980.

34 Coehlo, A.M., J.; Bramblett, C.A.: Interobserver agreement on a molecular ethogram of the genus *Papio.* Anim. Behav. in press.

35 Corley, K.C.; Shiel, F. O'M.; Mauck, H.P.; Clark, L.S.; Barber, J.V.: Myocardial degeneration and cardiac arrest in squirrel monkey: physiological and psychological correlation. Psychophysiology *14:* 322–328 (1977).

36 Corley, K.C.; Shiel, F. O'M.; Mauck, H.P.; Geenhoot, J.: Electrocardiographic and cardiac morphological changes associated with environmental stress in squirrel monkeys. Psychosom. Med. *35:* 361–364 (1973).

37 Dahl, L.K.; Heine, M.; Tassinari, L.J.: Role of genetic factors in susceptibility to experimental hypertension due to chronic excess salt ingestion. Nature, Lond. *194:* 480–482 (1962).

38 Dahl, L.K.; Heine, M.; Tassinari, L.J.: Effects of chronic excess salt ingestion: role of genetic factors in both Doca-salt and renal hypertension. J. exp. M. *118:* 605–617 (1963).

39 Dahl, L.K.; Heine, M.; Tassinari, L.J.: Effects of chronic salt ingestion. Further demonstration that genetic factors influence the development of hypertension: evidence from experimental hypertension due to cortisone and to adrenal regeneration. J. exp. Med. *122:* 533–545 (1965).

40 Danon, D.; Skutelsky, E.: Endothelial surface charge and its possible relationship to thrombogenesis. Ann. N.Y. Acad. Sci. *275:* 47–63 (1976).

41 Day, M.D.; Roach, A.G.: Centrally mediated cardiovascular effects of propranolol and other β-adrenoceptor antagonists in the conscious cat; in Reid, Davies, Central action of drugs in blood pressure regulation (Pitman Medical, London 1975).

42 DeChamplain, J.: Experimental aspects of the relationships between the autonomic nervous system and catecholamines in hypertension; in Genest, Koiw, Kuchel, Hypertension: physiopathology and treatment (McGraw-Hill, New York 1977).

43 DeChamplain, J.; Van Ameringen, M.R.: Role of sympathetic fibers and of adrenal medulla in the maintenance of cardiovascular homeostasis in normotensive and hypertensive rats; in Usdin, Snyder, Frontiers in catecholamine research (Pergamon Press, New York 1973).

44 Dembroski, T.M.; MacDougall, J.M.; Herd, J.A.; Shields, J.L.: Effect of level of challenge on pressor and heart rate responses in type A and type B subjects. J. appl. soc. Psychol. *9:* 209–228 (1979).

45 Deming, Q.B.; Mosbach, E.H.; Bevans, M.D.; Daly, M.M.; Akell, L.L.; Martin, E.; Kaplan, R.: Blood pressure, cholesterol content of serum and tissues and atherosclerosis in the rat. J. exp. Med. *107:* 581–590 (1958).

46 Dewanjee, M.K.; Kahn, P.C.: Mechanism of localization of ^{99m}Tc-labeled pyrophosphate and tetracycline in infarcted myocardium. J. nucl. Med. *17:* 639–646 (1976).

47 Dimsdale, J.E.; Moss, J.M.: Plasma catecholamines in stress and exercise. J. Am. med. Ass. *243:* 340–342 (1980).

48 Dittmar, C.: Über die Lage des sogenannten Gefässzentrums in der Medulla oblongata. Ber. Sachs. Ges. Wiss. Mat. Phys. Kl. *25:* 449–479 (1873).

49 Djojosugito, A.M.; Folkow, B.; Klystra, P.; Lisander, B.; Tuttle, R.S.: Differentiated interaction between the hypothalamic defense reaction and baroreceptor reflexes. 1. Effects on heart rate and regional flow resistance. Acta physiol. scand. *78:* 376–383 (1970).

50 Doba, N.; Reis, D.J.: Role of central and peripheral adrenergic mechanisms in neurogenic hypertension produced by brainstem lesions in rat. Circulation Res. *34:* 293–301 (1974).

51 Dykman, R.A.; Gantt, W.A.: Experimental psychogenic hypertension: blood pressure changes conditioned to painful stimuli. Bull. Johns Hopkins Hosp. *107:* 72–89 (1960).
52 Ehrstrom, M.D.: Psychogene Kriegshypertonien. Acta med. scand. *122:* 546–570 (1945).
53 Eliot, R.S.: Stress and the major cardiovascular disorders (Futura, New York 1979).
54 Eliot, R.S.; Todd, G.L.: Stress-induced myocardial necrosis. J. S.C. med. Ass. *72:* suppl., pp.33–37 (1976).
55 Eliot, R.S.; Todd, G.L.; Clayton, F.C.; Pieper, G.M.: Experimental catecholamine-induced acute myocardial necrosis; in Manninen, Halonen, Adv. Cardiol., vol. 25 (Karger, Basel 1978).
56 Engel, G.: Sudden and rapid death during psychological stress. Annls intern. Med. *74:* 771–782 (1971).
57 Engel, B.T.; Bickford, A.F.: Response specificity: stimulus-response and individual-response specificity in essential hypertensives. Archs gen. Psychiat. *5:* 479–484 (1961).
58 Esler, M.; Julius, S.; Zweifler, A.; Randall, O.; Harburg, E.; Gardiner, H.; De Quattro, V.: Mild high-renin essential hypertension – neurogenic hypertension? New Engl. J. Med. *296:* 405–411 (1977).
59 Falk, J.L.: Production of polydipsia in normal rats by an intermittend food schedule. Science *133:* 195–196 (1961).
60 Falk, J.L.; Tang, M.; Forman, S.: Schedule-induced chronic hypertension. Psychosom. Med. *39:* 252–263 (1977).
61 Falkner, B.; Onesti, G.; Angelakos, E.T.; Fernandes, M.; Langman, C.: Cardiovascular response to mental stress in normal adolescents with hypertensive parents. Hemodynamics and mental stress in adolescents. Hypertension *1:* 23–30 (1979).
62 Farris, E.J.; Yeakel, E.H.; Medoff, H.: Development of hypertension in emotional gray Norway rats after air blasting. Am. J. Physiol. *144:* 331–333 (1945).
63 Feigl, E.O.: Control of myocardial oxygen tension by sympathetic coronary vasoconstriction in the dog. Circulation Res. *37:* 88–95 (1975).
64 Ferrans, V.J.; Hibbs, R.G.; Black, W.C.; Weilbaecher, D.G.: Isoproterenol-induced myocardial necrosis: a histochemical and electron microscopic study. Am. Heart J. *68:* 71–90 (1964).
65 Ferrans, V.J.; Hibbs, R.G.; Walsh, J.J.; Burch, G.E.: Histochemical and electron microscopical studies on the cardiac necroses produced by sympathomimetic agents. Ann. N.Y. Acad. Sci. *156:* 309–332 (1969).
66 Fleckenstein, A.; Janke, J.; Doring, H.J.; Leder, O.: Key role of Ca in the production of noncoronarogenic myocardial necroses; in Fleckenstein, Rona, Recent advances in studies on cardiac structure and metabolism, vol. 6 (University Park Press, Baltimore 1975).
67 Folkow, B.: Vascular changes in hypertension: review and recent animal studies; in Berglund, Hansson, Werkö, Pathophysiology and management of arterial hypertension (Lindren & Söner, Mölndal 1975).
68 Folkow, B.; Grimby, G.; Thulesius, O.: Adaptive structural changes of the vascular walls in hypertension and their relation to the control of the peripheral resistance. Acta physiol. scand. *44:* 255–272 (1958).
69 Folkow, B.; Hallbäck, M.: Physiopathology of spontaneous hypertension in rats; in Genest, Koiw, Kuchel, Hypertension: physiopathology and treatment (McGraw-Hill, New York 1977).
70 Folkow, B.; Neil, E.: Circulation (Oxford University Press, London 1971).

71   Folkow, B.; Uvnäs, B.: Distribution and functional significance of sympathetic vasodilators to the hind limb of the cat. Acta physiol. scand. *15:* 389–400 (1948).

72   Forsyth, R.P.: Blood pressure and avoidance conditioning. Psychosom. Med. *30:* 125–135 (1968).

73   Forsyth, R.P.: Blood pressure responses to long-term avoidance schedules in the restrained rhesus monkey. Psychosom. Med. *31:* 300–309 (1969).

74   Forsyth, R.P.: Regional blood flow changes during 72-hour avoidance schedules in the monkey. Science *173:* 546–548 (1971).

75   Franco-Morselli, R.; De Mendonca, M.; Baudouin-Legros, M.; Guicheney, P.; Meyer, P.: Plasma catecholamines in essential human hypertension and in Doca-salt hypertension of the rat; in Meyer, Schmitt, Nervous system and Hypertension (Wiley, New York 1979).

76   Friedman, M.: The pathogenesis of coronary artery disease (McGraw-Hill, New York 1969).

77   Friedman, R.; Dahl, L.K.: The effect of chronic conflict on the blood pressure of rats with a genetic susceptibility to experimental hypertension. Psychosom. Med. *37:* 402–416 (1975).

78   Friedman, R.; Iwai, J.: Genetic predisposition and stress-induced hypertension. Science *193:* 161–162 (1976).

79   Friedman, R.; Iwai, J.: Dietary sodium, psychic stress, and genetic predisposition to experimental hypertension. Proc. Soc. exp. Biol. Med. *155:* 449–452 (1977).

80   Friedman, M.; Manwaring, J.H.; Rosenman, R.H.; Donlon, G.; Ortega, P.; Grube, S.M.: Instantaneous and sudden deaths: clinical and pathological differentiation in coronary artery disease. J. Am. med. Ass. *225:* 1319–1328 (1973).

81   Friedman, B.; Oester, Y.T.; Davis, O.F.: The effect of arterenol and epinephrine on experimental arteriopathy. Archs int. Pharmcodyn. Thér. *102:* 226–234 (1955).

82   Friedman, M.; Rosenman, R.H.: Association of specific overt behavior pattern with blood and cardiovascular findings. J. Am. med. Ass. *169:* 1286–1296 (1959).

83   Friedman, M.; Rosenman, R.H.; Straus, R.; Wurm, M.; Kositchek, R.: The relationship of behavior pattern A to the state of the coronary vasculature: a study of 51 autopsied subjects. Am. J. Med. *44:* 525–537 (1968).

84   Friedman, R.; Tassinari, L.M.; Heine, M.; Iwai, J.: Differential development of salt-induced and renal hypertension in Dahl hypertension-sensitive rats after neonatal sympathectomy. Clin. exp. Hypertens. *1:* 779–799 (1979).

85   Fuller, G.; Langer, R.: Elevation of aortic proline hydroxylase: a biochemical defect in experimental atherosclerosis. Science *168:* 987–989 (1970).

86   Gellman, M.; Schneiderman, N.; Wallach, J.; LeBlanc, W.: Cardiovascular responses elicited by hypothalamic stimulation in rabbits reveal a medio-lateral organization. J. autonom. nerv. Syst. (in press).

87   Genest, J.: Basic mechanisms of essential hypertension; in Genest, Koiw, Kuchel, Hypertension: physiopathology and treatment (McGraw-Hill, New York 1977).

88   Gill, J.R., Jr.; Casper, A.G.T.: Role of the sympathetic nervous system in the renal response to hemorrhage. J. clin. Invest. *48:* 915–922 (1969).

89   Glass, D.C.; Krakoff, L.R.; Contrada, R.; Hilton, W.F.; Kehoe, K.; Mannucci, E.G.; Collins, C.; Snow, B.; Elting, E.: Effect of harassment and competition upon cardiovascular and plasma catecholamine responses in type A and type B individuals. Psychophysiology *17:* 453–463 (1980).

90   Goldblatt, H.J.; Lynch, R.F.; Hanzal, R.F.; Summerville, W.W.: Studies on experimental

hypertension. I. The production of persistent elevation of systolic blood pressure by means of renal ischemia. J. exp. Med. *59:* 347 (1934).

91 Goldstein, J.L.; Brown, M.S.: Lipoprotein receptors, cholesterol metabolism and atherosclerosis. Arch. Path. *99:* 181–192 (1975).

92 Goldstein, D.S.; Harris, A.H.; Brady, J.V.: Baroreflex sensitivity during operant blood pressure conditioning. Biofeedback Self-Regul. *2:* 127–137 (1977).

93 Goldstein, D.S.; Harris, A.H.; Izzo, J.L.; Turkkan, J.S.; Keiser, H.R.: Plasma catecholamines and renin during operant blood pressure conditioning in baboons. Physiol. Behav. (in press).

94 Goth, A.; Johnson, A.R.: Current concepts on the secretory function of mast cells. Life. Sci. *16:* 1201–1214 (1975).

95 Graham, J.D.P.: High blood pressure after battle. Lancet *248:* 239–240 (1945).

96 Green, J.H.: Physiology of baroreceptor function: mechanism of receptor stimulation; in Kezdi, Baroreceptors and hypertension (Pergamon, Oxford 1967).

97 Groover, M.E.; Seljeskog, L.L.; Haglin, J.J.; Hitchcock, C.R.: Myocardial infarction in the Kenya baboon without demonstrable atherosclerosis. Angiology *14:* 409–416 (1963).

98 Guideri, G.; Barletta, M.; Chau, R.; Green, M.; Lehr, D.: Method for the production of severe ventricular dysrhythmias in small laboratory animals; in Roy, Rona, The metabolism of contraction (University Park Press, Baltimore 1975).

99 Guyton, A.C.: Personal views on mechanisms of hypertension; in Genest, Koiw, Kuchel, Hypertension: physiopathology and treatment (McGraw-Hill, New York 1977).

100 Haft, H.I.; Fani, K.: Intravascular platelet aggregation in the heart induced by stress. Circulation *48:* 164–169 (1973).

101 Hall, C.E.; Hall, O.: Augmentation of hormone-induced hypertensive cardiovascular disease by simultaneous exposure to stress. Acta endocr., Copenh. *30:* 557–566 (1959).

102 Hall, C.E.; Hall, O.: Enhancement of somatotrophic hormone-induced hypertensive vascular disease by stress. Am. J. Physiol. *197:* 702–704 (1959).

103 Hallbäck, M.: Consequences of social isolation on blood pressure, cardiovascular reactivity and design in spontaneously hypertensive rat. Acta physiol. Scand. *93:* 455–465 (1975).

104 Hallbäck, M.; Folkow, B.: Cardiovascular response to acute mental 'stress' in spontaneously hypertensive rats. Acta physiol. scand. *90:* 684–693 (1974).

105 Hallbäck-Norlander, M.; Lundin, S.: Background of hyperkinetic circulatory state in young spontaneously hypertensive rats; in Meyer, Schmitt, Nervous system and hypertension (Wiley, New York 1979).

106 Hamilton, R.B.; Ellenberger, H.; Liskowsky, D.; Schneiderman, N.: Parabrachial area as mediator of bradycardia in rabbits. J. autonom. nerv. Syst. (in press).

107 Han, J.; Detraglia, J.; Millet, D.; Moe, G.K.: Incidence of ectopic beats as a function of basic rate in the ventricle. Am. Heart J. *72:* 632–637 (1966).

108 Han, J.; Millet, D.; Chizzoniti, B.; Moe, G.K.: Temporal dispersion and recovery of excitability in atrium and ventricle as a function of heart rate. Am. Heart J. *71:* 481–486 (1966).

109 Han, J.; Moe, G.K.: Nonuniform recovery of excitability in ventricular muscle. Circulation Res. *14:* 44–60 (1964).

110 Hansen, C.T.: A genetic analysis of hypertension in the rat; in Okamoto, Spontaneous hypertension (Igaku Shoin, Tokyo 1972).

111 Harburg, E.; Erfurt, J.C.; Havenstein, L.S.; Chape, C.; Schull, W.J.; Schork, M.A.: Socio-ecological stress, suppressed hostility, skin color, and black-white male blood pressure: Detroit. Psychosom. Med. *35:* 276–296 (1973).

112   Harris, A.H.; Brady, J.V.: Long-term studies of cardiovascular control in primates; in Schwartz, Beatty, Biofeedback: theory and research (Academic Press, New York 1977).

113   Harris, A.H.; Gilliam, W.J.; Brady, J.V.: Operant conditioning of large magnitude, 12-hour duration, heart rate elevations in the baboon. Pavlov. J. biol. Sci. *11:* 86–92 (1976).

114   Harris, A.H.; Gilliam, W.J.; Findley, J.D.; Brady, J.V.: Instrumental conditioning of large-magnitude, daily, 12-hour blood pressure elevations in the baboon. Science *182:* 175–177 (1973).

115   Heindel, J.J.; Orci, L.; Jenarenaud, B.: Fat mobilization and its regulation by hormones and drugs in white adipose tissue; in Masoro, International encyclopedia of pharmacology and therapeutics. Pharmacology of lipid transport and atherosclerotic processes, vol. 1, pp. 175–373 (Pergamon Press, Oxford 1975).

116   Heitz, D.C.; Brody, M.J.: Possible mechanism of histamine release during active vaso-dilation. Am. J. Physiol. *228:* 1351–1357 (1975).

117   Henning, M.; Rubenson, R.: Evidence that the hypotensive action of methyldopa is mediated by central actions of methyl noradrenaline. J. Pharm. Pharmac. *23:* 407–413 (1971).

118   Henry, J.P.; Ely, D.L.; Stephens, P.M.: Changes in catecholamine-controlling enzymes in response to psychosocial activation of the defence and alarm reactions. Physiology, emotion and psychosomatic illness. Ciba Fdn Symp. *8:* 225–251 (1972).

119   Henry, J.P.; Ely, D.L.; Stephens, P.M.; Ratcliffe, H.L.; Santisteban, G.A.; Shapiro, A.P.: The role of psychosocial factors in the development of arteriosclerosis in CBA mice. Atherosclerosis *14:* 203–218 (1971).

120   Henry, J.P.; Meehan, J.P.; Stephens, P.M.: The use of psychosocial stimuli to induce pro-longed systolic hypertension in mice. Psychosom. Med. *29:* 408–432 (1967).

121   Henry, J.P.; Stephens, P.M.: Stress, health and the social environment: a sociobiologic approach to medicine (Springer, New York 1977).

122   Henry, J.P.; Stephens, P.M.; Axelrod, J.; Mueller, R.A.: Effect of psychosocial stimulation on the enzymes involved in the biosynthesis and metabolism of noradrenaline and adrenaline. Psychosom. Med. *33:* 227–237 (1971).

123   Henry, J.P.; Stephens, P.M.; Santisteban, G.A.: A model of psychosocial hypertension showing reversibility and progression of cardiovascular complications. Circulation Res. *36:* 156–164 (1975).

124   Herd, J.A.; Morse, W.H.; Kelleher, R.T.; Jones, L.G.: Arterial hypertension in the squirrel monkey during behavioral experiments. Am. J. Physiol. *217:* 24–29 (1969).

125   Hess, W.R.: Functional organization of the diencephalon (Grune & Stratton, New York 1957).

126   Higgs, E.A.; Moncada, S.; Vane, J.R.: Effect of prostacyclin (PGI_2) on platelet adhesion to rabbit arterial subendothelium. Prostaglandins *16:* 17–22 (1978).

127   Hilton, S.M.: Ways of viewing the central nervous control of the circulation – old and new. Brain Res. *87:* 213–219 (1975).

128   Hilton, S.M.; Spyer, K.M.; Timms, R.J.: Hind limb vasodilation evoked by stimulation of the motor cortex. J. Physiol., Lond. *252:* 22P–23P (1975).

129   Hines, E.A.; Brown, G.E.: The cold pressor test for measuring the reactibility of the blood pressure: data concerning 571 normal and hypertensive subjects. Am. Heart J. *11:* 1–9 (1936).

130   Hollander, W.: Biochemical pathology of atherosclerosis and relationship to hyperten-

sion; in Genest, Koiw, Kuchel, Hypertension: physiopathology and treatment (McGraw-Hill, New York 1977).

131 Ikeda, T.; Tobian, L.; Iwai, J.; Goosens, P.: Central nervous system pressor response in rats susceptible and resistant to NaCl hypertension; in Meyer, Schmitt, Nervous system and hypertension (Wiley, New York 1979).

132 Jonsson, L.; Johansson, G.: Cardiac muscle cell damage induced by restraint stress. Virchows Arch. Abt. B Zellpath. *17:* 1–12 (1974).

133 Johansson, G.; Jonsson, L.; Lannek, N.; Blomgren, L.; Lindberg, P.; Poupa, O.: Severe stress-cardiopathy in pigs. Am. Heart J. *87:* 451–457 (1974).

134 Jordan, D.; Khalid, M.; Schneiderman, N.; Sper, K.M.: The inhibitory control of vagal cardiomotor neurons. J. Physiol., Lond. *301:* 54P (1979).

135 Julius, S.; Esler, M.: The nervous system in arterial hypertension (Thomas, Springfield 1975).

136 Kabat, H.; Magoun, H.; Ranson, S.: Electrical stimulation of points in the forebrain and midbrain. Arch. Neurol. Psychiat. *34:* 931–955 (1935).

137 Kannel, W.B.; Gordon, T.: The Framingham Study: an epidemiological investigation of cardiovascular disease, sect. 27, No. 1740-0329 (US Government Printing Office, Washington 1971).

138 Kaplan, K.L.; Brockman, J.; Chernoff, A.; Lesznik, G.R.; Drillings, M.: Platelet alpha granule proteins. Studies on release and subcellular localization. Blood *53:* 604–618 (1979).

139 Kaplan, J.R.; Manuck, S.B.: Stress-induced heart rate reactivity and atherosclerosis in monkeys. Psychosom. Med. *43:* 189 (1981).

140 Kaplan, J.R.; Manuck, S.B.; Clarkson, T.B.: Social factors and coronary artery atherosclerosis in cynomolgus monkeys. Proc. Annu. Meet. of the Am. Heart Ass., Dallas 1981.

141 Kaufman, M.; Hamilton, R.; Wallach, J.; Petrik, G.; Schneiderman, N.: Lateral subthalamic area as mediator of bradycardia responses in rabbits. Am. J. Physiol. *236:* H471–H479 (1979).

142 Kelleher, R.; Morse, W.; Herd, J.A.: Effects of propranolol, phentolamine, and methylatropine on cardiovascular function in the squirrel monkey during behavioral experiments. J. Pharmac. exp. Ther. *182:* 204–207 (1972).

143 Klose, K.J.; Augenstein, J.S.; Schneiderman, N.; Manas, K.; Abrams, B.; Bloom, L.J.: Selective autonomic blockade of conditioned and unconditioned cardiovascular changes in rhesus monkeys. J. comp. physiol. Psychol. *89:* 810–818 (1975).

144 Kobinger, W.: Central α-adrenergic systems as targets for hypotensive drugs. Ergebn. Physiol. biol. Chem. exp. Pharmak. *81:* 40–100 (1978).

145 Koch, E.: Die reflektorische Selbststeuerung des Kreislaufes (Steinkopf, Leipzig 1931).

146 Korner, P.I.: Integrative neural cardiovascular control. Physiol. Rev. *51:* 312–367 (1971).

147 Krantz, D.S.; Sanmarco, M.I.; Selvester, R.H.; Matthews, K.A.: Psychological correlates of progression of atherosclerosis in men. Psychosom. Med. *41:* 467–475 (1979).

148 Lamb, L.E.; Hiss, R.G.: Influences of exercise on premature contractions. Am. J. Cardiol. *10:* 209–216 (1962).

149 Lang, C.M.: Effects of psychic stress on atherosclerosis in the squirrel monkey *(Saimiri sciureus)*. Proc. Soc. exp. Biol. Med. *126:* 30–34 (1967).

150 Lapin, B.; Cherkovich, G.M.: Environmental change causing the development of neuroses and corticovisceral pathology in monkeys; in Levi, Society, stress and disease: the psychosocial environment and psychosomatic diseases (London 1971).

151 Lawler, J.E.: Effects of behavioral stress on electrophysiological properties of the heart. Proc. Annu. Meet. of the Society for Psychophysiological Research, Toronto 1975.

152 Lawler, J.E.; Barker, G.F.; Hubbard, J.W.; Allen, M.T.: The effects of conflict on tonic levels of blood pressure in the genetically borderline hypertensive rat. Psychophysiology *17:* 363–370 (1980).

153 Lawler, J.E.; Barker, G.F.; Hubbard, J.W.; Schaub, R.G.: Pathophysiological changes associated with stress-induced hypertension in the borderline hypertensive rat. Proc. 7th Scientific Meet. Int. Society of Hypertension, New Orleans 1980.

154 Lawler, J.E.; Botticelli, L.J.; Lown, B.: Changes in cardiac refractory period during signalled avoidance in dogs. Psychophysiology *13:* 373–377 (1976).

155 Lawler, J.E.; Obrist, P.A.; Lawler, K.A.: Cardiovascular function during pre-avoidance, avoidance, and post-avoidance in dogs. Psychophysiology *12:* 4–11 (1975).

156 Lessem, J.; Pollimeni, P.; Page, F.: Tc-99m pyrophosphate image of rat ventricular infarcts: correlation of time course with microscopic pathology. Am. J. Cardiol. *39:* 279–285 (1977).

157 Levy, M.N.: Neural mechanisms in cardiac arrhythmias. J. Lab. clin. Med. *90:* 589–591 (1977).

158 Lew, E.A.: High blood pressure, other risk factors and longevity: the insurance viewpoint; in Laragh, Hypertension manual: mechanisms, methods, and management (Yorke Medical Books, New York 1973).

159 Lewis, P.J.: Propranolol – an antihypertensive drug with a central action; in Davies, Reid, Central action of drugs in blood pressure regulation (Univ. Park Press, Baltimore 1976).

160 Lipman, R.L.; Shapiro, A.: Effects of a behavioral stimulus on the blood pressure of rats with experimental pyelonephritis. Psychosom. Med. *29:* 612–618 (1967).

161 Liskowsky, D.; Ellenberger, H.; Haselton, J.; Schneiderman, N.; Hamilton, R.B.: Descending bradycardia pathways between the parabrachial nucleus and the medulla in the rabbit. Neurosci. Abstr. (in press, 1981).

162 Lown, B.: Sudden cardiac death: the major challenge confronting contemporary cardiology. Am. J. Cardiol. *43:* 313–328 (1979).

163 Lown, B.; DeSilva, R.A.; Reich, P.; Murawski, B.J.: Psychophysiologic factors in sudden cardiac death. Am. J. Psychiat. *137:* 1325–1335 (1980).

164 Lown, B.; Verrier, R.L.; Corbalan, R.: Psychologic stress and threshold for repetitive ventricular response. Science *132:* 834–836 (1973).

165 Malliani, A.; Lombardi, F.: Neural reflexes associated with myocardial ischemia; in Schwartz, Brown, Malliani, Zanchetti, Neural mechanisms in cardiac arrhythmias (Raven Press, New York 1978).

166 Malliani, A.; Schwartz, P.J.; Zanchetti, A.: A sympathetic reflex elicited by experimental coronary occlusion. Am. J. Physiol. *217:* 703–709 (1969).

167 Manuck, S.B.; Kaplan, J.R.: Behaviorally induced heart rate reactivity and coronary artery atherosclerosis in monkeys. Proc. Annu. Meet. of the Society for Psychophysiological Research, Washington 1981.

168 Mason, J.W.; Mangan, G.F.; Brady, J.V.; Conrad, D.; Rioch, D.M.: Concurrent plasma epinephrine, norepinephrine, and 17-hydroxycorticosteroid levels during conditioned emotional disturbances in monkeys. Psychosom. Med. *23:* 344–353 (1961).

169 Mason, J.W.; Tolson, W.W.; Brady, J.V.; Tolliver, G.A.; Gilmore, L.I.: Urinary epinephrine and norepinephrine responses to 72-hour avoidance sessions in the monkey. Psychosom. Med. *31:* 300–309 (1969).

170 Matta, R.J.; Verrier, R.L.; Lown, B.: The repetitive extrasystole threshold as an index of vulnerability to ventricular fibrillation. Am. J. Physiol. *230:* 1469–1473 (1976).

171 Medoff, H.S.; Bongiovanni, A.M.: Blood pressure in rats subjected to audiogenic stimulation. Am. J. Physiol. *143:* 300–305 (1945).

172 Meyers, A.; Dewar, H.A.: Circumstances attending 100 sudden deaths from coronary artery disease with coroner's necropsies. Br. Heart J. *37:* 1133–1143 (1975).

173 Miller, D.G.: Effect of signaled versus unsignaled stress on rat myocardium. Psychosom. Med. *40:* 432–434 (1978).

174 Miller, G.J.: High density lipoproteins and atherosclerosis. A. Rev. Med. *31:* 97–108 (1980).

175 Miller, D.G.; Gilmour, R.F.; Grossman, E.D.; Mallov, S.; Wistow, B.W.; Rohner, R.F.: Myocardial uptake of Tc-99m skeletal agents in the rat after experimental induction of microscopic foci of injury. J. nucl. Med. *18:* 1005–1009 (1977).

176 Miller, D.G.; Mallov, S.: The quantitative determination of stress-induced myocardial damage in rats. Pharmacol. Biochem. Behav. *7:* 139–145 (1977).

177 Moses, C.: Development of atherosclerosis in dogs with hypercholesterolemia and chronic hypertension. Circulation Res. *2:* 243–248 (1954).

178 Moss, A.J.: Prediction and prevention of sudden cardiac death. A. Rev. Med. *31:* 1–14 (1980).

179 Myasnikov, A.L.: Significance of disturbances in higher nervous activity in the pathogenesis of hypertensive disease; in Cort, Fennel, Hejl, Jirka, Symp. on the Pathogenesis of Essential Hypertension (Pergamon Press, New York 1962).

180 Myers, A.; Dewar, H.A.: Circumstances attending 100 sudden deaths from coronary disease with coroner's necropsies. Br. Heart J. *37:* 1133–1143 (1975).

181 McCarty, R.; Chiveh, C.C.; Kopin, I.J.: Spontaneously hypertensive rats: adrenergic hyper-reactivity to anticipation of electric shock. Behav. Biol. *23:* 180 (1978).

182 McCarty, R.; Chiveh, C.C.; Kopin, I.J.: Behavioral and cardiovascular responses of spontaneously hypertensive and normotensive rats to inescapable footshock. Behav. Biol. *22:* 405 (1978).

183 McCarty, R.; Kopin, I.J.: Alterations in plasma catecholamines and behavior during acute stress in spontaneously hypertensive and Wistar-Kyoto normotensive rats. Life Sci. *22:* 997 (1978).

184 McCarty, R.; Kopin, I.J.: Patterns of behavioral development in spontaneously hypertensive rats and Wistar-Kyoto normotensive controls. Dev. Psychobiol. *12:* 239 (1979).

185 McCarty, R.; Kventnansky, R.; Lake, C.R.; Thoa, N.B.; Kopin, I.J.: Sympathoadrenal activity of SHR and WKY rats during recovery from forced immobilization. Physiol. Behav. *21:* 951 (1978).

186 Nathan, M.A.; Reis, D.J.: Fulminating arterial hypertension with pulmonary edema from release of adrenomedullary catecholamines after lesions of the anterior hypothalamus in the rat. Circulation Res. *37:* 226–235 (1975).

187 Nathan, M.A.; Reis, D.J.: Chronic labile hypertension produced by lesions of the nucleus tractus solitarii in the cat. Circulation Res. *40:* 72–81 (1977).

188 Nathan, M.A.; Tucker, L.W.; Severini, W.H.; Reis, D.J.: Enhancement of conditioned arterial pressure responses in cats after brainstem lesions. Science *201:* 71–73 (1978).

189 Nerem, R.M.; Levesque, M.J.; Cornhill, J.F.: Social environment as a factor in diet-induced atherosclerosis. Science *208:* 1475–1476 (1980).

190 Nestel, P.J.; Verghese, A.; Levell, R.R.H.: Catecholamine secretion and sympathetic nervous responses to emotion in men with and without angina pectoris. Am. Heart J. *73:* 227–234 (1967).

191 Öberg, B.; Thorén, P.: Circulatory responses to stimulation of left ventricular receptors in the cat. Acta physiol. scand. *88:* 8–22 (1973).

192 Obrist, P.A.: Cardiovascular Psychophysiology (Plenum Publishing, New York 1981).

193 Okamoto, K.; Aoki, K.: Development of a strain of spontaneously hypertensive rat. Jap. Circul. J. *27:* 282–293 (1963).

194 Osborne, M.W.: On the genesis of essential hypertension – the possible role of central dopaminergic neurons; in Scriabine, Sweet, New antihypertensive drugs (Spectrum, New York 1976).

195 Owsjannikow, P.: Die tonischen und reflectorischen Centern der Gefässnerven. Ber. Sachs. Ges. Wiss. Mat-Phys. Kl. *23:* 135–147 (1871).

196 Page, I.H.: Pathogenesis of arterial hypertension. J. Am. med. Ass. *140:* 451–458 (1949).

197 Page, I.H.: Some regulatory mechanisms of renovascular and essential hypertension; in Genest, Koiw, Kuchel, Hypertension: physiopathology and treatment (McGraw-Hill, New York 1977).

198 Paré, W.P.; Rothfeld, B.; Isom, K.E.; Varady, A.: Cholesterol synthesis and metabolism as a function of unpredictable shock stimulation. Physiol. Behav. *11:* 107–110 (1973).

199 Parkey, R.W.; Bonte, F.J.; Meyer, S.L.; Graham, D.D.: A new method for radionuclide imaging of acute myocardial infarction in humans. Circulation *50:* 540–546 (1974).

200 Perhach, J.L.; Ferguson, H.C.; McKinney, G.R.: Evaluation of antihypertensive agents in the stress-induced hypertensive rats. Life Sci. *16:* 1731–1736 (1976).

201 Peterson, E.A.; Augenstein, J.S.; Tanis, D.C.; Augenstein, D.G.: Noise raises blood pressure without impairing auditory sensitivity. Science *211:* 1450–1452 (1981).

202 Pickering, T.G.; Johnston, J.; Honour, A.J.: Suppression of ventricular extrasystoles during sleep and exercise, and effects of autonomic drugs; in Schwartz, Brown, Malliani, Zanchetti, Neural mechanisms in cardiac arrhythmias (Raven Press, New York 1978).

203 Pickering, T.G.; Miller, N.E.: Learned voluntary control of heart rate and rhythm in two subjects with premature ventricular contractions. Br. Heart J. *49:* 152–159 (1977).

204 Powell, J.R.; Brody, M.J.: Identification and specific blockade of two receptors for histamine in the cardiovascular system. J. Pharmac. exp. Ther. *196:* 1–14 (1976).

205 Powell, D.A.; Goldberg, S.R.; Dauth, G.W.; Schneiderman, E.; Schneiderman, N.: Adrenergic and cholinergic blockade of cardiovascular responses to subcortical electrical stimulation in unanesthetized rabbits. Physiol. Behav. *8:* 927–936 (1972).

206 Raab, W.: Emotional and sensory stress factors in myocardial pathology. Am. Heart J. *72:* 538–564 (1966).

207 Raab, W.: Cardiotoxic biochemical effects of emotional-environmental stressors – fundamentals of psychocardiology; in Levi, Society, stress and disease (Oxford University Press, London 1971).

208 Raab, W.; Chaplin, J.P.; Bajusz, E.: Myocardial necroses produced in domesticated rats and in wild rats by sensory and emotional stresses. Proc. Soc. exp. Biol. Med. *116:* 665–669 (1964).

209 Rahe, R.L.: Stress and strain in coronary heart disease. J. S.C. med. Ass. *72:* suppl., pp. 7–14 (1976).

210 Randall, D.C.; Hasson, D.M.: Incidence of cardiac arrhythmias in monkey during classic

aversive and appetitive conditioning; in Schwartz, Brown, Malliani, Zanchetti, Neural mechanisms in cardiac arrhythmias (Raven Press, New York 1978).

211 Ratcliffe, H.L.: Environment, behavior, and disease; in Stellar, Sprague, Physiological psychology, vol. 2 (Academic Press, New York 1968).

212 Ratcliffe, H.L.; Luginbuhl, H.; Schnarr, W.R.; Chacko, K.: Coronary arteriosclerosis in swine. J. comp. physiol. Psychol. 68: 385–392 (1969).

213 Ratcliffe, H.L.; Snyder, R.L.: Arteriosclerotic stenosis of the intramural coronary arteries of chickens: further evidence of a relation of social factors, pp. 357–365 (Penrose Research Laboratory, Zoological Society of Philadelphia and the Department of Pathology, University of Pennsylvania, Philadelphia 1967).

214 Reich, P.; DeSilva, R.A.; Lown, B.; Murawski, B.J.: Acute psychological disturbances preceding life-threatening ventricular arrhythmias. J. Am. med. Ass. 246: 233–235 (1981).

215 Reichenbach, D.D.; Benditt, E.P.: Myofibrillar degeneration: a response of the myocardial cell to injury. Archs Path. 85: 189–199 (1968).

216 Reid, I.A.; Ganong, W.F.: Control of aldosterone secretion; in Genest, Koiw, Kuchel, Hypertension: physiopathology and treatment (McGraw-Hill, New York 1977).

217 Richter, C.P.: On phenomenon of sudden death in animals and man. Psychosom. Med. 19: 191–198 (1957).

218 Rissanen, V.; Romo, M.; Siltanen, P.: Premonitory symptoms and stress factors preceding sudden death from ischemic heart disease. Acta med. scand. 204: 389–396 (1978).

219 Rona, G.; Chappel, C.I.; Balasy, T.; Caudry, R.: An infarct-like myocardial lesion and other toxic manifestations produced by isoproterenol in the rat. Archs Path. 67: 443–455 (1959).

220 Rosenman, R.H.; Brand, R.J.; Jenkins, C.D.; Friedman, M.; Straus, R.; Wurm, M.: Coronary heart disease in the Western Collaborative Group Study: final follow-up experience of 8½ years. J. Am. med. Ass. 233: 872–877 (1975).

221 Ross, R.; Glomset, J.A.: The pathogenesis of atherosclerosis. New Engl. J. Med. 295: 369–377 (1976).

222 Ross, R.; Harker. L.: Hyperlipidemia and atherosclerosis. Science 193: 1094–1100 (1976).

223 Rothlin, E.; Cerletti, A.; Emmenegger, H.: Experimental psychoneurogenic hypertension and its treatment with hydrogenated ergot alkaloids (hydergine). Acta med. scand. suppl. 312, pp. 27–35 (1956).

224 Ruskin, A.; Beard, O.W.; Schaffer, R.L.: Blast hypertension: elevated arterial pressure in victims of the Texas City disaster. Am. J. Med. 4: 228–236 (1948).

225 Russek, H.I.: Emotional stress as a cause of coronary heart disease. J. Am. Coll. Hlth Ass. 22: 120–123 (1973).

226 Saul, L.J.: Hostility in cages of essential hypertension. Psychosom. Med. 1: 153–161 (1939).

227 Scade, D.; Eaton, R.: The regulation of plasma ketone body concentration by counter regulatory hormones in man. I. Effect of norepinephrine in diabetic man. Diabetes 26: 989 (1977).

228 Schlant, R.C.: Altered cardiovascular physiology of coronary atherosclerotic heart disease; in Hurst, Logue, Schlant, Wenger, The heart (McGraw-Hill, New York 1978).

229 Schmitt, H.; The pharmacology of clonidine and related products; in Gross, Handbook of experimental pharmacology: antihypertensive agents, vol. 39 (Springer, Berlin 1977).

230 Schmitt, H.; Schmitt, H.: Localization of the hypotensive effect of 2-(2-6-dichlorophenylamine)-2-imidazoline hydrochloride (St, 155, Catapresan). Eur. J. Pharmacol. 6: 8–12 (1969).

231   Schneiderman, N.: Animal models relating behavioral stress and cardiovascular pathology; in Dembroski, Weiss, Shields, Haynes, Feinleib, Coronary-prone behavior (Springer, New York 1978).

232   Schonfeld, G.; Pfleger, B.: Utilization of exogenous free fatty acids for the production of very low density lipoprotein triglyceride by livers of carbohydrate-fed rats. J. Lipid Res. *12:* 614–621 (1971).

233   Schwaber, J.; Schneiderman, N.: Aortic nerve activated cardioinhibitory neurons and interneurons. Am. J. Physiol. *229:* 783–789 (1975).

234   Schwartz, P.J.; Foreman, R.D.; Stone, H.L.; Brown, A.M.: Effect of dorsal root section on the arrhythmias associated with coronary occlusion. Am. J. Physiol. *231:* 923–928 (1976).

235   Selye, H.: The general adaptation syndrome and the diseases of adaptation. J. clin. Endocr. *6:* 117–230 (1946).

236   Selye, H.: The chemical prevention of cardiac necroses (Roland Press, New York 1958).

237   Selye, H.: The pluricausal cardiopathies (Thomas, Springfield 1961).

238   Shipley, R.E.; Study, R.S.: Changes in renal blood flow, extraction of inulin, glomerular filtration rate, tissue pressure, and urine flow with acute alterations of renal artery blood pressure. Am. J. Physiol. *167:* 676–682 (1951).

239   Sideroff, S.; Elster, A.J.; Schneiderman, N.: Cardiovascular conditioning in rabbits using appetitive or aversive hypothalamic stimulation as the US. J. comp. physiol. Psychol. *81:* 501–508 (1972).

240   Sigurdsson, G.; Nicoll, A.; Lewis, B.: Conversion of very low density lipoprotein to low density lipoprotein. J. clin. Invest. *56:* 1481–1490 (1975).

241   Skinner, J.E.; Lie, J.T.; Entman, M.L.: Modification of ventricular fibrillation latency following coronary artery occlusion in the conscious pig: the effects of psychological stress and beta-adrenergic blockade. Circulation *51:* 655–667 (1975).

242   Smookler, H.H.; Goebel, K.H.; Siesel, M.I.; Clark, D.E.: Hypertensive effects of prolonged auditory, visual, and motion stimulation. Fed. Proc. *32:* 2105–2110 (1973).

243   Sprague, E.A.; Troxler, R.G.; Peterson, D.F.; Schmidt, R.E.; Young, J.T.: Effect of cortisol on the development of atherosclerosis in cynomolgus monkeys; in Kalter, The use of nonhuman primates in cardiovascular diseases (University of Texas Press, Austin 1980).

244   Stamler, J.; Epstein, F.: Coronary heart diesease. Risk factors as guides to preventive action. Prev. Med. *1:* 27–36 (1970).

245   Sudakov, K.V.; Yumatov, E.A.: Acute psychosocial stress as the cause of sudden death. USA-USSR 1st Symp. on Sudden Death, Yalta 1978, pp. 405–416.

246   Takeshita, A.; Mark, A.L.: Neurogenic mechanisms contributing to vasoconstriction during high sodium intake in Dahl strain genetically hypertensive rat. Circulation Res. *43:* suppl., pp. 86–92 (1978).

247   Tarazi, R.C.; Dustan, H.P.: Beta-adrenergic blockade in hypertension. Am. J. Cardiol. *29:* 633–640 (1972).

248   Thorén, P.: Vagal depressor reflexes elicited by left ventricular C-fibers during myocardial ischemia in cats; in Schwartz, Brown, Malliani, Zanchetti, Neural mechanisms in cardiac arrhythmias (Raven Press, New York 1978).

249   Thorgeirsson, G.; Robertson, A.L.: The vascular endothelium-pathobiologic significance. Am. J. Path. *93:* 803–848 (1978).

250   Titus, J.L.: Pathology of sudden cardiac death. USA-USSR 1st Symp. on Sudden Death, Yalta 1978, pp. 309–318.

251   Troxler, R.G.; Sprague, E.A.; Albanese, R.A.; Fuchs, R.; Thompson, A.J.: The association

of elevated plasma cortisol and early atherosclerosis as demonstrated by coronary angiography. Atherosclerosis 26: 151–162 (1977).

252 Uhley, H.N.; Friedman, M.: Blood lipids, clotting and coronary atherosclerosis in rats exposed to a particular form of stress. Am. J. Physiol. 197: 396–398 (1959).

253 Ulyaninsky, L.S.; Stepanyan, E.P.; Krymsky, L.D.: Cardiac arrhythmia of hypothalamic origin in sudden death. USA-USSR 1st Symp. on Sudden Death, Yalta 1978, pp. 417–429.

254 Uvnäs, B.: Cholinergic vasodilator nerves. Fed. Proc. 25: 1618–1622 (1966).

255 Vander, A.J.; Henry, J.P.; Stephens, P.M.; Kay, L.L.; Mouw, D.R.: Plasma renin activity in psychosocial hypertension of CBA mice. Cirulcation Res. 42: 496–502 (1978).

256 Van Zwieten, P.A.: The central action of antihypertensive drugs mediated via central receptors. J. Pharm. Pharmac. 25: 89–95 (1973).

257 Vatner, S.F.; Higgins, C.B.; Braunwald, E.: Effects of norepinephrine on coronary circulation and left ventricular dynamics in the conscious dog. Circulation Res. 34: 812–823 (1975).

258 Viveros, O.H.; Garlick, D.G.; Renkin, E.M.: Sympathetic beta adrenergic vasodilation in skeletal muscle of the dog. Am. J. Physiol. 215: 1218–1225 (1968).

259 Volle, R.L.; Koelle, G.B.: Ganglionic stimulating and blocking agents; in Goodman, Gilman, The pharmacological basis of therapeutics; 5th ed. (MacMillan, New York 1975).

260 Von Holst, D.: Renal failure as the cause of death in Tupaia belangeri (tree shrews) exposed to persistent social stress. J. comp. Physiol. 78: 236–273 (1972).

261 Wall, R.T.; Harker, L.A.: The endothelium and thrombosis. A. Rev. Med. 31: 361–371 (1980).

262 Wallach, J.; Ellenberger, H.; Schneiderman, N.; Liskowsky, D.; Hamilton, R.; Gellman, M.: Preoptic-anterior hypothalamic area as mediator of bradycardia responses in rabbits. Neurosci. Abstr. 5: 52 (1979).

263 Weber, H.W.; Van der Walt, J.J.: Cardiomyopathy in crowded rabbits: a preliminary report. S. Afr. med. J. 47: 1591–1595 (1973).

264 Webb, S.W.; Adgey, A.A.J.; Partridge, J.R.: Autonomic disturbance at onset of acute myocardial infarction. Br. med. J. 3: 89–92 (1972).

265 Weiss, J.M.: Effects of coping behavior on development of gastroduodenal lesions in rats. Proc. 75th Annu. Convention of the Am. Psychological Association. Convention, APA, 1968, pp. 263–264.

266 Wiggers, L.J.; Wegria, R.: Ventricular fibrillation due to single, localized induction and condenser shocks applied during the vulnerable phase of ventricular systole. Am. J. Physiol. 128: 500–508 (1939/1940).

267 Williams, L.T.; Lefkowitz, R.J.; Watanabe, A.M.; Hathaway, D.R.; Besch, H.R.: Thyroid hormone regulation of beta-adrenergic receptor number: possible biochemical basis for the hyperadrenergic state in hyperthyroidism. Clin. Res. 25: 458 (1977).

268 Yamori, Y.; Matsumoto, M.; Yamabe, H.; Okamoto, K.: Augmentation of spontaneous hypertension by chronic stress in rats. Jap. Circul. J. 33: 399–409 (1969).

269 Zieler, K.L.; Maseri, A.; Klassen, D.; Rabinowitz, D.; Burgess, J.: Muscle metabolism during exercise in man. Trans. Ass. Am. Phys. 81: 266–268 (1968).

270 Zilversmit, D.B.: Mechanisms of cholesterol accumulation in the arterial wall. Am. J. Cardiol. 35: 559–566 (1975).

271 Zweiman, F.E.; Joman, B.L.; O'Keefe, A.; Idoine, J.: Selective uptake of ^{99m}Tc and ^{67}Ga in acutely infarcted myocardium. J. nucl. Med. 16: 975–979 (1975).

20 Coronary Heart Disease and Arousal of the Adrenal Cortical Axis[1]

James P. Henry

The Sympathetic Adrenal Medullary and the Pituitary Adrenal Cortical Systems

Mason [30] has argued that: 'In about 20 years, we have moved from a view of endocrine systems as controlled largely by humoral self-regulatory mechanisms to the view that a wide range of psychologic influences can profoundly affect hormonal balance on both a short- and a long-term basis.' He argues that: 'The superimposition of such complex and idiosyncratic psychological factors as emotions, defensive styles, and neurotic processes on virtually all bodily functions via the neuroendocrine machinery deserves prime suspicion in our search for fallibility or proneness to disease ... psychoendocrine approaches now provide us with new leverage in getting at the bodily mechanisms that play a mediating role between the psychosocial input and the diseased peripheral tissue.'

It is now more than 14 years since *Mason* [28, 29] published his classic reviews of psychoendocrine research on the pituitary adrenal cortical system and on the sympathetic adrenal medullary system. Evidence has since accumulated indicating that these two systems represent separate emotional responses of great importance to animal behavior. The first involves the fight-flight response which is evoked when the power to control access to food, water, shelter, mates, dependents, and significant others is challenged. On the high side, it ranges from extreme anger to fear-tinged alertness and action-proneness. This arousal is accompanied by high levels of catecholamines. The opposite end of the scale is relaxation, which is accompanied by subnormal levels of these hormones and occurs when the individual perceives that all is under control and no challenge in sight.

By contrast, the second system mediates depression which finds full expression when the individual perceives that he may be helpless to defend

[1] The support of our work over the years by the National Heart, Lung, and Blood Institute, National Institutes of Health, Bethesda, Md., is gratefully acknowledged.

himself and others to whom he is emotionally attached against challenge to their safety and status. The accompanying arousal of the pituitary adrenal cortical system involves release of the adrenocorticotropic hormone (ACTH), decreases aggression, and rapid learning of new patterns. The accompanying rise of corticosterone releases submissive behavior. The reverse of helplessness is a feeling of euphoria that comes with satisfying control over predictable challenge. The achievement of meeting the challenge results in a reinforcing sense of status. Adrenal cortical hormones decrease while gonadotropins increase [16].

Socialized mammals have a complex hierarchy and continuously compete for control and status; however, underneath this conflict is a certain commonality, and they achieve their goals by cooperative effort which is assisted by role specialization. The most basic of such specializations is the division into males and females. In primates, in general, but to an extraordinary degree in man, the hunter-gatherer, role differentiation reaches great complexity. To order the different activities so they mesh and so that those less skilled in any particular role help leaders at that particular task, there must be recognition of authority as expressed in the natural hierarchy. The expression of authority represents power. The acknowledgment by others of position in the hierarchy represents status [23]. The sympathetic adrenal medullary system is aroused when the individual's power to control is challenged. If the challenge is successful and control is lost, the individual's status within his social group will change. *Price* [37] has presented the ethologic argument that the ensuing yielding and loss of status are associated with depression for good reason. Experimental studies have shown that the increased activity of the pituitary adrenal cortical axis is associated with enhanced learning of new patterns and more ready abandonment of old ones [11]. The consequence is that instead of being expelled from the group, the individual is co-opted. Such a mechanism is vital for a social animal which relies on group effort. We suggest that the adrenal medullary and the adrenal cortical responses are critically important in the evolution of the primate's and especially of the human's social behavior. There is a growing body of human and animal experimental data showing that, under appropriate conditions, the adrenal medullary and the adrenal cortical responses represent behavioral patterns that move in different directions [16, 25].

Lundberg and Frankenhaeuser [25] have measured adrenaline, noradrenaline, and cortisol excretion in students during the experimental state when they were performing a task and at baseline conditions. By factor analysis they have extracted a factor for distress which has positive loadings in those subjective variables indicative of negative affect and moderately high positive loading in cortisol excretion, and another factor for effort with high positive loadings in subjective variables indicative of action-proneness and adrenaline excretion. This study points to a dissociation between *Mason's* pituitary adrenal cortical and sympathetic adrenal medullary activities, which was illustrated by data from an unpleasantly monotonous vigilance task, involving both effort and distress, in which there was a concomitant increase of adrenaline and cortisol excretions. The results contrasted with those from a pleasant, self-paced, reaction-time task which induced effort but not distress. The pleasant task led to increased adrenaline excretion and an actual decrease in cortisol excretion. This dichotomy was consistent with that described by *Ursin* [52] in his identification of a cortisol factor in certain parachutists who proved vulnerable to fear, who defended by repression, and who tended to perform poorly. In a contrasting group, *Ursin* [52] found a catecholamine factor in those with type A behavior who were striving for achievement, were competitive, and were well-defended as long as they could cope.

Lundberg and Frankenhaeuser [25] also recognized that their results fit those derived by *Henry and Stephens* [16] from their animal model. *Ely and Henry* [12] who compared dominant and subordinate animals also incorporated separate observations made previously by other investigators who chose to work with only one of the systems. They showed that the dominant animal in a colony of male and female mice had increased blood pressure (BP) and greatly increased synthetic capacity for noradrenaline and adrenaline. The subordinate animals had significantly less change in catecholamine synthesis; but for a brief period while they contested the developing hierarchy, their plasma corticosterone was higher than that of the dominants. *Candland and Leshner's* [8] studies with squirrel monkeys give results compatible with those for rodents.

One would expect that if the dichotomy between the adrenal medullary and the adrenal cortical axes is of biobehavioral significance, related patterns should have been independently observed by other disciplines. This has in fact occurred. For instance, separate 'power' and 'status' axes have been selected by sociologist *Kemper* [23] as pivotal parameters in his study of emotions. Psychoanalyst *Bakan* [3] has made a related distinction between an 'agentic masculine' and a 'communal feminine' principle. The meaning he attached to agentic is close to *Kemper's* [23] concept of power, this is, self-protective, self-assertive, and self-expansive. *Bakan's* [3] idea of communal emphasizes contact, cooperation, and affection [19]. The emphasis on togetherness represents the opposite of the behavioral characteristic of depression.

Social psychologist *Bem* [4] has used these distinctions to good effect in developing independent masculine and feminine measures for her scale of androgyny.

Pituitary Adrenal Cortical System and Depression

We now arrive at the question of an animal behavioral equivalent of the type A personality so vulnerable to coronary heart disease (CHD). *Glass* [15] has pointed out the need for an animal model in which the patterns responsible for type A behavior can be reproduced. One adavantage of such a model would be that arteriosclerosis could be reproduced in a form readily available to experimentation. *Henry and Stephens* [16] have suggested that from the point of view of the animal behaviorist, the pattern is the same as that in which an animal is attempting to achieve or maintain control in the face of challenge. The essence of this pattern is that to the subject the challenge threatens to be effective and he perceives any control he has achieved as tenuous.

In his discussion of the human situation *Glass* [15] has analyzed the situation thus: Once an individual perceives a threat to his sense of environmental control, he struggles to reestablish and maintain better control. During this period, we may expect active coping efforts and concomitant elevations in circulating noradrenaline. As long as there is no fear, adrenaline should remain unchanged, or, perhaps, even show a decline. In appraising the situation thus far, any pathophysiological changes would be explained by activation of the sympathetic adrenal axis. *Glass* [15], however, makes the crucial suggestion that at intervals the type A struggling in a competitive milieu will sense a threat to his control, and with this realization, he will become passive. His noradrenaline is likely to decline and 'central cholinergic dominance may prevail'. He now posits that the resulting alternation of control efforts followed by giving up is repeated over and over again during the lifetime of an individual. He finds it: 'Not unreasonable to suggest that the more frequently this cycle occurs, the more the coronary arteries are likely to be affected by atherosclerotic disease.' Thus, he sees atheroarteriosclerosis as requiring the influence of both adrenal medullary and adrenal cortical response patterns [15].

There is good evidence the type A coronary-prone man responds to threat to his sense of control of the environment with a vigorous effort to maintain it, and when challenged, he excretes more noradrenaline than the type B personality [14]. The type A will work on the treadmill closer to his maximum capacity, denying subjective feelings of fatigue in exaggerated efforts to achieve success [15]. But it is also true, as *Nixon and Bethell* [34] point out, that after a certain time, the chronic struggle often leads to exhaustion. As *Glass* [15] perceived it, type A subjects experience the alternation of active coping and giving up more frequently and more intensely than type B. This assumption seems reasonable if we recall that while type As vigorously engage in efforts to master the environment, nevertheless, many of these struggles end in failure and helplessness.

Evidence of Depression and Hostility in Coronary Heart Disease

Siegrist [45, p. 138] has recently quoted a current view which states that there is no evidence to date which bears on the interactive effects of depression and type A behavior on clinical CHD. Nevertheless, clinical evidence supports the idea of a connection between depression and CHD. *Appels* [2] has reported that he can confirm the finding of *Dreyfuss* that patients treated in a mental hospital for some form of depression have a significantly higher prevalence of myocardial infarction than those with nondepressive symptoms. *Thomas* et al. [50] noted that the Johns Hopkins medical students who 20–30 years later as practitioners developed CHD were from a subgroup that had been vulnerable to depression. In their famous observations of widowers, *Parkes* et al. [35] showed that for the first 6 months after bereavement, there was a sharp increase in the incidence of CHD, suggesting that the condition may be aggravated by depression. It is relevant that *Medalie and Goldbourt's* [31] study of the development of anginal symptoms of CHD in Israeli civil servants reports a significant increase in patients whose chronic anxiety was compounded by marital problems. Those who perceived their wives as loving and supportive had one half the incidence of anginal symptoms compared to those who did not (fig. 1).

Bruhn et al. [6] have described joyless striving as a typical characteristic of a person suffering from myocardial infarction – an effort-oriented person who struggles against odds but has very little sense of accomplishment or satisfaction. In a recent paper, *Jenkins* et al. [20] speak of anxiety and depression suffered by the coronary-prone. In their important report, *Williams* et al. [53] indicate that an attitudinal set, reflective of hostility toward people in general, is responsible for much of the variance in coronary atherosclerosis above that accounted for by the type A behavior pattern. These persons'

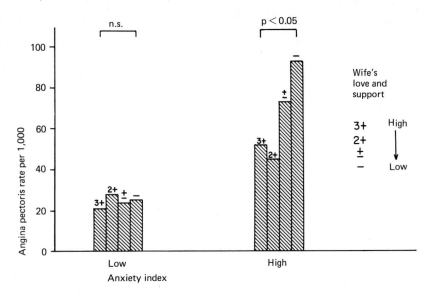

Fig. 1. The incidence of angina in Israeli civil servants having a good relationship with their spouses is contrasted with the incidence in those who perceive their relationship as non-supportive. Anxiety is an important cofactor [from ref. 31].

prevailing attitude was that others were inconsiderate, immoral, selfish, and deserving of punishment. There was a correlation between the severity of coronary atherosclerosis and this point of view. Such hostility could well be self-fulfilling. Eventually hostility gets on peoples' nerves eliciting antagonism and lack of support which could be a source of depression that has been observed in patients with coronary arteriosclerosis.

Such a trend should find biochemical expression in the pattern of hypothalamic pituitary axis overactivity which has now been established as typical of the depressed state [43] and, in fact, *Troxler* et al. [51] have shown a significant correlation between elevated, serial, morning plasma cortisols and moderate to severe coronary atherosclerosis (fig. 2). In their hands, plasma cortisol ranked close to serum cholesterol as a discriminator of the disease as verified by coronary angiography. These individuals were not examined for their noradrenaline and adrenaline levels, but there is every reason to suppose they had the same exaggerated responses as others with active CHD. Thus, *Troxler* et al. [51] had added evidence of activation of the adrenal cortical system to the biochemical picture of the coronary type A personality.

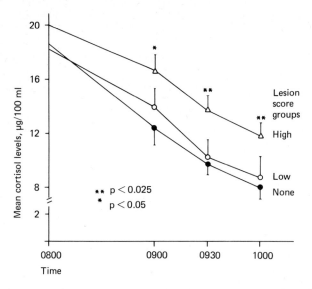

Fig. 2. Mean plasma cortisol levels during the period 8 to 10 a.m. are plotted in three conditions of coronary atherosclerotic involvement as measured by angiography: none = no lesions demonstrable; low = minimal disease; high = clinically more significant disease. Patients with one or few coronary lesions have a more rapid decline in plasma cortisol with time than patients with clinically significant disease [from ref. 51].

Protection against Coronary Heart Disease by Emotional Factors

In their discussion of hostility, *Williams* et al. [53] drew attention to the low incidence of clinical CHD among Japanese men living in California who cling to Japanese cultural patterns. They cited the data of *Marmot and Syme* [26] which indicate that the low incidence of heart disease is not due to the classical risk factors such as diet. *Marmot and Syme* [26] propose that an element of Japanese culture protecting the men against heart disease is the importance they place on group membership, interdependence, and mutual benevolence.

Supporting this view are the remarkable recent observations of *Nerem* et al. [33] who studied the effects of positive emotional factors on diet-induced atherosclerosis in young male New Zealand white rabbits. A one-to-one relationship between each animal and a female experimenter was established as follows. During an early morning half-hour visit, each animal was handled, stroked, talked to, and played with. The animal was also touched and talked to during an hour-long feeding period. In addition, rabbits received a

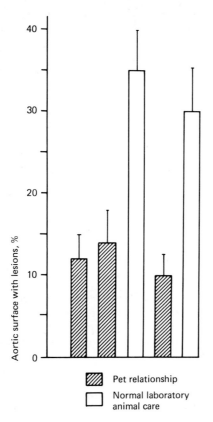

Fig. 3. The average percentage of aortic surface area exhibiting sudanophilia in rabbits exposed to a pet relationship (hatched columns) and rabbits exposed to normal laboratory animal care (open columns). Bars show SEM [from ref. 33].

number of 5-min visits during the day. Throughout this daily procedure, the rabbits quickly learned to recognize the experimenter and many even sought her personal attention. After a 2-week adaptation period during which the animal and the experimenter became acquainted, the rabbits were fed a regular diet supplemented by 2% cholesterol. After 5 weeks, the aortae were stained and the percent of the surface with sudanophilia was estimated. In the controls, it was approximately 2- to 3-fold of that in the petted animals ($p < 0.03$) (fig. 3).

Jevning et al. [21] have made a relevant observation that adrenal cortical activity, as measured by plasma cortisol, decreased significantly ($p < 0.03$) in

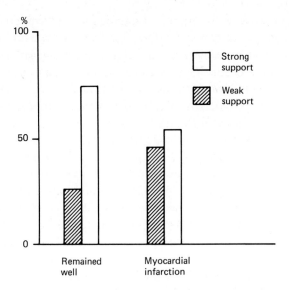

Fig. 4. All subjects had a heavy work load. Social support proved protective, and subjects who remained well received more social support than those who developed myocardial infarction [from ref. 46].

long-term practitioners during meditation. The work of *Cooper and Aygen* [9] showed that fasting serum cholesterol decreased significantly ($p < 0.005$) in hypercholesterolemic subjects who regularly practiced meditation during an 11-month period. The foregoing changes, including those in rabbits, may have been due to alteration in adrenal cortical function. These combined human and animal observations indicate that persons who, in addition to being driven to make great efforts, are also depressed and perceive themselves as helpless and without social support (fig. 4), are especially vulnerable to CHD, and that the opposite response of euphoria and perception of social support may be protective.

Acceleration of Atheroarteriosclerosis by Administration of Adrenal Cortical Hormones

The mechanisms by which sympathetic adrenal medullary arousal could lead to hyperlipidemia and platelet aggregation have been discussed by *Taggart and Carruthers* [49]. *Maseri* et al. [27] have pioneered the recent growing recognition of the importance of coronary vascular spasm in precipitating untoward myocardial events. *Lown and DeSilva* [24] have documented the importance of the autonomic nervous system in cardiac arrhythmias that so often precede sudden cardiac death. Our problem is the way adrenal cortical arousal could enhance factors leading to disease of the blood vessels. The pathogenesis of atherosclerosis underlying CHD is currently hypothesized by workers, such as *Ross and Glomset* [42], to occur as a response to various injuries that induce gaps in the lining of arterial endothelial cells. Such alterations provide an opportunity for the underlying smooth muscle cells to be exposed to degranulation of platelets and release of the platelet-derived growth factor. This factor controls the smooth muscle proliferation of arteriosclerosis and the formation and degradation of connective tissue matrix components and the binding and internalizing of lipoproteins. Platelets are known to transport the active factor to muscle cells in the injured region of the blood vessel. The factor, whose origin is as yet unknown, is a low molecular weight peptide which may have been manufactured by the pituitary gland or by megakaryocytes. Among the many questions awaiting solution is the possible role of the pituiatry adrenal cortical system in the activity of this crucial component of atherogenesis [41].

Another point at which adrenal cortical response could be of importance is in the development of the original injury to the arterial wall. Since *Minick* et al. [32] have made their basic observations, it has been clear that allergic injury to arteries can be synergic to the effects of a lipid-rich diet. They experimented with rabbits, giving them horse serum injections and dietary cholesterol supplements; the combination led to fatty proliferative lesions closely resembling coronary arteriosclerosis in man.

Hollander et al. [18] have followed the immunological aspects of atherosclerosis over the years. They note that the inflammatory reaction in the arterial wall produced by a foreign protein, such as horse serum, is associated with deposition of immune complexes in the involved areas of the artery. They have also studied the soluble proteins in spontaneously occurring human atherosclerotic plaques and suggest that the γ-G immunoglobulin (IgG) contained and synthesized by it may represent an immune response to an antigen associated with plaque collagen. The IgG alone or in the form of an immune complex may change the removal rate of debris from plaques, influencing the course of atherosclerosis. Their data indicate that there are autoantibodies directed against the fibrous proteins of the artery. Immune responses to the continued presence of antigen in the artery wall could maintain disease by providing antigen antibody complexes, stimulating further proliferation in the artery [17]. *Parums and Mitchinson* [36] have recently shown that the degree of inflammatory cellular infiltration of atherosclerotic plaques correlated with its severity. Thus, the inflammation seems to be the result of atherosclerosis, and the local production of IgG suggests that autoallergy and inflammation with plasma cells and lymphocytes may contribute to the enlargment of plaques.

A well-established association exists between the administration of corticosterone, for conditions such as rheumatoid arthritis [22], and the acceleration of arteriosclerosis. In animals it is known that ACTH and cortisone induce increased serum lipids [47] and coagulation of blood [10, 38]. *Rosenfeld* et al. [40] showed that ACTH enhances experimental atherosclerosis in dogs on a high cholesterol diet. Dogs treated with ACTH for about a year showed higher serum cholesterol and more vascular damage than the controls on the diet alone. The experiment took advantage of clinical observations of the development of hypercholesterolemia during cortisone and ACTH therapy. In 1950 *Adlersberg* et al. [1] reported a 30–30% increase in the total serum cholesterol of patients being treated with cortisone or ACTH; 36% attained levels in excess of 280 mg/100 ml. This earlier work has been confirmed by *Stern* et al. [48] who reported on increased cholesterol and triglyceride and pre-β-lipoprotein turnover in patients with rheumatic diseases receiving steroid treatment. They comment on the development of severe atheroma in 18 months in the transplanted heart of a patient treated with adrenal cortical steroids to prevent rejection. Still more recently *Bulkley and Roberts* [7] have commented on the deleterious effects of corticosteroids on the hearts of patients being treated for systemic lupus erythematosus. Systemic hypertension was twice as common in patients receiving corticosteroids for 12 months and was 5 times as common in patients with lupus erythematosus before steroids were used. In addition, congestive cardiac failure occured 8 times more frequently in patients treated with corticosteroids than in those who were not [34].

The Effect of the Adrenal Cortical System on the Immune Response

In the first place, when considering the mechanism of the adrenal cortical system's effect on the immune system, glucocorticoids increase the number of dead or injured cells in the arterial endothelium, as *Björkerud* [5] has reported. He regarded it as a possible factor in the formation of arteriosclerosis. Another important factor is the possibility of disturbing immunocompetence. In a recent review, *Riley* [39] has shown that the increase of adrenal cortical hormones in response to psychosocial stress has an easily demonstrable effect on the specific cells and tissues required for optimum immunological defense. The organism becomes less capable of defending itself against those diseases responsive to cell-mediated immunity. *Riley* [39] confines himself to evidence from experiments in his laboratories dealing with the effects of psychosocial arousal associated with activation of the adrenal cortex. The crucial effects involve T cells and thymic components. An elevation of corticosterone concentration in blood plasma leads to lymphocytopenia, involution of thymus, and loss of tissue mass of the spleen and of peripheral lymph nodes. All these effects can be associated with adverse changes in immunocompetence. It is true that psychosocial stimuli induce other biochemical changes, particularly in catecholamines, but they primarily affect the cardiovascular system. Thus, the influence of psychosocial stress on immune mechanisms appears more closely related to changes in the adrenal cortical hormones [39].

The basic observations of *Schömig* et al. [44] showed that raised cortisol increases the response of the vascular bed to catecholamines and points to synergy between the adrenal cortical and the adrenal medullary systems. The association between adrenal cortical activity and the immune response makes it plausible to extend this synergy to higher levels of integration. The vulnerability of the type A patient to depression involves adrenal cortical activation which adds fuel to the fire of his driven sympathetic system and exacerbates his tendency to atheroarteriosclerosis.

Conclusion

Psychoendocrine changes involving the hippocampal pituitary-adrenal axis range between the extremes of euphoria and distress (fig. 5). In euphoria, the individual feels secure and in control of critical variables. Gonadotropins are elevated and reproduction and parenting are actively pursued. Distress, at the other end of the scale, involves a perception of loss of control and helplessness. Distress involves conservation-withdrawal, submissive behavior accompanied by elevated plasma cortisol, and an ACTH-activated relearning of behavioral patterns.

The sympathetic adrenal medullary system is presented in figure 5 as a relaxation-effort axis. At the active end, the fight-flight response is elicited by defense of status and aggressive territorial control. Fight is associated with

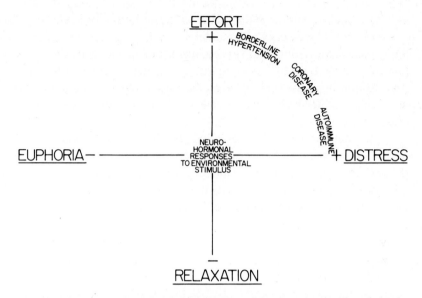

Fig. 5. Responses to challenging situations involve arousal of several hormonal patterns. The horizontal axis represents adrenal cortical activity, ranging from self-confidence, with euphoria and suppressed corticoids, to helpless depression, with increased response of the pituitary adrenal cortical axis. The vertical axis represents sympathetic adrenal medullary activity, ranging from relaxation, with decrease in catecholamines, to effort, with a mixture of noradrenaline (hostility) and adrenaline (anxiety). The coronary type A personality combines arousal of both medullary and cortical patterns.

the vascular bed hormone, noradrenaline, whose release relates to anger. On the other hand, flight is associated with release of the metabolic hormone, adrenaline, and anxiety, i.e. uncertainty as to how things will go. The individual is in doubt about the efficacy of his control.

Differing perceptions of the possibilities of action will give rise to relatively pure responses of one system or the other or a mixture of the two.

(1) Situations which the individual perceives can be met by effective coping elicit a feeling of mastery which, with resistance, turns to anger. The sympathetic system is activated by a brief release of catecholamines during the period of acute exposure. Labile high-renin hypertension is found in individuals who are angry and have elevated catecholamines, but suppress awareness of this anger (fig. 5).

(2) Demanding situations which are distressing, causing feelings of inadequacy and fear of failure, produce cortisol release in addition to

increased catecholamines. One victim is the anxious overachiever with a coronary type A personality. Threatened even by forced inactivity [13] with loss of control, he is vulnerable to depression and increased corticoids. At the same time, his striving burdens him with sympathetic arousal. Often suppressing awareness of his involvement, he falls under the influence of the neuroendocrinologically adverse ends of both the distress and effort axes (fig. 5).

(3) Situations which the individual perceives as out of control in which he cannot act effectively are associated with suppressed or conscious helplessness. There can be a marked and prolonged elevation of corticosteroid release. This pattern of passive distress may be associated with diseases involving disturbances of immunocompetence (fig. 5).

References

1   Adlersberg, D.; Schaefer, L.; Drachman, S.R.: Development of hypercholesteremia during cortisone and ACTH therapy. J. Am. med Ass. *144:* 909–914 (1950).
2   Appels, A.: Myocardial infarction and depression. A crossvalidation of Dreyfuss' findings. Activitas nerv. sup. *21:* 65–66 (1979).
3   Bakan, D.: The duality of human existence. An essay on psychology and religion, chap. 4, pp. 102–153 (Rand McNally, Chicago 1966).
4   Bem, S.L.: Beyond androgyny: some presumptuous prescriptions for a liberated sexual identity; in Sherman, Denmark, The psychology of women: future directions in research, chap. 1, pp. 4–23 (Psychological Dimensions, New York 1978).
5   Björkerud, S.: Effect of adrenocortical hormones on the integrity of the rat aortic endothelium; in Schettler, Weizel, Atherosclerosis III. Proc. 3rd Int. Symp., pp. 245–249 (Springer, New York 1974).
6   Bruhn, J.G.; Paredes, A.; Adsett, C.A.; Wolf, S.: Psychological predictors of sudden death in myocardial infarction. J. psychosom. Res. *18:* 187–191 (1974).
7   Bulkley, B.H.; Roberts, W.C.: The heart in systemic lupus erythematosus and the changes induced in it by corticosteroid therapy. A study of 36 necropsy patients. Am. J. Med. *58:* 243–264 (1975).
8   Candland, D.K.; Leshner, A.I.: A model of agonistic behavior: endocrine and autonomic correlates; in DiCara, Limbic and autonomic nervous systems research, chap. 4, pp. 137–163 (Plenum Press, New York 1974).
9   Cooper, M.J.; Aygen, M.M.: A relaxation technique in the management of hypercholesterolemia. J. hum. Stress *5:* 24–27 (1979).
10 Cosgriff, S.W.; Dienfenbach, A.J.; Vogt, W., Jr.: Hypercoagulability of the blood associated with ACTH and cortisone therapy. Am. J. Med. *9:* 752–756 (1950).
11 De Wied, D.; Delft, A.M. van; Gispen, W.H.; Weijnen, J.A.W.M.; Wimersma Greidanus, Tj. B. van: The role of pituitary-adrenal system hormones in active avoidance conditioning; in Levine, Hormones and behavior, pp. 135–171 (Academic Press, New York 1972).

12   Ely, D.L.; Henry, J.P.: Neuroendocrine response patterns in dominant and subordinate mice. Horm. Behav. *10:* 156–169 (1978).

13   Frankenhaeuser, M.; Lundberg, U.; Forsman, L.: Note on arousing type A persons by depriving them of work. J. psychosom. Res. *24:* 45–47 (1980).

14   Friedman, M.; Byers, S.O.; Diamant, J.; Rosenman, R.H.: Plasma catecholamine response of coronary-prone subjects (type A) to a specific challenge. Metabolism *24:* 205–210 (1975).

15   Glass, D.C.: Behavior patterns, stress, and coronary disease (Erlbaum, Hillsdale/Wiley, New York 1977).

16   Henry, J.P.; Stephens, P.M.: Stress, health, and the social environment. A sociobiologic approach to medicine (Springer, New York 1977).

17   Hollander, W.; Colombo, M.A.; Kirkpatrick, B.; Paddock, J.: Soluble proteins in the human atherosclerotic plaque. With spectral reference to immunoglobulins, C_3-complement component, α_1-antitrypsin and α_2-macroglobulin. Atherosclerosis *34:* 391–405 (1979).

18   Hollander, W.; Colombo, M.A.; Kramsch, D.M.; Kirkpatrick, B.: Immunological aspects of atherosclerosis; in Symp. Comparative Pathology of the Heart, Boston 1973. Adv. Cardiol., vol. 13, pp. 192–207 (Karger, Basel 1974).

19   Hoyenga, K.B.; Hoyenga, K.T.: The question of sex differences. Psychological, cultural, and biological issues (Little, Brown, Boston 1979).

20   Jenkins, C.D.; Tuthill, R.W.; Tannenbaum, S.I.; Kirby, C.: Social stressors and excess mortality from hypertensive diseases. J. hum. Stress *5:* 29–40 (1979).

21   Jevning, R.; Wilson, A.F.; Davidson, J.M.: Adrenocortical activity during meditation. Horm. Behav. *10:* 54–60 (1978).

22   Kalbak, K.: Incidence of arteriosclerosis in patients with rheumatoid arthritis receiving long-term corticosteroid therapy. Ann. rheum. Dis. *31:* 196–200 (1972).

23   Kemper, T.D.: A social interactional theory of emotions (Wiley & Sons, New York 1978).

24   Lown, B.; DeSilva, R.A.: Roles of psychologic stress and the autonomic nervous system changes in provocation of ventricular premature complexes. Am. J. Cardiol. *41:* 979–985 (1978).

25   Lundberg, U.; Frankenhaeuser, M.: Pituitary-adrenal and sympathetic-adrenal correlates of distress and effort. J. psychosom. Res. *24:* 125–130 (1980).

26   Marmot, M.G.; Syme, S.L.: Acculturation and coronary heart disease in Japanese-Americans. Am. J. Epidemiol. *104:* 225–247 (1976).

27   Maseri, A.; L'Abbate, A.; Baroldi, G.; Chierchia, S.; Severi, S.; Parodi, O.; Biagini, A.; Distante, A.: Coronary vasospasm as a possible cause of myocardial infarction; in Mason, Neri Serneri, Oliver, Int. Meet. on Myocardial Infarction, Florence 1979, vol. 2, pp. 67–74 (Excerpta Medica, Amsterdam 1979).

28   Mason, J.W.: A review of psychoendocrine research on the pituitary-adrenal cortical system. Psychosom. Med. *30:* 576–607 (1968).

29   Mason, J.W.: A review of psychoendocrine research on the sympathetic-adrenal medullary system. Psychosom. Med. *30:* 631–653 (1968).

30   Mason, J.W.: Psychologic stress and endocrine function; in Sachar, Topics in psychoendocrinology, pp. 1–18 (Grune & Stratton, New York 1975).

31   Medalie, J.H.; Goldbourt, U.: Angina pectoris among 10,000 men. II. Psychosocial and other risk factors as evidenced by a multivariate analysis of a five-year incidence study. Am. J. Med. *60:* 910–921 (1976).

32   Minick, C.R.; Murphy, G.E.; Campbell, W.G., Jr.: Experimental induction of athero-
     arteriosclerosis by the synergy of allergic injury to arteries and lipid-rich diet. I. Effect of
     repeated injections of horse serum in rabbits fed a dietary cholesterol supplement. J. exp.
     Med. *12:* 635–655 (1966).

33   Nerem, R.M.; Levesque, M.J.; Cornhill, J.F.: Social environment as a factor in diet-
     induced atherosclerosis. Science *208:* 1475–1476 (1980).

34   Nixon, P.G.F.; Bethell, H.J.N.: Preinfarction ill health. Am. J. Cardiol. *33:* 446–449
     (1974).

35   Parkes, C.M.; Benjamin, B.; Fitzgerald, R.G.: A broken heart: a statistical study of
     increased mortality among widowers. Br. med. J. *i:* 740–743 (1969).

36   Parums, D.; Mitchinson, M.J.: Demonstration of immunoglobulin in the neighbourhood
     of advanced atherosclerotic plaques. Atherosclerosis *38:* 211–216 (1981).

37   Price, J.: The dominance hierarchy and the evolution of mental illness. Lancet *ii:* 243–246
     (1967).

38   Rich, A.R.; Cochran, T.H.; McGoon, D.C.: Marked lipemia resulting from the adminis-
     tration of cortisone. Johns Hopkins med. J. *88:* 101–109 (1951).

39   Riley, V.: Psychoneuroendocrine influences on immunocompetence and neoplasia.
     Adverse effects of stress upon immunocompetence and the consequences for cancer and
     other pathologies. Science (in press).

40   Rosenfeld, S.; Marmorston, J.; Sobel, H.; White, A.E.: Enhancement of experimental ath-
     erosclerosis by ACTH in the dog. Proc. Soc. exp. Biol. Med. *103:* 83–86 (1960).

41   Ross, R.: The pathogenesis of atherosclerosis. Mech. Age. Dev. *9:* 435–440 (1979).

42   Ross, R.; Glomset, J.A.: The pathogenesis of atherosclerosis (parts 1 and 2). New Engl.
     J. Med. *295:* 369–377, 420–425 (1976).

43   Schlesser, M.A.; Winokur, G.; Sherman, B.M.: Hypothalamic-pituitary-adrenal axis
     activity in depressive illness. Archs gen. Psychiat. *37:* 737–743 (1980).

44   Schömig, A.; Lüth, B.; Dietz, R.; Gross, F.: Changes in vascular smooth muscle sensitivity
     to vasoconstrictor agents induced by corticosteroids, adrenalectomy, and differing salt
     intake in rats. Clin. Sci. mol. Med. *51:* 51–63 (1976).

45   Siegrist, J.: Myocardial infarction and psychosocial risks: concluding remarks; in Siegrist,
     Halhuber, Myocardial infarction and psychosocial risks, pp. 133–147 (Springer, Berlin
     1981).

46   Siegrist, J.; Dittmann, K.; Rittner, K.; Weber, I.: Soziale Belastungen und Herzinfarkt.
     Eine medizinsoziologische Fall-Kontroll-Studie, p. 178 (Enke, Stuttgart 1980).

47   Skanse, B.; Studnitz, W. von; Skoog, N.: The effect of corticotrophin and cortisone on
     serum lipids and lipoproteins. Acta endocr., Copenh. *31:* 442–450 (1959).

48   Stern, M.P.; Kolterman, O.G.; Fries, J.F.; McDevitt, H.O.; Reaven, G.M.: Adrenocortical
     steroid treatment of rheumatic diseases. Effects on lipid metabolism. Archs intern. Med.
     132: 97–101 (1973).

49   Taggart, P.; Carruthers, M.: Behavior patterns and emotional stress in the etiology of coro-
     nary heart disease: cardiological and biochemical correlates; in Wheatley, Stress and the
     heart: interactions of the cardiovascular system, behavioral state, and psychotropic drugs;
     2nd ed., pp. 25–37 (Raven Press, New York 1981).

50   Thomas, C.B.; Ross, D.C.; Duszynski, K.R.: Youthful hypercholesteremia: its associated
     characteristics and role in premature myocardial infarction. Johns Hopkins med. J. *136:*
     193–208 (1975).

51   Troxler, R.G.; Sprague, E.A.; Albanese, R.A.; Fuchs, R.; Thompson, A.J.: The association

of elevated plasma cortisol and early atherosclerosis as demonstrated by coronary angiography. Atherosclerosis 26: 151–162 (1977).

52   Ursin, H.: Personality, activation and somatic health. A new psychosomatic theory; in Levine, Ursin, Coping and health (NATO Conf. Ser.), ser. III, vol. 12, pp. 259–279 (Plenum Press, New York 1980).

53   Williams, R.B., Jr.; Haney, T.L.; Lee, K.L.; Kong, Y.-H.; Blumenthal, J.A.; Whalen, R.E.: Type A behavior, hostility, and coronary atherosclerosis. Psychosom. Med. 42: 539–549 (1980).

21 Physiological Changes in Male *Tupaia belangeri* under Different Types of Social Stress

D. v. Holst, E. Fuchs, W. Stöhr

Our research program on social behavior and social stress in tree shrews *(Tupaia belangeri)* can be subdivided with respect to three major questions [for details see 1, 3, 4]: (1) Which social situations, or stimuli originating in conspecifics, cause social stress? (2) How are acute and chronic social stresses reflected in the behavior and physiological state of the animals and how does an organism recover from prior stress? (3) Wherein lies the significance – or selective advantage – of these stress responses, in view of the fact that they harm the individual itself?

In the following, we will concentrate on experiments which should help to identify the behavioral and physiological reactions of male Tupaias to social conflict in order to understand their biological significance.

Tree shrews are diurnal mammals, about the size of a squirrel, distributed throughout Southeast Asia. Their systematic position is unclear. Many consider them primates, but it now seems likely that, rather than providing a living model for the ancestral primate, tree shrews probably provide a better indication of the characteristics of the common ancestor of all living placental mammals. They are thus usually classified as a separate order: Scandentia or Tupaiidae [6, 7]. In nature, they live singly or in pairs in territories defended vigorously against strange conspecifics of the same sex [5]. In laboratory enclosures (ca $7 m^2$) adult tree shrews of both sexes also immediately attack strange conspecifics and normally defeat them within a few minutes. Shortly after fighting has ended, the victor shows no further sign of arousal and pays virtually no attention to the submissive animal. The subordinate tree shrew, however, cowers in a corner, which it leaves only to feed and drink. It hardly moves at all, spending more than 90% of the daily activity phase lying motionless in its hiding place and following the movements of the victor with its head. During the following days, agonistic encounters between the 2 animals are very rare or completely lacking. Nevertheless, the subordinate animal dies within 20 days.

The death does not result from the physical exertions of fighting or from wounds received, but rather from the continued presence of the victor as the following results show: If an adult male is placed into the cage of an unknown male conspecific, it is usually attacked instantly and subdued in less than 2 min. Following separation of the 2 animals by an opaque partition, the loser recovers from the fight nearly as rapidly as the winner. Under such conditions, even when the subordinate animal is subjected to an encounter every day for more than 2 weeks, it hardly loses any body weight and does not die prematurely. If the 2 animals are separated after their first fight by a partition of wire mesh, so that the loser cannot be attacked but sees the victor constantly, however, it dies within a few days. Thus, death is not a (direct) result of social interactions and their physiological consequences, but rather results from central nervous system processes in the subordinate animal based on experience (being defeated) and learning (to recognize the victor). To put it anthropomorphically, the subordinate dies of constant 'anxiety'.

To determine the cause of death or more generally the physiological reactions of subordinate male tree shrews to the continued presence of their victors, the following parameters were determined: various hormones (by radioimmunoassays or radioenzymatically) and other clinically important parameters in the blood and urine; the activity of tyrosine hydroxylase (TH) from the adrenal glands (radioenzymatically) as well as that of other biologically important enzymes; the histology and histochemistry of various organs, and the heart rates of some individuals (telemetrically: the transmitters were developed in our laboratory; size: $15 \times 8 \times 4$ mm; weight including battery: 1.5 g, duration of continuous registration: 4–5 months).

All experimental animals were maintained under constant conditions with food and water ad libitum [for details see 2]. The experimental procedure was as previously described: A male was placed in the cage of an unknown conspecific of the same sex, which subjugated him completely within less than 2 min. Afterwards, both animals were separated by a partition of wire mesh (fig. 1). Every 1–2 days the fights were repeated. Some ($n = 38$) of the submissive animals died in this situation, generally during the night; but most ($n = 64$) were sacrificed for analysis within 1–16 days after their first defeat.

From the time of first submission, the animals showed a progressive decrease in body weight and died within 2–20 days. The daily weight loss was more or less constant for any animal throughout the entire experiment, but differed considerably between individuals (fig. 2).

There was a good correlation between number of days between initial confrontation and death and daily weight loss (fig. 3): Daily weight loss is thus a good index of the intensity of an animal's stress responses – at least during acute stress.

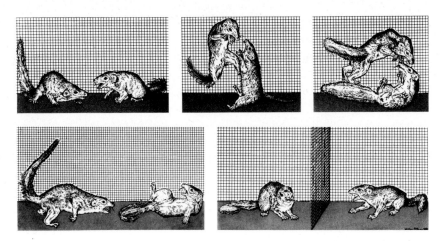

Fig. 1. Submission sequence of a male Tupaia introduced into the cage of a conspecific (from photographs).

Submissive animals may be classified in two distinct group – those that live less than 8 days (type I) and those that live longer (type II). Differences in behavior, central nervous and peripheral physiological parameters support this classification. After their first submission, animals of type I sat in a corner of the cage for practically the whole day and hardly responded to external stimuli. Even the threats and attacks of the dominants were accepted without the animals attempting to flee or defend themselves. Type II submissive animals, in contrast, showed a high locomotor activity and attempted, at least during the first few days, to escape this situation. During fights they fled from the attacking dominant or even fought back.

As can be seen from figure 4, the kidney function of the type I submissives was severely impaired, leading to death from uremia. Histological examination showed that this was due to a more or less reduced blood circulation through the kidneys. Hormonal data showed a dramatic increase in adrenocortical activity and a corresponding decrease in activities of the thyroidal and gonadal systems. In type II submissives, the concentrations of most hormones and other parameters in the blood changed correspondingly but at a slower rate. In contrast to the type I submissives, their urea-N content in the serum did not increase to uremic levels. The cause of death of these animals is not yet known [further details see 2, 4].

The introduction of an individual into the cage (territory) of a strange conspecific is an extremely intense form of stress in a territorial animal such

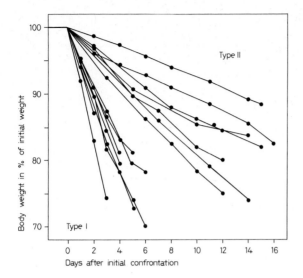

Fig. 2. Decrease of body weight of some submissive Tupaias after initial confrontation.

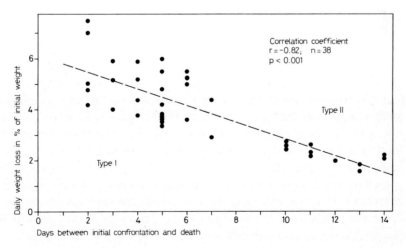

Fig. 3. Correlation between daily loss of body weight of submissive Tupaias and survival time under persistent social stress.

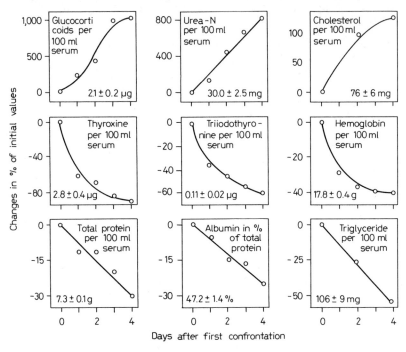

Fig. 4. Physiological changes of some parameters in the serum (or blood) of type I submissives (n = 25). Blood samples were taken before and every 1–2 days after the beginning of
social confrontation (always about 2 h before the beginning of the light phase). The absolute
initial values are given, along with their mean errors. All parameters differ significantly
(p < 0.001) from the initial value within 1–2 days (triglycerides after 4 days).

as the tree shrew. To obtain physiological data on less severe forms of stress
and even on adaptation to it, 2 male Tupaias which were unknown to each
other were put together in a strange cage. In some cases this led to high intensity fights and the establishment of a clear dominance relationship between
the 2, resulting in the death of the submissive within a few days. In many
cases, however, this situation did not result in intensive fighting. After
approximately 2 days and subsequent to low-intensity attacks, however, a
dominance structure was established in which the subordinate, by active
avoidance behavior, withdrew from situations which could lead to more
intense fights. Under these conditions, a subordinate – in contrast to a submissive – was capable of living in a dominant's cage, albeit with a very
reduced sphere of action, for weeks.

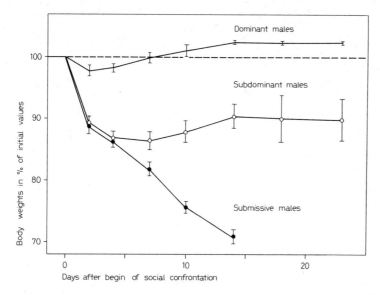

Fig. 5. Body weight (M ± SE) of dominant, subdominant and submissive male Tupaias after the beginning of social confrontation (n = 22).

The body weight of dominant animals remained more or less constant throughout the experimental period. Subdominants and submissives showed a drastic decrease in body weight up to the fourth day of the experiment. Whereas, however, the subdominant animals stabilized at the levels, the body weight of the submissive Tupaias progressively decreased; the daily weight loss was about 2.5% of the initial weight, which is within the upper range of the values for type II submissives in the first experiment (fig. 5). Correspondingly, there was no apparent difference in the physiological reactions between the latter and the submissives in the second experiment.

The first (preliminary) results show (fig. 6): Hormone concentrations (as well as other physiological parameters) in the serum of dominant Tupaias largely correspond to those of control animals without direct social contact (n = 10). There is even a tendency of dominants to increase their testosterone levels.

The concentrations of thyroidal and gonadal hormones in submissives are significantly lower than those of dominants. The values for subdominants are between those of the other groups. Cortisol concentrations in the serum of dominants and subdominants are within the range of controls, while those of the submissives are increased. The TH activity of the adrenal glands in sub-

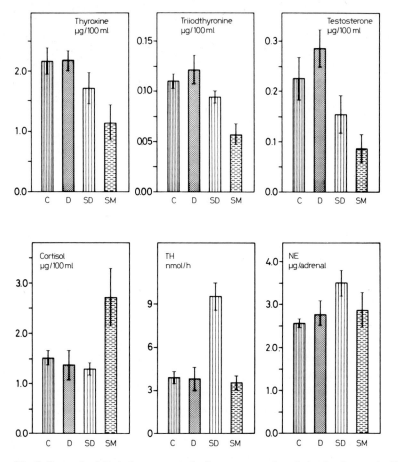

Fig. 6. Some physiological parameters in the serum or adrenal glands of controls (C), dominant (D), subdominant (SD), and submissive (SM) male Tupaias. All values are given with their standard errors. The data are from animals that were sacrificed 4–16 days after begin of social confrontation. Since, with these preliminary data, no significant time dependence with regard to the changes was found, all values are pooled.

missives does not differ from that of dominants, but in subdominants it is about 150% higher. The norepinephrine content of the adrenals in the three groups shows similar changes. This indicates an increased sympathetic activity in subdominant animals, but not in the dominant or submissive Tupaias.

The heart rates of 10 tree shrews were measured telemetrically over months. Before social confrontation all animals showed similar marked

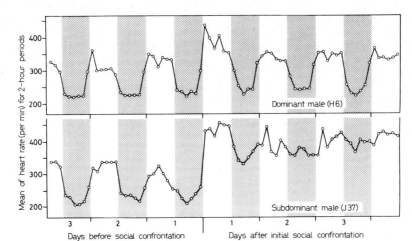

Fig. 7. Mean heart rate of 2 male Tupaias before and after social confrontation.

day/night variation. After onset of social confrontation the heart rate of dominant males (n = 5) remained more or less as it had previously. The heart rate of the subdominants (n = 5), however, showed a dramatic increase in the mean frequency of day values, and even more so of the night values, thereby reaching night values significantly higher than the daily mean before confrontation. This points to a constant high activation of the subordinate's sympathetic nervous system in this situation (fig. 7). Submissives have not been examined yet, but we have the impression that, in contrast to subdominants, they have a decreased heart rate (as well as a very low blood pressure).

To summarize: A social confrontation leading to dominance relationships has apparently no negative effects on dominant Tupaias, even if the position is maintained by fighting. Subordinate and submissive animals, however, show distinct stress reactions in all physiological parameters measured in our laboratory. In general, the physiological reactions are qualitatively the same, differing only in degree. There is, however, a clear qualitative distinction between subdominant and submissive animals with respect to their adrenal functions. In relation to dominant animals, submissives show no change in sympathetic-adrenomedullary activity but an increase in adrenocortical function. Subdominants, in contrast, show no change in adrenocortical function but an increase in sympathetic-adrenomedullary activity.

References

1   Holst, D. v.: Sozialer Stress bei Tupajas *(Tupaia belangeri).* Die Aktivierung des sym-
     pathischen Nervensystems und ihre Beziehung zu hormonal ausgelösten ethologischen
     und physiologischen Veränderungen. Z. vergl. Physiol. *63:* 1–58 (1969).
2   Holst, D. v.: Renal failure as the cause of death in *Tupaia belangeri* exposed to persistent
     social stress. J. comp. Physiol. *78:* 236–273 (1972).
3   Holst, D. v.: Social stress in the tree-shrew: its causes and physiological and ethological
     consequences; in Martin, Doyle, Walker, Prosimian biology, pp. 389–411 (Duckworth,
     London 1974).
4   Holst, D. v.: Social stress in the tree shrews: problems, results, and goals. J. comp. Physiol.
     120: 71–86 (1977).
5   Kawamichi, T.; Kawamichi, M.: Spatial organization and territory of tree shrews *(Tupaia
     glis).* Anim. Behav. *27:* 381–393 (1979).
6   Martin, R.D.: Towards a new definition of primates. Man *3:* 377–401 (1968).
7   Starck, D.: Vergleichende Anatomie der Wirbeltiere auf evolutionsbiologischer Grund-
     lage, Bd 1 (Springer, Berlin 1978).

22 Social Behavior of Rats as a Model for the Psychophysiology of Hypertension[1]

J.M. Koolhaas, T. Schuurman, D.S. Fokkema

A considerable amount of evidence indicates that, under certain conditions, psychosocial factors affect somatic health [4]. Many clinical observations, psychological and psychiatric studies, and animal experiments, suggest that the development of essential hypertension might also be of psychosocial origin. *Groen* et al. [6] formulate this more specifically: (a) 'Essential hypertension is a disturbance of the homeostasis of the blood pressure (BP) caused by an exaggeration in time and intensity of the same mechanisms which produce a temporary rise in BP in normal individuals during certain interpersonal conflict situations. (b) Certain individuals are predisposed to react by a certain behavior in certain conflict situations with key figures in their environment.' These two aspects of the psychosomatic hypothesis of hypertension need further experimental evidence. Also, the underlying mechanisms and causes of the exaggerated pressure response and the higher susceptibility of certain individuals for the hemodynamic effects of social stimuli are largely unexplained. These psychophysiological aspects of hypertension can be studied very well in animal experiments. Although much animal research is devoted to the effects of stress on the development of hypertension, there is only a vague, if any, relationship between the stressors used in these experiments and the stimuli the animal might meet in its everyday life in a more natural social setting. Ideally one should study the relationship between psychosocial factors and hypertension in situations that are biologically meaningful to the experimental animal. A few animal models fulfil this condition.

In a number of elegant studies, *Henry* et al. [8] and *Henry and Cassel* [7] extensively studied in mice the relationship between BP and various aspects of the social structure such as population size, familiarity, dominance,

[1] Part of this work was supported by a grant from the Netherlands Organization for the Advancement of Pure Research to Dr. *Schuurman*, and by a grant from the Dutch Heart Foundation to Dr. Fokkema.

etc. Similar work has been done in the tree shrew *Tupaia belangeri*. This work involves the physiological changes in subordinate animals due to the prolonged presence of their victor [9, 14, 15]. Although these studies are highly relevant to a better understanding of the psychophysiology of hypertension, it is beyond the scope of this paper to review the results thoroughly. Characteristic of these studies is the fact that they report the behavioral and physiological changes resulting from a more or less prolonged social stimulation.

None of these studies investigated these processes while a social interaction is going on. Such a detailed analysis is necessary if we want to obtain more experimental evidence for the psychosomatic hypothesis of hypertension as formulated above. In this article we want to demonstrate that social behavior of rats might be a suitable animal model for a further investigation in this direction. The model combines techniques derived from two scientific disciplines. In the first place, ethological methods for manipulating, observing, and analyzing social behavior under seminatural conditions allow for a detailed analysis of the way in which various social factors affect behavior in individual animals. Secondly, several methods are available to monitor and continuously manipulate various physiological processes during social interactions in relatively free-moving animals. Finally, some data will be presented that show that this combined ethological and physiological approach might be fruitful in the study of the psychophysiology of hypertension.

Social Behavior of Male Rats

The behavior of rats has been described by a number of authors [1, 3, 12]. In the wild, they live in burrows around which a male dominates a small group of females and other, often younger, male rats. In this social structure, several roles can be distinguished. There is usually one dominant or alpha male, which attacks intruder males and which is dominant over all other members of the group. There is a large group of so-called beta males, the behavior of which is adapted in such a way that they live quite peacefully in the presence of the alpha male. Finally, there is a small group of omega males, that are in fact the outcasts of the social structure. These animals are often attacked by other members of the group and have a marginal existence on the border of the colony. This social structure of the colony is established and maintained by a wide variety of separate social behavior elements (movements and postures).

These elements can be easily recognized by a trained observer, and they are defined in such a way that the animal always performs one of these elements, and only one at a time. More extensive descriptions of the behavior of rats can be found in *Grant and Mackintosh* [5], *Lehman and Adams* [10], and *Timmermans* [18]. In our experiments we distinguished a repertoire of 20 elements. This repertoire can be easily observed in domesticated male rats and does not differ essentially from that of wild rats. By counting frequencies and durations of these separate elements, a quantitative picture of the behavior of an animal in a certain social situation can be obtained.

Ways to Manipulate Social Situations

The colony structure just described is to complex to allow for a detailed analysis of the behavioral and physiological processes during social interactions. However, part of the processes that occur in the complex social structure can be easily studied in a more simple dyadic interaction in small observation cages ($85 \times 60 \times 60$ cm). A male rat of 3 months of age or more, that lives in such a cage, will readily perform aggressive behavior when an unfamiliar male intruder of the same weight and strain is introduced into its cage. In order to prevent any artifacts of social isolation, and to promote the development of this territorial aggressive behavior, the home cage animal should always live together with a female (sterilized by ligation of the oviducts). This territorial aggressive behavior can be easily used to manipulate the social situation of the experimental animal under study. A male rat is always dominant when tested in its home cage in the presence of a male intruder of the same weight and strain, whereas the same animal will be subordinate when tested in the home cage of another male rat of the same weight and strain. Variation in this basic scheme can be made by using opponents of different weights or strains. For example, an animal can be defeated in its home cage by a heavy and highly experienced male of the same strain or by using an intruder male of a more aggressive strain of rats.

Although other strains may also be suitable for this purpose, good results can be obtained using Tryon Maze Dull S3 rats as the highly aggressive strain, WEzob (TNO breeding colony) as the intermediate strain and Wistar as the low aggressive strain. The social situation can be manipulated in even more detail by varying the time and frequency of exposure to an opponent, by presenting only odors of dominant or subordinate opponents, or by introducing opponents in a small wire mesh cage.

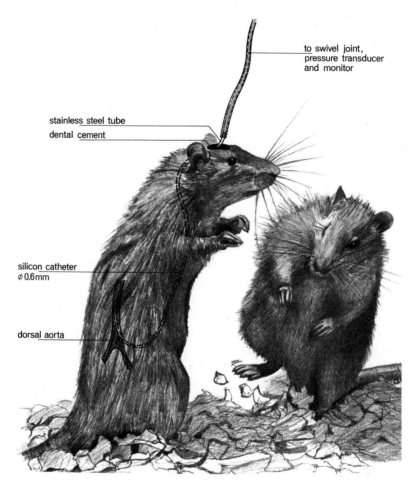

to swivel joint,
pressure transducer
and monitor

stainless steel tube

dental cement

silicon catheter
⌀ 0.6mm

dorsal aorta

Fig. 1. Canulation technique used for continuous blood pressure recording in free moving rats. The canulated rat adopts the defensive upright posture, and the opponent the sideways posture.

Physiological Measurements

The method used for physiological measurements and manipulations during a direct social interaction between 2 animals is based upon a technique for chronic canulation of blood vessels originally designed by *Steffens* [17] (fig. 1).

Characteristic of this method is that the distal end of the catheter goes to a connector which is fixed to the skull of the animal. During an experiment this connector can be coupled to a polyethylene tube leading to a blood sampling device, an infusion pump or a BP monitor. In order to give the animal as much freedom as possible, and to prevent torsion of the tubing, two swivel joints are included in the system as well as a spring which keeps the tube tight during vertical movements of the animal. In the social situations described above, animals provided with this equipment perform social behavior which is indistinguishable from that of intact animals.

For frequent blood sampling or continuous infusion of various substances during social behavior we usually canulate the jugular vein. For a continuous recording of the BP we use a free indwelling catheter implanted directly into the abdominal aorta.

Aspects of Coronary-Prone Behavior in Rats

Using the methods just described we have extensively studied the endocrine processes underlying victory and defeat in male rats [16]. In these studies, we obtained evidence that even in male rats, there are striking differences between individual animals' physiological responses to certain social interactions.

Although the experiments were not designed for this purpose, the results made us realize that the animal model we used might be relevant for the study of the psychophysiology of hypertension. These results were based upon experiments in which we studied the behavioral and endocrine changes in a situation in which the experimental animal meets an opponent of the same weight and strain in an area that is unfamiliar to both animals. In such a situation, there is an initial period of exploration after which an aggressive interaction follows. The final result is that the experimental animal is either the winner or the loser of this combat.

Figure 2 shows how the plasma testosterone (T) concentration changes during this social interaction, both in the case of victory and defeat. In victors, after an initial rise, plasma T returned to baseline levels after the aggressive encounter. In the defeated animals, however, the initial rise of plasma T was significantly lower, and after this, the T concentration dropped to a level which was significantly below baseline concentrations. All defeated rats maintained this lowered baseline plasma T level on the first day after the defeat.

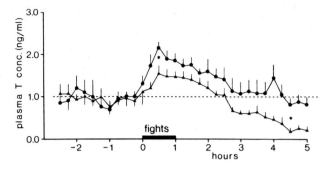

Fig. 2. Plasma T concentrations of victors (n = 6, ●) and losers (n = 8, ▲) before during and after the 1-hour encounter. Bars = SEM. * $p < 0.01$, victors vs losers; ** $p < 0.001$, victors vs losers.

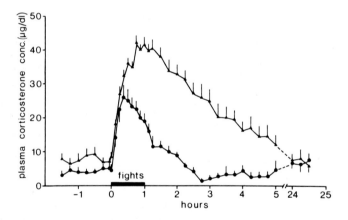

Fig. 3. Plasma corticosterone concentrations of victors (n = 6, ●) and losers (n = 9, ▲) during and after the 1-hour encounter. Bars = SEM. * $p < 0.05$, victors vs losers; ** $p < 0.005$, victors vs losers.

The corticosterone response of winners and losers is presented in figure 3. In the case of victory, after an initial rise, plasma corticosterone (C) started to decline even during the social interaction, and reached baseline levels within 3 h after the fight. In the defeated animals plasma C did not start to decrease until the end of the interaction, and was still significantly higher than baseline levels after 5 h.

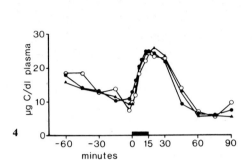 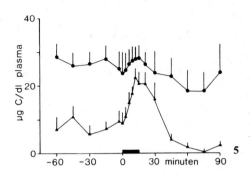

Fig. 4. Corticosterone response of victors (n = 6) to tests in unfamiliar cages. ○ = Before victory; ● = 1, 2 days after victory; ▲ = 7, 8 days after victory.

Fig. 5. Two different types of plasma corticosterone response in previously defeated rats during unfamiliar cage test 1 week after the defeat. ● = n = 4; ▲ = n = 5; ▬ = presence of stimulus rat; bars = SEM. * p < 0.01 (● vs ▲).

The second part of the hypothesis formulated in the introduction postulates that certain individuals are more susceptible to the effects of social stimuli. It is relevant therefore, to see how each experimental animal recovers behaviorally and physiologically from its serious combat. To illustrate this, both winners and losers were tested daily during 15 min, again in an unfamiliar area, but now in the presence of a subordinate male opponent.

All victors of the first combat spontaneously attacked the subordinate opponent even at the first day in this situation. Plasma T changed in a similar way as during the first combat (fig. 2), and there was only a small and short-lasting rise in plasma C (fig. 4) which did not change in the course of the days.

In the losers, however, two types of animals developed in the course of the experiments. One group of animals gradually recovered physiologically from the defeat within a few days. They exhibited a corticosterone response during the social interaction which was similar to that of the winners (fig. 5).

On the first day after the defeat, plasma T did not show an increase during the confrontation, but this response gradually returned in the course of the experiments. About half of the group of defeated male rats, however, developed more consistent changes in their physiological reaction pattern during the confrontations with the subordinate opponent. In these animals baseline plasma T did not return to predefeat levels, and there was hardly any rise in plasma T during the social interaction.

Plasma C was strongly elevated from the introduction of the experimental animal into the unfamiliar cage onwards, and there was no rise in plasma C during the confrontation with the subordinate opponent (fig. 5). In most animals, this pattern developed in the course of days after the defeat. In a few animals, however, plasma C did not decrease after the defeat and remained high over the next 24 h. These latter animals were also strongly hypoglycemic.

These data suggest that one strongly negative social experience is sufficient to induce, at least in some animals, a more permanent change in the appreciation of what is in itself a rather harmless social situation. This is also reflected in the behavioral change after a serious combat. The behavior of the victors did not change notably, i.e. they performed as much offensive behavior towards the opponent as before the serious combat. In the losers, however, remarkable behavioral changes were observed, which seem to be correlated with the physiological changes. Offensive behavior disappeared almost completely immediately after the defeat and, instead, these animals behaved defensively when being approached by the opponent. Those animals that showed the gradual recovery of the physiological responses, replaced this defensive behavior for offense in the course of the days. The chronically changed animals with the high plasma C concentrations and the low plasma T levels maintained the defensive behavioral strategy.

We have shown now that a single social interaction has considerable physiological and behavioral consequences, especially in the defeated animals. There is some evidence that the physiological changes can be considered as a causal factor for the changes in behavior. The plasma T concentration strongly influences offensive behavior, especially when tested in an unfamiliar area [16]. This means that the decrease in testosterone in the losers reduces the chance of being involved in another serious combat. *Leshner and Politch* [11] demonstrated that corticosterone facilitates submissive behavior and possibly also defensive behavior in mice. This suggests that the corticosterone response reduces the chance of severe injury when being attacked. It seems likely, therefore, that the pattern of physiological change helps the animal to cope not only physically, but also behaviorally with the changing social situation.

Since our data show that some animals develop an increased susceptibility for certain social stimuli, it is clear that it is an important question why these animals react so differently from other losers to the same social experience. These differences must have a genetic or an ontogenetic basis [2, 13] which may be expressed in an inadequate behavioral response in certain social situations. In that case one should be able to predict the differential results on the basis of a detailed ethological analysis of the animal's behavior prior to the negative social experience. Unfortunately our data do not allow such an analysis of the behavioral differences between individuals, but in a recently started project we are trying to relate the results of a detailed ethological analysis to the BP response in a variety of social situations.

Finally it is tempting to consider the possibility that the differences between individuals that we observe in dyadic interaction are the basis of the different social roles that have been described in more complex rat societies [1, 3].

Although our experiments are far from conclusive, it seems that the model described here makes it possible to study in more detail the two aspects of the psychosomatic hypothesis of hypertension mentioned in the introduction.

References

1   Barnett, S.A.: The rat, a study in behavior (University of Chicago Press, Chicago 1963).
2   Bronstein, P.M.; Hirsch, S.M.: Ontogeny of defensive reactions in Norway rats. J. comp. physiol. Psychol. *90:* 620–629 (1976).
3   Calhoun, J.B.: The ecology and sociology of the Norway rat (US Department of Health, Education and Welfare, Bethesda 1962).
4   Dohrenwend, B.S.; Dohrenwend, B.P.: Stressful life events: their nature and effects (Wiley & Sons, New York 1974).
5   Grant, E.C.; Mackintosh, J.H.: A comparison of the social postures of some common laboratory rodents. Behavior *21:* 246–259 (1963).
6   Groen, J.J.; Valk, J.M. van der; Welner, A.; Ben-Ishay, D.: Psychobiological factors in the pathogenesis of essential hypertension. Psychotherapy Psychosomatics *19:* 1–26 (1974).
7   Henry, J.P.; Cassel, J.C.: Psychosocial factors in essential hypertension. J. Epidemiol. *90:* 171–200 (1969).
8   Henry, J.P.; Mehan, J.P.; Stephens, P.M.: The use of psychosocial stimuli to induce prolonged systolic hypertension in mice. Psychosom. Med. *29:* 408–432 (1967).
9   Holst, D. v.: Renal failure as the cause of death in *Tupaia belangeri* exposed to persistent social stress. J. comp. Physiol. *78:* 236–273 (1972).
10   Lehman, M.N.; Adams, D.B.: A statistical and motivational analysis of the social behaviors of the male laboratory rat. Behavior *61:* 238–275 (1977).
11   Leshner, A.I.; Politch, J.A.: Hormonal control of submissiveness in mice: irrelevance of androgens and relevance of the pituitary-adrenal hormones. Physiol. Behav. *22:* 531–534 (1979).
12   Lore, R.L.; Flanelly, K.: Rat societies. Sci. Am. *236:* 106–116 (1977).
13   Price, E.O.; Belanger, P.L.: Maternal behavior of wild and domesticated stocks of norway rats. Behav. Biol. *20:* 60–69 (1977).

14   Raab, A.: Der Serotoninstoffwechsel in einzelnen Hirnteilen vom Tupaia *(Tupaia belan-geri)* bei soziopsychischem Stress. Z. vergl. Physiol. *72:* 54–66 (1971).

15   Raab, A.; Storz, H.: A long-term study on the impact of sociopsychic stress in tree shrews *(Tupaia belangeri)* on central and peripheral tyrosine hydroxylase activity. J. comp. Physiol. *108:* 115–131 (1976).

16   Schuurman, T.: Hormonal correlates of agonistic behavior in adult male rats. Progr. Brain Res. *53:* 415–420 (1980).

17   Steffens, A.B.: A method for frequent sampling of blood and continuous infusion of fluids in the rat without disturbing the animal. Physiol. Behav. *4:* 833–836 (1969).

18   Timmermans, P.J.A.: Social behaviour in the rat; thesis, Nijmegen (1978).

23 Central Nervous System Mechanisms in Experimental Hypertension[1]

F. Lamprecht

During the last decade, numerous findings have emerged to underline the importance of the role the central nervous system (CNS) plays in initiating and maintaining hypertension. For a long period of time, easy accessibility to the peripheral circulation via venipuncture has led to an overemphasis of peripheral mechanisms and to the neglect of what might be going on in the CNS. CNS activity could lead to changes in the circulating pressor amines, in receptor sensitivity and in the renin-angiotensin-aldosterone system, and vice versa, primary changes within peripheral mechanisms could be followed by altered CNS function. The interpretation of data becomes increasingly difficult since the composition of the pathogenic factors varies during initiation, maintenance, and fixation of hypertension. Thus, the question always arises: What are the predisposing, precipitating and maintaining factors on the one hand, and what are the secondary alterations due to the elevated blood pressure (BP) on the other? One of the pioneers in hypertension research, *Page* [38] has stated the dilemma as follows: 'Physicians tend either to oversimplify it prescribing a regimen and then letting the office or a visiting nurse take over, or at the other extreme to subject all patients to a searching and extensive analysis involving measurements of renin, catecholamine, aldosterone, and blood volume as well as other difficult technical procedures. Unfortunately, when the results are all in, few physicians have any clear idea what they mean.' In addition, methodological pitfalls have to be taken into account. For instance, taking plasma norepinephrine (NE) as an example, *Goldstein* [16] recently reviewed 32 studies published since 1973. In only 40% of the studies statistically significant hypertensive-normotensive differences in plasma NE were found. These 'positive' studies, however, had lower values within the control group and frequently had used fluorimetric assays instead of radioenzymatic assays. Moreover, a negative correlation was found between hypertensive-normotensive differences and mean patient age [16]. How these factors exert their effects, however, remains unanswered.

---

[1] Dedicated to Prof. Dr. med. *F. Gross* on the occasion of his 70th birthday.

At least it seems advisable to be very cautious with premature interpretations. In this chapter, I would like to select four lines of evidence for CNS involvement in hypertension by giving some examples of each: (a) manipulations within the CNS which could prevent experimental or genetic hypertension; (b) manipulations within the CNS which would lead to hypertension; (c) the pharmacological effects upon receptors within the CNS by agents used in the treatment of hypertension, and (d) neurochemical, morphological, and physiological changes observed in the CNS before, during, and after the development of hypertension under experimental conditions. To discuss the central catecholaminergic neurons involved in neuroendocrine regulation, which in turn could contribute to BP elevation, would be beyond the scope of this brief chapter. The results will be discussed with regard to the possible meaning they might have for essential hypertension in humans.

(a) With the development of 6-hydroxydopamine (6-OHDA), a substance which selectively destroys noradrenergic neurons [51], a very useful tool has become available for investigating the role that these noradrenergic neurons might play in the development of hypertension. In some investigations, intravenously applied 6-OHDA showed either no effect [4, 10], or only a delay in onset of hypertension after DOCA-salt [35]. The varied results might be explained by different degrees of sympathetic nerve destruction achieved within the blood vessels which are responsible for peripheral vascular resistance, and this might account for the failure of this procedure to prevent or to reverse hypertension. The increased turnover of noradrenalin in heart, intestine and spleen found by de Champlain et al. [2], and the decreased turnover of noradrenaline in the brain stem of rats made hypertensive with DOCA-salt have been interpreted as compensatory inhibition by central adrenergic action of peripheral sympathetic nerve activity [36]. Therefore, the time was right to destroy the central inhibiting adrenergic neurons by intraventricularly applied 6-OHDA, an idea which was carried out by several research groups independently of each other in the early 1970s [18, 29, 33, 34]. When 6-OHDA was given intraventricularly 7 days prior to the experimental manipulation, it was possible to prevent renal hypertension [18, 34] and DOCA-salt hypertension [18, 29, 33]. Two intraventricular injections of 6-OHDA in 7-week-old spontaneously hypertensive rats caused a drop in BP and prevented a further rise [18]. By intracisternal administration of 6-OHDA, it was possible to reverse neurogenic hypertension induced by buffer nerve section in rabbits [3]. Since intracisternal pretreatment with 6-OHDA in one study [34] had only a minimal protecting effect in DOCA-salt hypertension, we examined different patterns of depletion of central NE

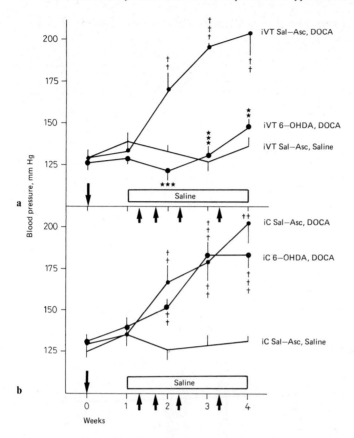

Fig. 1. Mean tail blood pressure was measured at weekly intervals, Intracerebral injections of 6-OHDA or the saline-ascorbic vehicle were made at the large arrows above the abscissa (intraventricular injections in **a**, intracisternal injections in **b**). From week 1 to week 4, 1% saline was provided as the only source of drinking water and subcutaneous injections of DOCA or saline were made at 3- to 7-day intervals as indicated by the small arrows under the abscissa. Data points ($\bar{x} \pm$ SEM) significantly different (t-test) from non-DOCA controls are indicated by †† = p < 0.01; ††† = p < 0.001. Data points significantly different from non-6-OHDA controls are indicated by ** = p < 0.01; *** = p < 0.001 [from 31].

produced by two different administration routes of 6-OHDA [31]. The results are shown in figure 1 and table I. NE depletion was significantly more pronounced in connection with the intraventricular application route, except for the spinal cord and the locus coeruleus, thus eliminating these structures for the preventive effect of intraventricularly given 6-OHDA. In this study [31] the depletion of NE in various subcortical structures by intraventricularly

Table I. Norepinephrine content in different areas of the rat brain 5 weeks after 6-hydroxy-dopamine treatment

Area	Intraventricular injection, %	Intracisternal injection, %
Cortex	10	41
Septal area	26	74
Neostriatum	48	82
Lateral hypothalamus	25	42
Dorsomedial hypothalamus	16	40
Ventromedial hypothalamus	19	50
Locus ceruleus	41	41
Rest of brain	13	43
Spinal cord	8	8

Animals received 250 µg 6-hydroxydopamine injected intracisternally or intraventricularly as described in the text; results are expressed as percentage of controls.

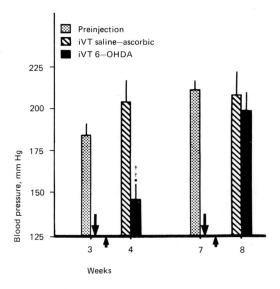

Fig. 2. Mean tail blood pressure was measured after 2 and 6 weeks of DOCA-salt treatment. An intraventricular injection of 6-OHDA or the vehicle was made at the large arrows above the abscissa. The rats were maintained for an additional week on the DOCA-salt treatment. The small arrows under the abscissa indicate a subcutaneous DOCA or saline injection. Data points ($\bar{x} \pm$ SEM) significantly different from preinjection levels are indicated by †† = $p < 0.01$. Data points significantly different from iVT vehicle injection group are indicated by * = $p < 0.02$ [from 31].

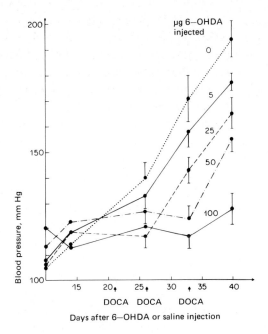

Fig. 3. DOCA-salt-induced hypertension in rats pretreated with different doses of 6-OHDA in the third ventricle [from 30].

given 6-OHDA might disrupt the development of hypertension by preventing the increased impulse traffic from the neostriatum, the septal area or the hypothalamus to peripheral sympathetic nerves. The ability of 6-OHDA to reverse hypertension established by DOCA-salt seems to depend very much on the time of administration. Only during the early stage (2 weeks after DOCA-salt treatment) was it possible to reverse hypertension by intraventricular application of 6-OHDA, whereas the same procedure showed no effect following 6 weeks of DOCA-salt treatment (fig. 2), indicating a different role of central noradrenergic neurons during the early and later phase of DOCA-salt hypertension. Since the 6-OHDA was applied in this study in the lateral ventricle, we thought that limitation of the destruction by 6-OHDA in the region adjacent to the third ventricle would give further hints for the areas involved in the development of DOCA-salt hypertension. Figure 3 shows the protective effect of various doses of 6-OHDA given directly in the third ventricle [30]. The histological examination of these brains showed that the cannular tip was localized in the medial hypothalamus in the region of the ventral medial nucleus dorsal of the arcuate nucleus. A reduced number of fluorescent fibers was apparent on the side of drug placement in the paraventricular, periventricular, and dorsomedial nuclei of the hypothalamus, in the septal nuclei, and in the nucleus interstitialis stria terminalis. In addition, probably due to reflux, there was a striking reduction in the number of dopaminergic cell bodies of the substantia nigra at the site of the lesion [30]. Since electrical stimulation of the posterior hypothalamus [40] leads to a rise in BP, and since the anterior hypothalamus is seen as the rostral end of the baroreceptor depressor reflex arch [20], the preventative drug effect could be exerted by destruction of the noradrenergic neurons within these structures. Furthermore, since the hypothalamus is also involved in thirst regulation, one could have assumed that diminished salt intake after centrally applied 6-OHDA is responsible for the protective effect against DOCA-salt, but this is not the case. *Reid* et al. [41] showed that the saline intake of 6-OHDA-pretreated rats is indeed reduced compared to that of vehicle-treated controls, but when the saline intake of the control rats was reduced to a similar level, they still developed hypertension after DOCA-salt treatment.

(b) On a general level, central manipulations leading to BP elevation include two different approaches: one is to facilitate the discharge of pressor centers by submitting animals to chronic stress [19, 32] at the same time increasing the sensory input, or by direct chronic electrical stimulation [12]; the other is by inhibition of inhibitory pathways. Sinoaortic denervation [22] leads to labile hypertension, whereas deafferentiation of the cells of the nucleus tractus solitarii (NTS) [6] and bilateral destruction of the NTS by electrolytic lesions [42, 43] leads to sustained hypertension. The NTS is seen as the primary site of the termination of baroreceptor afferents but the rostral end of the integrative center of the baroreceptor reflex seems to be the anterior hypothalamus [20] and destruction leads to an increased peripheral resistance due to enhanced preganglionic sympathetic discharge as a consequence of the release of central sympathetic vasomotor neurons from inhibition. The close neuroanatomical connections of the vasomotor centers in the brain stem with the cortical areas, particularly the frontal lobe [39] and the functional relationship to the nucleus amygdalae [50], make the vasomotor center in the anterior hypothalamus extremely sensitive to sensory inputs and to what we experience. This will be of importance when we discuss the meaning of these findings for essential hypertension in humans.

(c) Two therapeutic agents used in the treatment of hypertension are taken as an example to make the point that the mechanism of action lies within the CNS: one is α-methyldopa and the other clonidine. α-Methyldopa becomes decarboxylated to α-methyldopamine and then β-hydroxylated to α-methylnoradrenalin. This was first demonstrated by *Carlsson and Lindquist* [1]. This discovery led to the formulation of the false transmitter hypothesis, which states that α-methylnoradrenalin would replace noradrenalin in the available storage pool and compete with NE for the postsynaptic receptor site and that, due to the lower intrinsic activity, vasopressor activity would be decreased. α-Methyldopa can cross the blood-brain barrier, whereas α-methyldopamine cannot. Therefore, it was possible to demonstrate that a simultaneous inhibition of peripheral dopadecarboxylase led to an enhancement of the BP lowering effect of α-methyldopa [5]. Intraventricular application of the drug was 100 times as effective as systemic application and the effect could be diminished when central dopamine-β-hydroxylase was inhibited [5], thus indicating that central α-methylnoradrenalin is responsible for the antihypertensive effect. In another investigation [9], it was possible to abolish the antihypertensive effect of α-methyldopa in spontaneously hypertensive rats by destruction of central noradrenergic neurons (by 6-OHDA) or by centrally applied phentolamine, an α-blocking agent, thus giving credence to the assumption that the drug action is mediated by central α-adrenergic receptors [9]. The same seems to be true for the α-agonist clonidine [52], a substance which inhibits secretion of ACTH, vasopressin, and renin [14]. The inhibition of renin secretion is central and neurally mediated [14]. As shown by several investigators [24], the concept of presynaptic α-receptors which are now called α_2-receptors would explain how noradrenalin could regulate its own release by a local feedback loop. α-Methylnoradrenalin has been shown to have a higher affinity to presynaptic than postsynaptic α-receptors. *Häusler* [17] has seen the activation of adrenergic interneurons in the NTS at which the first synapse of the baroreceptor reflex ends, as a possible mechanism of the hypotensive action of clonidine. Activation of these interneurons would lead to an increased inhibitory tone in the vasomotor center and an increased stimulation of the vagus center.

(d) Some of the first findings in the CNS during experimental hypertension came from turnover studies [36, 37] in DOCA-salt and genetic hypertension. Whereas in DOCA-salt hypertension, the NE turnover in the brain stem was found to be delayed reciprocally to the acceleration in the periphery, in genetic hypertension, the central NE turnover was unchanged in the prehypertensive and hypertensive states [37]. In rats made temporarily hypertensive by immobilization [31], there was an increase in hypothalamic tyrosine-hydroxylase [39] and NE content (fig. 4). This increase in NE content was not seen in the brain stem and the remainder of the brain. The increase of hypo-

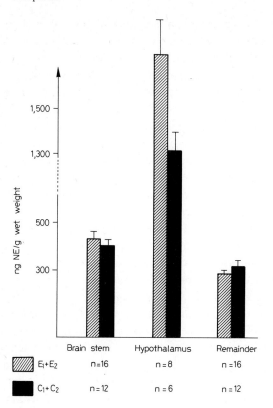

Fig. 4. Norepinephrine content determined radioenzymatically in brains obtained from rats exposed to 4 weeks of immobilization 2 h daily $(E_1 + E_2)$ and from the corresponding control rats $(C_1 + C_2)$ [*Lamprecht, Williams and Kopin*, unpublished observation].

thalamic tyrosine hydroxylase persisted when examined 4 weeks after the last immobilization, accompanied by increased fighting behavior, although the BP had by then returned to normal control levels. This persisting increase of hypothalamic tyrosine hydroxylase could not account for the foregoing BP elevation but might be responsible for the sensitivity of the baroreceptor-depressor response due to an increased activity in inhibitory adrenergic inter-neurons (fig. 5). *Folkow* [11] discussed the central neurohormonal mechanisms in spontaneously hypertensive rats in comparison to essential hypertension in humans, stressing the exaggerated defense reaction even in the pre-hypertensive stage, which reminds me of *Alexander's* formulation that a hypertensive patient is constantly prepared for a fight which never takes place.

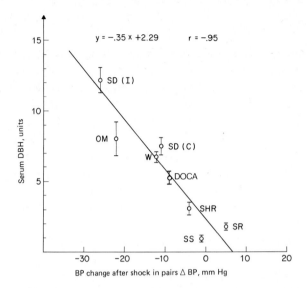

Fig. 5. Relationship of serum dopamine-β-hydroxylase (DBH) levels (units) to blood pressure (mmHg) changes after shock in different rat strains. SD (I) = Sprague-Dawley immobilized rats; SD (C) = Sprague-Dawley control rats; OM = Osborne-Mendel rats; W = NIH Wistar rats; DOCA = DOCA-salt-hypertensive rats; SHR = spontaneously hypertensive rats; SS = salt-sensitive rats (Dahl); SR = salt-resistant rats (Dahl); BP = blood pressure. The experiment with the DOCA-salt-hypertensive rats was done by the author in completion of another study [from 28].

The interplay between dispositional factors and environmental stimuli leads to a close relationship in the sense that neurohormonal pressor influences are highly dependent on environmental stimuli [11]. *Folkow* [11] sees in the structural changes of large arteries a probable contribution to the resetting of the baroreceptor reflex, which then would help maintain hypertension. The behavioral hyperreactivity of spontaneously hypertensive rats and the increased life-long hyperarousal and aggressiveness [47] led to conditioning methods which modified the development of high BP in this animal model of essential hypertension [48]. The changes in central catecholaminergic neurons and spontaneously hypertensive rats [45] includes reduced NE content in the anterior hypothalamic nucleus and increased phenylethanolamine-N-methyltransferase (PNMT) during the early and prehypertensive stage in the A_1 and A_2 region. The A_1 area in the rat brain contains catecholaminergic cell bodies that send axons to the spinal cord, and A_2 corresponds partially to the terminating point of the carotid sinus nerve fibers in the NTS [13].

Discussion

Most of the findings we have mentioned so far interfered in one way or another with the regulation of the baroreceptor-depressor reflex mechanism. However, particularly the supramedullary modulation of this autonomic reflex makes it extremely sensitive to events in the outer and inner (visceral) world. *Lacey* [23] has conceived a classification of behavior between the two polar extremes of pure attention to external stimuli on the one hand and motivated inattention on the other. Along this hypothetical continuum, psychophysiological reaction profiles could be classified as *Richter-Heinrich* et al. [44] have described for hypotensive and hypertensive patients. *Lacey's* [23] pure attention certainly has a relationship to *Cannon's* 'flight-fight-response' and goes along with a sympathetic activation, which enables the organism to behave against a threatening environmental stimulus. *Lacey's* motivated inattention has a certain resemblance to *Engel and Schmale's* [7] 'conservation withdrawal' and goes along with a parasympathetic activation. This behavior enables the organism to retreat and to save energy and this leads to a disengagement with a threatening stimulus. However, to behave in one way or another requires a decision. In this context, it is worth mentioning that the Greek word crisis characterizes a state in which a decision has to be made. In a situation in which a decision cannot be made in reality or tried out in fantasy life, the organism will activate the autonomic nervous system in a planless fashion, alternating very rapidly between its two branches, with concomitant symptoms of trembling, piloerection, salivation, vomiting, urination, defecation, etc. In case this persists for a longer period of time the reciprocity between the two systems may break down [15]. The organism is somehow in a state of psychological immobilization and does not know whether to fight, flee, or to ignore the threatening stimulus. The uncertainty in humans how to use these phylogenetic mechanisms has to do with the development of the limbic system and the neocortex and their numerous connections to the autonomic centers within the CNS. These connections at least partially dismiss vegetative functions from their so-called autonomy. In humans it is difficult to differentiate whether the vasomotor tonus is stimulated by higher cortical areas or inhibited by the carotid sinus. The latter could be counteraffected by central stimulation. This goes along with the clinical experience that simple bed rest leads to a significant drop in BP in most cases. This clinical impression is explained by the fact that the effectiveness of baroreceptor inputs depends on the state of cortical arousal. During sleep, for instance, a lower pressure stimulus gives rise to a greater baroreceptor

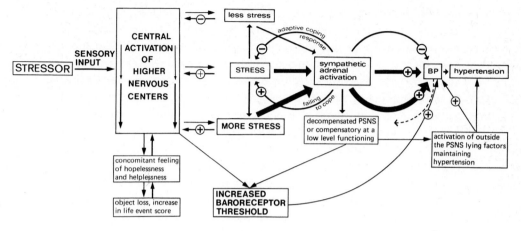

Fig. 6. The immobilized rat is seen as a stressed individual, which at the beginning of its restraint tries to cope through activation of the sympathetic adrenal system which, challenged too often, either decompensates or is functioning at a lower level to compensate for hypertension maintaining factors lying outside the peripheral sympathetic nervous system (PSNS). This latter state seems to be psychologically characterized as being helpless and hopeless in the sense that the forcefully restrained animal could do nothing about it.

reflex response [49]. Moreover, it has recently been shown that mild psychological stimuli [8] lead to increased CNS-mediated adrenergic activity in patients with labile hypertension or with a genetic risk of it. In still another study [21], it was found that a mild psychological stimulus did produce a much more pronounced change in renal blood flow, and correspondingly in plasma renin activity, in patients with essential hypertension than in the normotensive control subjects. The resetting of the baroreceptor reflex in essential hypertension, as in different animal models including renal hypertension, is now widely acknowledged. This has led to the concept of baroreceptor stimulation devices as treatment in otherwise untreatable hypertension [46], and thereby overcoming the increased threshold to triggering of the reflex.

Thus, the adaptation of the threshold for the depressor reflex that is seen in essential hypertension might be due to an imbalance between the sympathetic and vagal components of the autonomic nervous system due to contradicting inputs from cortical areas and the limbic system upon the hypothalamic depressor area, which is seen as the rostral end of the integrative center for the carotid-sinus depressor mechanisms. Such a contradicting input might be the result of interpersonal conflicts in the sense that decisions have to be made but neither way seems to be a sensible way out – neither in fantasy life nor in reality. Thus, the individual seems to be psychologically immobilized. In this connection, animal experiments are reexamined which showed immobilized rats to become temporarily hypertensive, to become aggressive, and to show an increase in hypothalamic tyrosine hydroxylase, and a lowering of the threshold for the baroreceptor-depressor reflex (fig. 5). In the beginning of stress exposure (fig. 6), increased sympathetic nervous activity is seen as an adaptive response, thereby enabling the animal to cope, but if the attempts to cope meet with constant failure, the stress becomes unbearable. The attitude of giving up is accompanied by low-level functioning of the sympathetic nervous system. This goes along with an adaptation of the baroreceptor depressor mechanism [for more details see 25–28]. As a consequence, any kind of additional stress would not lead to a fall in BP as we have shown under different experimental conditions. By integrating psychological, neurochemical, and physiological processes that are concurrent with the BP regulation, the increased threshold for the baroreceptor depressor mechanism might be the fundamental link and therefore a small stone in the mosaic of hypertension theory.

References

1   Carlsson, A.; Lindquist, M.: In vivo decarboxylation of α-methyldopa and α-methyl-*meta*-tyrosine. Acta physiol. scand. *54:* 87–96 (1972).
2   Champlain, J. de; Müller, R.A.; Axelrod, J.: Turnover and synthesis of norepinephrine in experimental hypertension in rats. Circulation Res. *25:* 285–291 (1969).
3   Chalmers, J.P.; Reid, J.L.: Participation of central noradrenergic neurones in arterial baroreceptor reflexes in the rabbit. A study with intracisternally administered 6-hydroxy-dopamine. Circulation Res. *31:* 789–804 (1972).
4   Clarke, D.E.; Schmookler, H.H.; Barry, H.: Sympathetic nerve function and DOCA-salt induced hypertension. Life Sci. *9:* 1097–1108 (1970).
5   Day, M.D.; Roach, A.G.; Whiting, R.L.: The mechanism of the antihypertensive action of α-methyldopa in hypertensive rats. Eur. J. Pharmacol. *21:* 271–280 (1973).
6   De Jong, W.; Palkovits, M.: Hypertension after localized transection of brain stem fibres. Life Sci. *18:* 61–64 (1976).
7   Engel, G.L.; Schmale, A.H.: Conservation-withdrawal: a primary regulatory process for organismic homeostasis. Physiology, emotion, psychosomatic illness. Ciba Fdn Symp. *8:* 57–75 (1972).
8   Falkner, B.; Onesti, G.; Angelakos, E.T.; Fernandes, M.; Langman, C.: Cardiovascular response to mental stress in normal adolescents with hypertensive parents. Hemodynamics and mental stress in adolescents. Hypertension *1:* 23–30 (1979).
9   Finch, L.; Häusler, G.: Further evidence for a central hypertensive action of alpha-methyl-dopa in both the rat and cat. Br. J. Pharmacol. *47:* 217–228 (1973).

10 Finch, L.; Leach, G.D.H.: The contribution of the sympathetic nervous system to the development and maintenance of experimental hypertension in the rat. Br. J. Pharmacol. *39:* 317–324 (1970).

11 Folkow, B.: Central neurohormonal mechanisms in spontaneously hypertensive rats compared with human essential hypertension. Clin. Sci. molec. Med. *48:* 205–214 (1975).

12 Folkow, B.; Rubenstein, E.H.: Cardiovascular effects of acute and chronic stimulation of the hypothalamic defense area in the rat. Acta physiol. scand. *68:* 48–57 (1966).

13 Fuxe, K.: Evidence for the existences of monoamine containing neurons in the central nervous system. IV. Distribution of monoamine terminals in the central nervous system. Acta physiol. scand. suppl. 247, *64:* 36–85 (1965).

14 Ganong, W.F.; Jones, H.; Chalett, J.: The role of peripheral and central catecholamines in the regulation of renin secretion; in Catecholamines: basic and clinical frontiers. Proc. 4th Int. Catecholamine Symp., Pacific Grove 1978, pp. 1431–1433 (Pergamon Press, Oxford 1979).

15 Gellhorn, E.: Principles of autonomic-somatic integration. (University of Minnesota Press, Minneapolis 1967).

16 Goldstein, D.S.: Plasma norepinephrine in essential hypertension. A study of the studies. Hypertension *3:* 48–51 (1981).

17 Häusler, G.: Activation of the central pathway of the baroreceptor reflex, a possible mechanism of the hypotensive action of clonidine. Arch. Pharmacol. *278:* 231–246 (1973).

18 Häusler, G.; Finch, L.; Thoenen, H.: Central adrenergic neurons and the initiation and development of experimental hypertension. Experientia *28:* 1200–1203 (1972).

19 Henry, J.P.; Stephens, P.M.; Axelrod, J.: Effect of psychosocial stimulation on the enzymes involved in the biosynthesic and metabolism of noradrenaline and adrenaline. Psychosom. Med. *33:* 227–237 (1971).

20 Hilton, S.M.; Spyer, K.M.: Participation of the anterior hypothalamus in the baroreceptor reflex. J. Physiol., Lond. *218:* 271–293 (1971).

21 Hollenberg, N.K.; Williams, G.H.; Adams, D.F.: Essential hypertension: abnormal renal vascular and endocrine responses to a mild psychological stimulus. Hypertension *3:* 11–17 (1981).

22 Krieger, E.M.: Neurogenic hypertension in the rat. Circulation Res. *15:* 511–521 (1964).

23 Lacey, J.I.: Some cardiovascular correlates of sensorimotor behavior: examples of visceral afferent feedback? in Limbic system mechanisms and autonomic function, pp. 175–201 (Thomas, Springfield 1972).

24 Langer, S.Z.: Presynaptic regulation of catecholamine release. Biochem. Pharmacol. *23:* 1773–1800 (1974).

25 Lamprecht, F.: Serum dopamine-beta-hydroxylase and hypertension: implications for an integrative model of hypertension. Proc. 4th Congr. of the Int. College of Psychosomatic Medicine, Kyoto 1977, 383–388.

26 Lamprecht, F.: Der Barorezeptorenreflex und seine Beziehung zur Hochdruckentstehung. Z. psycho-somat. Med. (in press, 1981).

27 Lamprecht, F.; Eichelmann, B.; Thoa, N.B.; Williams, H.B.; Kopin, I.J.: Rat fighting behavior: serum dopamine-β-hydroxylase and hypothalamic tyrosine hydroxylase. Science *177:* 1214–1215 (1972).

28 Lamprecht, F.; Eichelman, B.S.; Williams, R.B.; Wooten, C.F.; Kopin, I.J.: Serum dopamine-beta-hydroxylase (DBH) activity and blood pressure response of rat strains to shock-induced fighting. Psychosom. Med. *36:* 298–303 (1974).

29   Lamprecht, F.; Henry, D.P.; Richardson, J.S.; Thomas, J.A.; Williams, R.; Bartter, F.C.:
     Central adrenergic neurons in DOCA-salt hypertension. Fed. Proc. *32:* 763 (1973).
30   Lamprecht, F.; Jacobowitz, D.M.; Richardson, J.S.; Kopin, I.J.: Central adrenergic
     neurons in DOCA-salt hypertension. J. Neurosci. Res. *1:* 227–234 (1975).
31   Lamprecht, F.; Richardson, J.St.; Williams, R.B.; Kopin, I.J.: 6-Hydroxydopamine
     destruction of central adrenergic neurones prevents or reverses developing DOCA-salt
     hypertension in rats. J. neural Transm. *40:* 149–158 (1977).
32   Lamprecht, F.; Williams, R.B.; Kopin, I.J.: Serum dopamine-β-hydroxylase during
     development of immobilization-induced hypertension. Endocrinology *92:* 953–956
     (1973).
33   Lewis, P.J.; Reid, J.; Chalmers, J.P.; Dollery, C.T.: Importance of central catecholaminer-
     gic neurones in the development and maintenance of renal hypertension. Clin. Sci. mol.
     Med. *45:* 115–118 (1973).
34   Mizogami, S.; Suzuki, M.; Sokabe, H.: Reactivity of norepinephrine receptors in the car-
     diovascular system of the hypertensive rats. Jap. Heart J. *13:* 428–437 (1972).
35   Müller, R.A.; Thoenen, H.: Effect of 6-hydroxydopamine hydrobromide and adrenal-
     ectomy on the development of desoxycorticosterone trimethylacetate-NaCl hypertension
     in rats. Fed. Proc. *29:* 546 (1970).
36   Nakamura, K.; Gerold, M.; Thoenen, H.: Experimental hypertension of the rat: reciprocal
     changes of norepinephrine turnover in heart and brain stem. Arch. Pharmakol. *268:* 125–
     139 (1971).
37   Nakamura, K.; Gerold, M.; Thoenen, H.: DOCA-salt and spontaneously hypertensive
     rats: comparative studies on norepinephrine turnover in central and peripheral adrenergic
     neurons; in Okamoto, Spontaneous hypertension, pp. 51–58 (Igaku Shoin, Tokyo 1972).
38   Page, I.H.: The continuing failure to understand and treat hypertension. J. Am. med. Ass.
     241: 1897–1898 (1979).
39   Palkovits, M.; Zaborszky, L.: Neuroanatomy of central cardiovascular control. Nucleus
     tractus solitarii: afferent and efferent neuronal connections in relation to the baroreceptor
     arc. Prog. Brain Res. *47:* 9–34 (1977).
40   Przuntek, H.; Guimaraes, S.; Philippu, A.: Importance of adrenergic neurons of the brain
     for the rise of blood pressure evoked by hypothalamic stimulation. Arch. Pharmakol. *271:*
     311–319 (1971).
41   Reid, J.L.; Zivin, J.A.; Kopin, I.J.: Central and peripheral adrenergic mechanisms in the
     development of deoxycorticosterone-saline hypertension in rats. Circulation Res. *37:*
     569–579 (1975).
42   Reis, D.J.; Doba, N.: The central nervous system and neurogenic hypertension. Prog. Car-
     diovasc. Dis. *17:* 51–71 (1974).
43   Reis, D.J.; Joh, T.H.; Nathan, M.A.; Renaud, B.; Snyder, D.W.; Talman, W.T.: The
     nucleus tractus solitarii, its catecholaminergic innervation and the normal and abnormal
     control of arterial pressure; in Schmitt, Meyer, Perspectives in nephrology and hyperten-
     sion, pp. 147–164 (Wiley, New York 1979).
44   Richter-Heinrich, E.; Borys, M.; Sprung, H.; Läuter, J.: Psychophysiologische Reaktions-
     profile von Hypo- und Hypertonikern. Dt. Gesundh Wes. *26:* 1481–1489 (1971).
45   Saavedra, J.M.; Grobecker, H.; Axelrod, J.: Changes in central catecholaminergic neurons
     in the spontaneously (genetic) hypertensive rat. Circulation Res. *42:* 529–534 (1978).
46   Sapru, R.N.; Krieger, A.J.: Rationale for the use of baroreceptor stimulators. J. surg. Res.
     25: 77–82 (1978).

47   Schaefer, C.F.; Brackett, D.J.; Gunn, C.G.; Wilson, M.F.: Behavioral hyperreactivity in the spontaneously hypertensive rat compared to its normotensive progenitor. Pavlov. J. *13:* 211–216 (1978).

48   Schaefer, C.F.; Brackett, D.J.; Wilson, M.F.; Gunn, C.G.: Lifelong hyperarousal in the spontaneously hypertensive rat indicated by operant behavior. Pavlov. J. *13:* 217–225 (1978).

49   Smyth, H.S.: Discussion remarks to P. Dell: Nucleus fasciculus solitarius activity visceral afferents and somatic functions; in Hockman, Limbic system mechanisms and autonomic function, pp. 139–151 (Thomas, Springfield 1972).

50   Stock, G.; Schlör, K.H.: Beitrag zur zentralen Kreislaufregulation – Experimente zur funktionellen Bedeutung des Mandelkerns; in Schiffter, Zentral-vegetative Regulationen und Syndrome, pp. 56–71 (Springer, Berlin 1980).

51   Tranzer, J.P.; Thoenen, H.: An electron microscopic study of selective, acute degeneration of sympathetic nerve terminals after administration of 6-hydroxydopamine. Experientia *24:* 155–156 (1968).

52   Van Zwieten, P.A.: Antihypertensive drugs with a central action. Prog. Pharmacol. *1:* 1–63 (1975).

24 A New Dimension in the Prevention of Coronary Heart Disease

Chandra Patel

'*Prevention better than a cure*' is probably more relevant to coronary heart disease (CHD) than any other condition today because it is the most common of all causes of death in middle-aged males in western countries. Approximately 40% of the deaths in men aged 45–64 years are attributed to CHD [99]. Although coronary care units and coronary bypass surgery have contributed to the quality of life in individual cases, it has generally been recognized that prevention only can reduce the great burden of mortality from CHD in our countries. Many studies conducted over the last 35 years have identified numerous risk factors: amongst them are high blood pressure (BP), raised serum cholesterol, cigarette smoking, diabetes, obesity, sedentary life and positive family history [31]. The first three are known as the major risk factors because of the stronger and more consistent association.

However, many studies reported in the literature also indicate the weakness in predicting future CHD from the level of risk factors. For example, *Gordon* et al. [21] compared incidence rate of CHD from studies which had used uniform methods in Framingham, Honolulu, and Puerto Rico. The incidence of CHD in Framingham was 2–3 times higher than that in Puerto Rico and Honolulu. Even when the studies were controlled for BP, serum cholesterol and smoking, the excess in Framingham persisted. In other words, the higher rate in Framingham could not be accounted for by the conventional risk factors. Smoking, for example, had no effect on the incidence rate of CHD in Puerto Rico. Similarly, in the Seven Countries Study [36], smoking was not found to be a significant risk factor.

There is no dearth of such discrepancies in the literature for every single conventional risk factor. Thus, it is reasonable to conclude that although the ability to predict CHD from the presence of these widely accepted risk factors is very impressive, a substantial proportion of CHD must occur for reasons other than these risk factors. Maybe it is because of this that a number of intervention trials using diets and drugs have consistently shown poor results.

Hypertension Intervention Trials

Earlier studies of drug treatment of hypertension were shown to reduce the incidence of uremia, strokes and heart failure, but not of myocardial infarction (MI) [3, 91, 92]. Recently, two studies [30, 40] from the USA and Australia respectively showed that drug treatment of mild hypertension reduces the incidence of all complications including MI, while at least one study [82] claimed that hypotensive therapy had not only failed to restrain the onset of CHD but it may even have been responsible for increased risk of precipitating MI in patients treated too energetically to bring their final diastolic BP (DBP) to less than 90 mm Hg.

It is also important to remember that if we are to treat all patients, including those with mild hypertension (DBP 90 mm Hg) up to a third of an adult population may qualify for a life-long treatment [25] and mild hypertensives constitute approximately 70% of the total hypertensive population [30]. We do not yet know whether the treatment will be acceptable by the patients and what the long-term safety record will be. Therefore, it is justifiable to explore a non-drug behavioural approach which can reduce high BP, prevent complications, is free from side effects, and is relatively inexpensive in view of the magnitude of the problem.

Lipid Intervention Trials

A number of international trials using dietary methods showed conflicting results [8, 37, 47, 71, 72]. Either they did not show significant reduction in mortality, or the benefits seen were marginal. In some trials, although the mortality from CHD was significantly reduced, the total mortality was not. Some of these dietary trials as well as cholesterol lowering drug trials [7, 10, 70] showed some disturbing side effects like increased incidence of cancer, gallbladder, liver and other intestinal diseases in intervention groups, in spite of the fact that most of them were effective in reducing serum cholesterol. An editorial article in *The Lancet* [6] summed up: 'The treatment was beneficial but unfortunately the patient died!'

Cigarette Smoking

Doll and Hill [9] observed encouraging results in a 10-year follow-up of British doctors who gave up smoking and this lower mortality in ex-smokers was observed in other observational studies [24, 32]. However, *Rose and*

Hamilton [75] pointed out the difficulties in interpreting that mortality was due to smoking cessation from these studies, as people who stop smoking often come from higher social classes and they probably change other behaviors at the same time. In a controlled trial of smoking cessation they failed to show a difference in mortality between the groups at 8-year follow-up. However, in a secondary prevention trial, smoking cessation was associated with reduction in the incidence of sudden death [94]. There is no doubt regarding the evils of smoking, and yet apart from selective groups, mainly from the upper social classes, there are no signs of a drop in the number of cigarettes smoked, pointing out the fact that merely telling people to stop smoking is not enough.

Other Risk Factors

Diabetes has been shown to be associated with ECG abnormality and increased arterial diesease in some studies [34, 56] both in England and the USA. On the other hand, it is remarkable that Japanese and Asian-Israelis, in spite of the low incidence of CHD, have relatively higher incidence of diabetes [1, 45, 46].

A large-scale trial revealed that treatment of diabetes with phenformin or tolbutamide may increase the incidence of CHD [87]. The Pooling Project Research Group [67] showed that obesity was shown to be important in men under the age of 50, while over 55 it was slightly beneficial! A general concensus is that diabetes or obesity might be important if associated with any of the major risk factors.

Physical activity was suggested to be a protective factor on the basis of lower incidence of CHD in people with active jobs like those of bus conductors and postmen [50, 51] or those who pursue vigorous leisure time sports and exercise [49]. On the other hand, it is well known that the CHD mortality in East Finns is the highest in the world, despite the fact that most of the men are farmers or lumberjacks involved in most strenuous exercise, often consuming over 4,000 cal a day and who are lean and tall.

Jogging has been widely advocated and enthusiastically pursued in North America but it is not without its dangers. *Burch* [4], a cardiologist from New Orleans, commented on jogging as a dangerous fad, quoting the American Automobile Association's reports of 8,300 joggers killed and over 100,000 injured by automobiles in 1977. He added: 'When automobiles kill thousands of joggers, their jogging becomes a serious and dangerous disease of the environment.' The reported incidence of sudden deaths in sportsmen [54], marathon runners [52] soldiers in action [14, 48, 89], or during diagnostic exercise testing [73] questions the wisdom of prescribing exercise in those who are already showing some signs of myocardial ischemia.

Multiple Risk Factor Intervention

When single risk factor intervention proved disappointing, it was suggested that as many risk factors as possible must be controlled together to have an appreciable effect. Accordingly, a comprehensive community program was started in North Karelia, a county in Finland with the highest CHD mortality in the world. It was relatively successful in reducing risk factor levels compared with those of the control county of Kuopio [68]. However, this did not result in greater reduction in mortality in North Karelia [81]. It was explained that this was due to general decline in CHD mortality in all counties of Finland [88].

In the UK, which is one of the countries participating in the European multifactorial intervention trial [98], the heart disease prevention project team randomly allocated 24 factories or occupational groups, comprising 18,210 men aged 45–59 years, into intervention or control groups. Men in the intervention groups received advice on dietary reduction of fat and cholesterol, stopping or reducing cigarette smoking, regular exercise and reducing weight in the overweight, while people with hypertension were treated with antihypertensive drugs. In addition to the group campaign, the top 10–15% of the higher risk group received personal counseling and personal letters of advice and follow-up. At the end of a 5-year follow-up, there were no clear differences between the intervention and control groups in the total risk estimates [76]. In a subanalysis of men with elevated risk factors, the estimated reduction in risk, calculated from the changes in risk factor levels using multiple logistic function, was 9% at the end of 5 years or an average of 11% over the last 3 years of follow-up. It was pointed out that the above trial does not have the statistical power to detect such small differences, and, thus, it is possible that when the trial is finally concluded, it may not show significant reduction in CHD mortality and miss a difference as important as 10–15% [41].

It is of crucial importance that every effort is made to elucidate other important etiological factors, so that future intervention trials not only show large enough differences in morbidity and mortality to be detected by the available statistical means, but also make an impressive contribution in eradicating the great burden of mortality from CHD. If nothing is done to prevent CHD, it has been projected that 1 man in 6 will get CHD before the age of retirement and half of these will be fatal [74]. When a disease is responsible for death of 1 in every 12 men under the age of retirement, when their families and communities need them most, the very least we can do is to mobilize all our resources and explore any new hypothesis. It is my aim to put forward a hypothesis and support it with the results of studies carried out so far. There is a lot of work that needs to be done before the hypothesis can be proven or the appropriate intervention can be shown to be successful, but at least a start has been made.

Stress Hypothesis

Psychosocial occupational stress has been considered by some to be an important risk factor, but there are more who strongly refute this. I suggest that psychosocial stress may be a causative factor (fig. 1) which, working through appropriate neuroendocrine stimulation and biochemical disturbances, leads to sudden death, probably throught the electrical disturbance of the conducting system. It may also lead to MI through gradual development of atherosclerosis, thrombosis or prolonged vasospasm of the coronary arteries. The disease can occur directly, or indirectly through a network of known and some yet unknown risk factors. It is well recognized that emotional stress can be one of the factors which lead to overeating, alcohol drinking or cigarette smoking. It may also lead to aggressive or type A behavior [15] and physical inactivity possibly by promoting early fatigue [53]. Overwhelming stress can result in production of stress hormones leading to decrease in insulin and increase in blood glucose and free fatty acids [11]. Its contribution to hypertension [23, 26] and hypercholesterolemia [17, 86] is gradually being revealed. The stress hypothesis is based on clinical observation, epidemiological studies, and experimental evidence.

Clinical Observation

Many astute physicians in the past have observed relevant and often profound details showing an association between psychosocial stress and symptoms of angina pectoris and MI. *William Haberden* in 1768 added to his vivid description of angina pectoris that the disease increased by the disturbance

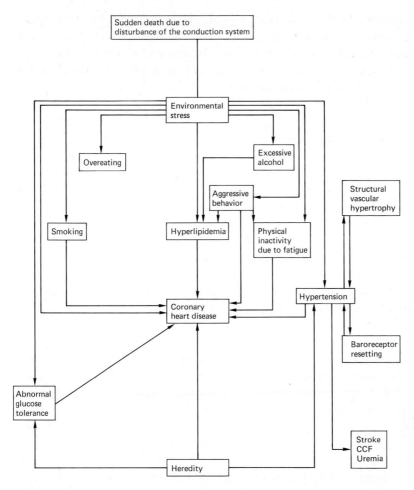

Fig. 1. Relationship between environmental stress and coronary heart disease: a hypothesis.

of the mind [5]. *John Hunter*, an English Surgeon of 18th century is quoted to have said 'my life is at the mercy of any fool who shall put me in passion' [5]. He died suddenly during a debate at St. George's Hospital's boardroom meeting. *Osler* [55] in one of his Lumlein lectures given at the Royal Society of Medicine in London said: 'A coronary-prone man is keen and ambitious man the indicator of whose engine is set full speed ahead.' *Kemple* [35] described him as an aggressive ambitious individual with an intense emotional drive, unable to delegate authority or responsibility with ease, possessing no hobbies and concentrating all his thoughts and energy in the narrow groove of his career. *Wolf* [95] described a coronary-prone person as one who not only meets a challenge by putting out extra effort, but who takes little satisfaction from his accomplishment.

Epidemiological Studies

Friedman and Rosenman [16] described an overt behavior pattern called 'type A' behavior characterized by intense ambition, competitive drive, constant preoccupation with occupational deadlines and a keen sense of time urgency. In a large prospective trial known as the Western Collaborative Group Study, [77, 78], they classified 3,524 men according to their behavior pattern and showed higher mortality from CHD in the type A group compared with the type B group over a period of 4.5 year follow-up. *Russek and Zohman* [80] and *Russek and Russek* [79] failed to recognize such an overt behavior pattern in a group of young patients with MI but remarked at their striking degree of self-control, dignified reserve and outward complacency.

In recent years, social scientists and epidemiologists have shown unfavorable effect on health, including increased rates of CHD, of difficulties of adjusting to new environment and strange cultures which people must face following changes in jobs, moving to new locations and moving upwards in social status [33, 83, 84], or emigrating to countries with a different culture [45, 46]. There is some evidence that social and cultural factors may interact with the conventional risk factors in an important manner which influences the incidence of CHD. *Gordon* [19, 20] and others [97] found an increasing gradient in mortality from CHD in Japanese living in Japan, Hawaii, and California, respectively, which persisted even when the data were compared controlling for differences in each risk factor separately [44].

Marmot and Syme [43] suggested that the greater emotional support the Japanese derive from strong family bonds and group cohesiveness might be protective and that, if this is so, the Japanese-Americans who have maintained the Japanese tradition would have lower rates of CHD compared with the Japanese-Americans who had changed their culture and adopted an American way of life. In a prevalence study, they showed that definite CHD, and indeed each characteristic (angina pectoris, pain of MI, and major ECG abnormality for each age group) was greater in the Americanized Japanese-

Americans compared with the traditional Japanese-Americans and that these differences could not be accounted for by changes in age, levels of BP, serum cholesterol, cigarette smoking, blood sugar, serum triglycerides and body weight.

Animal Experiments

In rabbits kept on high-fat, high-cholesterol diets, it was shown that the group receiving hypothalamic stimulation via implanted electrodes developed atherosclerotic lesions more rapidly and extensively [22]. Similarly, in chickens fed diets rich in animal fat, the quality and nature of social interactions were major determinants in the development of atherosclerosis. A 10-fold increase in CHD amongst mammals in Philadelphia Zoo without change in a dietary pattern was attributed to changes in housing arrangements which promoted increased aggressive behavior and competition between members of the species [69]. *Henry and Stephens* [27] showed that social deprivation by isolation from 2 weeks to maturity at 4 months produced mice which were unable to establish a stable social hierarchy, were aggressive, and if left in a colony, constantly fought, aged prematurely, and died from atherosclerosis and renal failure. There may be some analogy between these observations in experimental animals and civilized men, with the erosion of social hierarchy and exposure to similar psychosocial and environmental stimuli of urbanized, industrialized society which nurture aggressiveness and openly rewards competitiveness.

Future Intervention

It is apparent that conventional risk factors only account for part of the occurrence of CHD. The psychosocial stress hypothesis discussed in this paper suggests that the personality of the individual, his social, ecological and cultural environments might also be very important. If the hypothesis is right, we may expect to prevent CHD by dealing with psychosocial stress and increasing the individual's coping ability. The attraction of this hypothesis is that it can explain why some patients who get MI are overweight, while others have high serum cholesterol or high BP, depending upon their genetic susceptibility. It can also explain the cases who do not have any of the recognizable risk factors. It is a working hypothesis upon which we should gather evidence without joining any specific lobby or being overawed by the eminence of the authorities with differing views. The studies carried out so far show that hypertension may be reduced by behavioral methods aimed at counteracting environmental stress. There is some evidence that such methods may also reduce blood lipids and help smokers to give up smoking.

Proposed and Tested Therapeutic Behavior

A behavioral program based on theoretical grounds [61] and improved by practical experience in field studies consitst of the following:

Cognitive Restructuring. The patient is told that the intensity of the response depends upon his mental evaluation of a particular situation. The response is mobilized when a person perceives situations as threatening or overdemanding. Audiovisual methods are used to demonstrate appropriate and inappropriate responses in everyday life, as well as realistic and unrealistic fears and aggression. In other words, the patient is made more and more aware of his inappropriate responses and given the knowhow to correct them. He is encouraged to change his maladaptive habitual response to a more appropriate response by perseverance.

Breathing Exercise. He is taught simple breathing exercise at first. It is known that breathing is erratic when a person is excited, yet slow and regular when he is calm and composed. By a simple, rhythmic diaphragmatic breathing exercise, a certain amount of physical calmness is induced. This exercise can be performed anywhere and in any position without anybody even noticing it. This is followed by:

Deep Muscle Relaxation. The person is asked to lie down, close the eyes and systematically relax each part of the body. He is told that for full benefit he should do this exercise with an empty stomach and bladder. The fact that deep muscle relaxation reduces the intensity of the hypothalamic response is evident from animal experiments. For example, increase in proprioception through passive movements increases the intensity and a greater rise in BP, while a decrease in proprioception through curarization decreases the itensity and causes a smaller rise in BP when the hypothalamus is electrically stimulated [18, 28, 29]. It is thought that the intensity of the response is directly proportional to the amount of sensory input to the brain. In this context, it is also interesting to note that an increase in isometric contraction, such as a tight hand grip or the carrying of a heavy suitcase, a considerable rise in BP has been observed [38]. Maybe we live in a world with far too much sensory stimulation. It is assumed that a reduction in sensory input due to mental and physical relaxation would reduce the sympathetic responsiveness of the hypothalamus, and eventually lower BP.

Meditation. After a few sessions in breathing exercise and deep muscle relaxation, a type of mental relaxation is introduced in the form of passive concentration and eventually meditation. One definite advantage of meditation is that it at least prevents sleep. Relaxation is very conducive to sleep in accordance with the mechanisms of sleep [39]. But if the patient is allowed to sleep, the whole concept of voluntary control is nullified. Meditation is also known to change the EEG pattern into a more synchronized one with a high-amplitude, slow wave pattern of the relaxed brain not passing into sleep [93]. It is also known to increase coherence between two hemispheres as well as between the anterior and posterior parts of each hemisphere [2].

Biofeedback. In short, the points so far discussed in the program are aimed at reducing the levels of arousal. The biofeedback instruments are used to train patients to shift more efficiently into a low arousal state. One of two very simple instruments are used. A galvanic skin resistance measure, which by and large informs the patient about his level of skin resistance and indirectly of the level of his arousal or an electromyographic feedback machine, which continuously measures and displays his level of muscular tension. As the patient relaxes, the sound becomes fainter and the clicks become fewer until they stop. The sensitivity is then turned up to give further signals and the patients has to relax further to stop the signal and so on. The idea behind this procedure is that the knowledge of results reinforces the learning. In addition to this relaxation feedback, the patient is also given an overall feedback of his BP level at the end of each session. Every success the patient has is taken as an opportunity to raise his self-esteem and his motivation to continue the program on a long-term basis. Each session is about half an hour long. Originally, the patients had three training sessions per week, but experience as well as a more comprehensive educational program have shown that on the average one training session per week for 8 weeks may be adequate. In addition, the patient is asked to practice twice a day on his own for 15–20 min. Recent studies have included loaning the patient an instruction cassette tape for home practice.

Stress Management. The next point in the plan is deconditioning, or integrating the relaxation response into daily activities. It would be useful to know what situations in an individual's life contribute to hypertension or atherosclerosis – so that one could desensitize that individual against those situations. In practice, it is not possible to identify these situations in every individual. However, we know that environments of urbanized industrialized society are important. Therefore, we can assume that desensitization against situations of modern civilizations would be beneficial. Counterconditioning, or the method of reciprocal inhibition, is used in which the fear or aggression inducing stimulus is paired with another neutral stimulus, such as relaxation, which inhibits fear or aggression [96]. For example, car driving is one of the modern activities which raises BP in some individuals and causes aggression. What the patient is asked to do is to take one deep breath, relax and 'let go' at every red traffic light or intersection. He uses the same method before answering a telephone, speaking in public, during an interview, while waiting for a bus or in a dentist's surgery, and so on. This list is exhaustive and can be made up by an individual to suit his requirements. A tiny, colored paper disc is stuck to his wrist watch dial, so that every time he looks at the watch, he is reminded to relax, knowing how time pressure is considered to be one of the important risk factors [15].

Another way of integrating meditation in everyday life is through meditation in action. It is seen when a meditator becomes one with whatever he is doing at that point. For example, when an artist is painting or a sculpturist is sculpting or a dancer is dancing: when his mind is so concentrated on the thing he is doing that he becomes completely engrossed. It is a way of releasing or channelling emotional energy. We do not have to pursue higher arts for this. We can practice meditation in action during our everyday work or leisure activity, whether interviewing, washing up, or jogging, provided we could learn to concentrate on the activity at hand with our body and mind and shut out irrelevant ideas and associated anxieties.

Studies of Behavior Therapy in Hypertension: A Pilot Study

At first, a pilot study was carried out [57–59]. 20 hypertensive patients entered the trial as they came in for routine consultation. The only criterion was that they must be known to be hypertensive for at least a year. The hypertensive controls were added from the age and sex register kept in the group general practice. The groups were comparable with respect to mean duration of hypertension and severity of hypertension. Most were controlled on antihypertensive medication. At the end of a 3-month training program of three sessions per week, mean systolic BP (SBP) was reduced by 20.4 mm Hg, while the mean DBP was reduced by 14.2 mm Hg in the treatment group. In addition to this highly significant reduction in BP ($p = < 0.001$), it was also possible to reduce drugs in 12 patients, ranging from 33 to 100%. The control group patients also attended the same number of sessions and had the same number of BP measurements made but, instead to being trained in behavior modification, were asked to lie down and rest. The average reduction in SBP and DBP in this group were 0.5 and 2.1 mm Hg, respectively. These were not significant and their drug requirement remained unchanged.

In a parameter such as BP, where spontaneous fluctuation is so common, the value of any therapy can be assessed by its long-term effectiveness. The patients in both groups were followed up monthly up to 1 year. Except for some minor changes in BP and drug requirements in both the groups, the reduction obtained in the treatment group was maintained. In some patients, the BP started to go up. They turned out to be mostly those who could not continue the regular practice of relaxation. However, when restarting the relaxation practice, BP came down again. The lesson learnt during this follow-up study is the clear importance of motivating these patients for a lifelong discipline of practicing regularly and integrating relaxation into their daily activities.

Randomized Controlled Trial

Having seen fairly impressive results, it became important to conduct a controlled study. To avoid subjective and objective bias, all the BP measurements were made by an experienced nurse using a random zero sphygmomanometer [100]. 34 patients, known to be hypertensive for at least 6 months, with original DBP of 110 mm Hg or more before stabilizing them on medications, took part. The baseline BP was an average of nine measurements taken

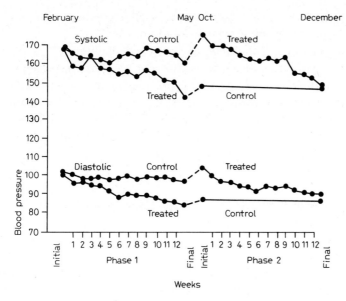

Fig. 2. Results of randomized controlled trial [60].

during three separate sessions (fig. 2). They were then randomly allocated to either treatment group or control group. Both the groups attended twice a week for 6 weeks for half-hour sessions. The treatment group patient was offered the treatment already described while the control group patient was asked to lie down and relax using whatever means he thinks is relaxing. The number of BP measurements were kept the same in both the groups. After the 6-week program, each patient was followed up once every fortnight, for 3 months. The average of all the measurements made during the follow-up is given as final values for each group (fig. 2). Antihypertensive drugs were kept constant.

The average drops in the treated group were 26 mm Hg SBP and 15 mm Hg DBP. The respective drops in the control group were 8 and 4 mm Hg. The differences between the groups were significant ($p = <0.005$). After 2 months all the patients were recalled. Surprisingly, the pressure in the control group had at least gone back to its original levels, while most of the reductions obtained in the treated group were maintained. The treated group was, of course, asked to continue with the practice of relaxation and its integration into everyday life. Perhaps the results in the control group are typical of a placebo group in the sense that the placebo effects persist only as long as placebo factors are operating, whatever they may be.

By chance, the random allocation had not divided all the independent variables; the study was extended to phase two, during which the behavioral modification program was offered to the previous control group over a 6-week period, while the already treated group now became the control group and attended once at the beginning and again at the end of phase 2 for reference purposes. The results showed reduction of both SBP and DBP, almost to the level of the groups previously treated.

Behavioral Methods in Reducing Stress in Hypertensive Patients

BP rises as a result of stress whether due to physical, emotional or painful stimuli in all of us. However, the rise is more acute and prolonged in hypertensive patients. The pressure load on the left ventricle or the vessel walls is an integrated average pressure over long periods. Therefore, cumulative benefit of reductions in magnitude, as well as duration of pressor responses, is obvious. 32 hypertensive patients were randomly allocated to treatment and control groups [59, 64]. All patients were subjected to two experimental stressors – an exercise test and a cold pressor test – and repeated 6 weeks later. During this interval, the treatment group patients were trained in the behavioral modification program outlined. The control group patients were exposed to an equivalent amount of attention placebo. The results showed significant reduction in the magnitude as well as duration of pressure increases in the treatment group compared with the control group.

Relaxation in Reducing Blood Lipids and Cigarette Smoking

Friedman et al. [17] have shown that occupational deadlines and increased pressure of work in a group of accountants prior to tax deadlines were associated with a small, but significant, increase in serum cholesterol. They have also shown in a prospective study that in people with an aggressive type A personality there is a higher level of serum cholesterol and higher mortality from CHD [77, 78]. Other investigators have also shown a rise in various blood lipids in association with experimental and other naturally occurring psychosocial stress [85, 86]. If relaxation-based behavioral modification can reduce high BP as well as emotional and occupational stress, it is possible that it may also reduce blood cholesterol and other lipids.

In a pilot study involving 14 hypertensive patients [62], the results over a 6-week period showed a highly significant reduction in mean SBP from 170.6 to 147.9 mm Hg and DBP from 102.5 to 89 mm Hg. The mean cholesterol level in this group of patients was reduced from 241.6 to 217 mg/100 ml (p= < 0.001). 13 out of 14 patients showed some decrease in serum cholesterol. However, this was an uncontrolled study.

In another pilot study [63], four groups of subjects were studied. A normotensive group of 18 subjects acted as control; another normotensive group of 18 subjects was treated by the biofeedback-relaxation-meditation-behavioral modification program; a group of 22 hypertensives and a group of 18 current smokers were similarly treated.

The results showed a significant reduction in BP in all the treated groups with no significant change in the control group. Plasma cholesterol, triglycerides and free fatty acids were reduced significantly in some, but not in all the treated groups, with no change in the control group. In smokers, the number of cigarettes smoked was reduced by 48% at the end of the first week, dropping gradually week by week until an approximate 80% reduction was achieved by the end of a 6-week training period. Obviously, not all the reduction was maintained, but at 6-month follow-up the total number of cigarettes smoked was still 60% less than the original. Most of these smokers wanted to give up smoking and had themselves approached the local antismoking clinic for help. There are dangers in extrapolating results from a volunteer group to the smoking population in general.

Multiple Risk Factor Intervention by Behavior Modification

Having seen fairly convincing evidence that relaxation-based behavioral modification can reduce hypertension, and some indication that it may also reduce serum cholesterol and cigarette smoking, a randomized controlled trial was set up to see if all the major risk factors can be reduced at once in an unselected group of people engaged in full-time jobs [65, 66]. 1,132 employees of a large manufacturing industry between 35 and 64 years of age were screened. Those with two or more risk factors were reexamined. Risk factors were defined as an average of two measurements of BP to be 140/90 or more; serum cholesterol of 6.3 mmol/l or more and current cigarette smoking of 10 or more cigarettes per day. If the person still qualified on the grounds of two or more risk factors at the second examination, he was invited to participate in the study. In a subgroup, a further sample of blood was withdrawn for plasma renin activity (PRA) and plasma aldosterone assays. 204 or 89% of those that qualified consented and were randomly allocated to treatment and control groups.

The groups were comparable at entry to the study. The mean BP in the treatment and control groups were 145/87 and 144/88, respectively, if we include all the subjects, or 160/100 and 160/98, respectively, if only those with an initial BP of 140/90 or more are included (high-risk group). The mean levels of cholesterol were 6.9 and 7.0, respectively. The mean number of cigarettes smoked per day by the smokers were 19 and 20, respectively.

The management for both groups consisted of 10 min of individual counseling about their risk factors and distribution of health education literature on BP, smoking or dietary fats. The treatment group, in addition, followed a behavior modification program consisting of a 1-hour group session once a week for 8 weeks and 3 h of stress-management education. The training was carried out in groups. The subjects were requested to practice relaxation-meditation twice a day as usual. They were further assessed at 8 weeks and again at 8 months.

The results (table I) show significantly greater reduction in SBP and DBP in the treatment group, whether the analysis included the whole group or was confined to the high-risk subgroups with initial pressure of 140/90 or more. These reductions were maintained at 8-month follow-up. Serum cholesterol was significantly lower in both groups at 8 weeks as well as at 8 months ($p = < 0.001$). However, the greater drop in the treatment group was only significant at 8 weeks and was confined to the high-risk subgroup ($p = < 0.025$).

Our dietary analysis showed that the groups were similar at entry in their intake of total calories and animal fats, and that both groups had reduced their intake of saturated fats and increased their intake of polyunsaturated fats. To the degree that the dietary assessment using the Heart Disease Prevention Project questionnaire [76] was accurate and unbiased, the control group had made a slightly greater change in dietary fat intake. Therefore, the greater reduction in serum cholesterol, evident at 8 weeks in the treatment group, is likely to be due to relaxation and not due to dietary changes. Body weight was measured at entry and at each follow-up examination. Despite the reported dietary changes, there was no significant change in either group. It is further evidence that BP and cholesterol differences between the groups were unrelated to dietary or weight changes.

Finally, of the people in the two groups who initially were smokers, 68%

Table I. Reductions in risk factors after 8 weeks and 8 months

Reduction in risk factors	At 8 weeks		At 8 months	
	biofeedback group mean ± SE	control group mean ± SE	biofeedback group mean ± SE	control group mean ± SE
SBP mm Hg				
Whole group	13.8 ± 1.34***	4.0 ± 1.30	15.3 ± 1.55***	6.1 ± 1.56
High-risk group[a]	19.6 ± 2.06	8.2 ± 1.64	22.4 ± 2.39***	11.4 ± 1.87
DBP mm Hg				
Whole group	7.2 ± 0.91***	1.4 ± 0.81	6.8 ± 0.09***	0.63 ± 0.91
High-risk group[a]	10.6 ± 1.40***	3.6 ± 1.10	11.5 ± 1.34***	2.7 ± 1.32
Cigarette smoking % reporting reduced smoking	67.9 ± 5.19***	39.1 ± 6.10	67.5 ± 5.34***	37.5 ± 6.47
Average number of cigarettes/ day less	5.8 ± 0.73**	2.6 ± 0.75	4.8 ± 0.77*	2.3 ± 0.74
Plasma cholesterol, mmol/l				
Whole group	0.71 ± 0.12	0.53 ± 0.11	0.63 ± 0.09	0.57 ± 0.10
High-risk group[b]	0.90 ± 0.12*	0.52 ± 0.12	0.77 ± 0.10	0.56 ± 0.11

[a] Initial BP ≥ 140/90. [b] Initial cholesterol ≥ 6.3 mmol/l. Between group difference significance (two tailed): * $0.01 < p < 0.05$; ** $0.001 < p < 0.01$; *** $p < 0.001$.

in the treatment group claimed to have reduced the number of cigarettes that they smoked per day, compared with 39% in the control group. The mean number of cigarettes consumed fell by six in the treatment group, compared with three in the control group. These differences were statistically significant. At 8 months, the differences between the groups were maintained, and 10% of the treatment group, compared with 5% of the control group, had stopped smoking, althogether. Although these differences were statistically significant, one might have hoped for a greater effect, judging from the results of our pilot study [63].

Plasma renin activity and aldosterone were analyzed in a subsample of 54 subjects. There were significantly greater reductions in both parameters in the treatment group at 8 weeks, but not at 8 months ($p = < 0.05$). There were no correlations between the changes in BP and changes in PRA in either group, but there were significant correlations between changes in aldosterone and changes in both SBP and DBP at 8 weeks. Plasma renin activity is mediated through β-adrenoreceptors, while it is possible that BP was reduced by a central mechanism involving both α- and β-adrenoreceptors as well as hormonal changes.

It was impractical to perform the study blind, when the subjects are expected to change their behaviors consciously. Therefore, attemps were made to standardize the measurements as closely as possible, using a trained nurse to take BP measurements with random-zero sphygmomanometer. This does not eliminate bias completely, but it does reduce it. Smoking was assessed by questionnaire rather than confronting the subjects face-to-face in order to minimize the tendency to please the experimentor. The treatment group may still have exaggerated their reduction. Therefore, caution is in order.

It is unlikely that laboratory measurements of cholesterol, PRA and aldosterone, which were carried out blind, were biased. Therefore, it is most likely that observed BP changes were neither the result of observer bias, nor merely short-term reactions at the time of measurement. However, reduction in biochemical measures were significant at 8 weeks only. This suggests that mechanisms of acute BP reduction might be different from those responsible for long-term reductions. It is a common experience of clinicians that BP control becomes easier with time and that BP of patients on long-term antihypertensive medications may not revert to its original levels for some weeks or months after the medications are stopped. This may be because of some adaptive changes which have been demonstrated in experimental studies [13, 90]. It is possible that a partial reversal of some of the factors responsible for maintaining and perpetuating hypertension and its persistance by limited practice of regular relaxation may be responsible for long-term maintenance of BP reduction.

Implications

Although the hypothesis that psychosocial stress is a causative factor of hypertension is not yet proven, there is enough evidence from the studies carried out so far that it is at least an important risk factor. Assuming that the greater reductions in BP, cigarette smoking and cholesterol achieved in this study would reduce mortality from CHD, we can calculate the potential reduction in mortality using the multiple logistic function from the London Whitehall Study [42]. The figure at 8 weeks is 21% reduction in the predicted risk of CHD death while at 8 months, the figure is 18%, which can be attributed to relaxation only. This may not sound very impressive, but when one considers the fact that subjects in this study had elevations of risk factors too mild to warrant the hazards of pharmacological intervention, and yet serious enough to increase their risk of dying from CHD, the results obtained may not be a mean achievement. It is possible that reduction in risk may occur through paths other than through the conventional risk factors, although it is not possible to estimate its magnitude from the present study. In fact, the results are quite encouraging when comparisons are made with other multiple risk factor intervention studies using conventional methods [12, 68, 76]. The predicted reductions in mortality from CHD in these studies followed up for up to 5-year periods have been estimated at 9–17.4%. The follow-up period in our study has been comparatively short. Therefore, we must remain cautious in making claims. However, there is no reason why relaxation therapy cannot be combined with conventional therapies, so that the future intervention trials not only show large enough differences in mor-bidity and mortality to be detected by the available statistical means, but also make an impressive contribution in eradicating the great burden of mortality from CHD in our communities.

References

1 Blackard, W.G.; Omor, Y.; Freedman, L.R.: The epidemiology of diabetes mellitus in Japan. J. chron. Dis. *18:* 415–427 (1965).

2 Banquet, J.P.: Spectral analysis of the EEG in meditation. Electroenceph. clin. Neuro-physiol. *35:* 143–151 (1973).

3 Breckenridge, A.; Dollery, C.T.; Parry, E.H.: Prognosis of treated hypertension. Q. Jl. Med. *39:* 411–429 (1970).

4 Burch, G.E.: Of jogging. Am. Heart J. *97:* 407 (1979).

5 Willins, F.A.; Keys, T.E. (eds): Cardiac classics (Mosby, St. Louis 1941).

6 Clofibrate: a final verdict. Lancet *ii:* 1131–1132 (1978).

7 Coronary Drug Projet Research Group: Gall bladder disease as a side effect of drugs influencing lipid metabolism. New Engl. J. Med. *296:* 1185–1190 (1977).

8 Dayten, S.; Pearce, M.I.; Hasimoto, S.; Dixon, W.J.; Tomiyasu, U.: A controlled clinical trial of a diet high in unsaturated fat. Circulation *39/40*: suppl. II (1969); Am. Heart Ass. Monogr. 25.

9 Doll, R.; Hill, A.B.: Mortality in relation to smoking: ten years' observation of British doc-tors. Br. med. J. *1:* 1339–1410 (1964).

10 Ederer, F.; Leren, P.; Turpeinen, O.; Frantz, D.: Cancer among men on cholesterol-lower-ing diets: experiments from five clinical trials. Lancet *ii:* 203–206 (1971).

11 Efendic, S.; Cerasi, E.; Luft, R.: Trauma: hormonal factors with special reference to diabetes mellitus. Acta anaesth. scand. suppl. 55, pp. 107–119 (1974).

12 Farquhar, J.W.; MacCoby, N.; Wood, P.D.; Alexander, J.K.; Breitrose, H.; Brown, B.W.; Haskell, W.L.; McAlister, A.L.; Meyer, A.J.; Nash, J.D.; Stern, M.D.: Community education for cardiovascular health. Lancet *i:* 1192–1195 (1977).

13 Folkow, B.; Hallback, M.; Lundgren, Y.; Sivertsson, R.; Weiss, L.: Importance of adaptive changes in vascular design for establishment of primary hypertension studied in man and in spontaneously hypertensive rats. Circulation Res. *32/33:* suppl. i, pp. 1.2–1.16 (1973).

14 French, A.J.; Dock, W.: Fatal coronary arteriosclerosis in young solders. J. Am. med. Ass. *124:* 1233–1237 (1944).

15 Friedman, M.; Rosenman, R.: Type A behaviour and your heart (Knopf, New York 1974).

16 Friedman, M.; Rosenman, R.H.: Association of specific overt behaviour pattern with blood and cardiovascular findings Blood cholesterol level, blood clotting time, incidence of archus senilis and clinical coronary artery disease. J. Am. med. Ass. *169:* 1286–1296 (1959).

17 Friedman, M.; Rosenman, R.H.; Carroll, V.: Changes in the serum cholesterol and blood clotting time in man subjected to cyclic variation of occupational stress. Circulation *1958:* 852–861.

18 Gellhorn, E.; Kiely, W.E.: Mystical states of consciousness: neurological and clinical aspects. J. nerv. ment. Dis. *154:* 399–405 (1972).

19 Gordon, T.: Mortality experience among the Japanese in the United States, Hawaii and Japan. Publ. Hlth Rep. *72:* 543–553 (1957).

20 Gordon, T.: Further mortality experience among Japanese Americans. Publ. Hlth Rep. *1967:* 973–984.

21 Gordon, T.; Garcia-Palmieri, M.R.; Kagan, A.; Kannel, W.B.; Schiffman, J.: Differences in coronary heart disease in Framingham, Honolulu and Puerto Rico. J. chron. Dis. *27:* 329–344 (1974).

22 Gunn, C.G.; Friedman, M.; Byers, S.O.: Effect of chronic hypothalamic stimulation upon cholesterol induced atherosclerosis in rabbits. J. clin. Invest. *39:* 1963 (1960).

23 Guttman, M.C.; Benson, H.: Interaction of environmental factors and systemic arterial blood pressure. Medicine, Baltimore *50:* 543–553 (1971).

24 Hammond, E.C.: Smoking in relation to the death rate of one million men and women. Natn. Cancer Inst. Monogr., No. 19, pp. 127–204 (1966).

25 Hawthorne, V.M.; Greaves, D.A.; Beevers, D.G.: Blood pressure in a Scottish town. Br. med. J. *iii:* 600–603 (1974).

26 Henry, J.P.; Cassel, J.C.: Psycho-social factors in essential hypertension. Recent epidemiological and animal experimental evidence. Am. J. Epidem. *90:* 171–200 (1969).

27 Henry, J.P.; Stephens, P.M.: Stress, health and the social environment. A sociobiologic approach to medicine (Springer, Berlin 1977).

28 Hess, W.R.: In Hughes, Functional organisation of diencephalon (Grune & Stratton, New York 1957).

29 Hodes, R.: Electroencephalographic synchronisation resulting from reduced proprioceptive drive caused by neuromuscular blocking agents. Electroenceph. clin. Neurophysiol. *14:* 220–232 (1962).

30 Hypertension Detection and Follow-up Program: Co-operative Group five-year findings of the hypertension detection and follow-up program. 1. Reduction in mortality of persons with high blood pressure, including mild hypertension. J. Am. med. Ass. *242:* 2562–2571 (1979).

31   Intersociety Commission for Heart Disease Resources: primary prevention of the atherosclerotic diseases. Circulation *42:* suppl. II, pp. A55–A95 (1970).

32   Kahn, H.A.: The Dorn Study of Smoking and Mortality among US Veterans: Report on 8½ years of observation. Natn. Cancer Inst. Monogr., No. 19, pp. 1–125 (1966).

33   Kaplan, B.H.; Cassel, J.C.; Tyroler, H.A.; Cornoni, J.C.; Kleinbaum, D.G.; Hames, C.G.: Occupational mobility and coronary heart disease. Archs intern. Med. *128:* 936–942 (1971).

34   Keen, H.; Rose, G.A.; Pyke, D.A.; Boyns, D.; Chlouverakis, C.; Mistoy, S.: Blood sugar and arterial disease. Lancet *ii:* 505–508 (1965).

35   Kemple, C.: Rorschach method and psychosomatic diagnosis. Psychosom. Med. *7:* 85–89 (1945).

36   Keys, A.: Coronary heart disease in seven countries. Circulation *41/42:* suppl. I (1970).

37   Laren, P.: The effect of plasma lowering diet in male survivors of myocardial infarction Acta med. scand. suppl. 466, pp. 5–92 (1962).

38   Lind, A.R.; Taylor, S.H.; Humphreys, P.W.; Kennelly, B.M.; Donald, K.W.: The circulatory effects of sustained voluntary muscle contraction. Clin. Sci. *27:* 229–244 (1964).

39   Magoun, H.W. (ed.): The waking brain; 2nd ed. (Thomas, Springfield 1963).

40   Management Committee: The Australian therapeutic trial in mild hypertension. Lancet *i:* 1261–1267 (1980).

41   Marmot, M.G.: Epidemiological basis for the prevention of coronary heart disease Bull. WHO *57:* 331–347 (1979).

42   Marmot, M.G.; Rose, G.; Shipley, M.; Hamilton, P.J.S.: Employment grade and coronary heart disease in British Civil Servants. J. Epidem. Community Hlth *32:* 244–249 (1978).

43   Marmot, M.G.; Syme, S.L.: Acculturation and coronary heart disease in Japanese-Americans. Am. J. Epidem. *104:* 225–246 (1976).

44   Marmot, M.G.; Syme, S.L.; Kagan, A.; Kato, H.; Cohen, J.B.; Belsky, J.: Epidemiologic studies of coronary heart disease and stroke in Japanese men living in Japan, Hawaii and California: prevalence of coronary and hypertensive heart disease and associated risk factors. Am. J. Epidem. *102:* 514–525 (1975).

45   Medalie, J.H.; Kahn, H.A.; Neufeld, H.N.; Riss, E.; Goldbourt, U.: Myocardial infarction over a five-year period. I. Prevalence incidence and mortality experience. J. chron. Dis. *26:* 63–83 (1973).

46   Medalie, J.H.; Kahn, H.A.; Neufeld, H.N.; Riss, E.; Goldbourt, U.: Five-year myocardial infarction incidence. II. Association of single variables to age and birthplace. J. chron. Dis. *26:* 329–349 (1973).

47   Miettinen, M.; Turpeinen, O.; Karvonen, M.J.; Elosuo, R.; Paavilainen, E.: Effect of cholesterol-lowering diet on mortality from coronary heart disease and other causes. Lancet *ii:* 835–838 (1972).

48   Moritz, A.R.; Zamcheck, N.: Sudden and unexpected deaths of young soldiers: diseases responsible for such deaths during World War II. Archs Path. *42:* 459 (1946).

49   Morris, J.N.; Everitt, M.G.; Polland, R.; Chave, S.P.W.; Semmence, A.M.: Vigorous exercise in leisure time: protection against coronary heart disease. Lancet *1:* 1207–1210 (1980).

50   Morris, J.N.; Heady, J.A.; Raffle, P.A.B.; Roberts, C.G.; Parks, J.W.: Coronary heart disease and physical activity of work. Lancet *ii:* 1053–1057 (1953).

51   Morris, J.N.; Kagan, A.; Pattison, D.C.; Gardner, M.J.; Raffle, P.A.B.: Incidence and prediction of ischaemic heart disease in London busmen, Lancet *ii:* 553–559 (1966).

52   Noakes, T.D.; Opie, L.H.; Rose, A.G.; Kleynhans, P.H.; Schepers, N.J.; Dowdeswell, R.:

Autopsy proved coronary atherosclerosis in marathon runners. New Engl. J. Med. *301:* 86–89 (1979).

53 Nixon, P.: Human function curve with special reference to cardiovascular disorders. Part I. Practitioner *217:* 765–770 (1976).

54 Opie, L.H.: Sudden death and sport. Lancet *i:* 263–266 (1975).

55 Osler, W.: The Lumlein lectures on angina pectoris. Lancet *i:* 839–844 (1910).

56 Ostrander, L.D., Jr.; Francis, T., Jr.; Hayner, N.S.; Kjelsberg, M.O.; Epstein, F.H.: The relationship of cardiovascular disease to hyperglycaemia. Ann. intern. Med. *62:* 1188–1198 (1965).

57 Patel, C.H.: Yoga and biofeedback in the management of hypertension. Lancet *ii:* 1053–1055 (1973).

58 Patel, C.: 12-month follow-up of yoga and biofeedback in the management of hypertension. Lancet *i:* 62–65 (1975).

59 Patel, C.: Yoga and biofeedback in the management of 'stress' in hypertensive patients. Clin. Sci. mol. Med. *48:* suppl., pp. 171s–174s (1975). Proc. 3rd Symp. of the Int. Society of Hypertension, Milan 1974 (Blackwell, Oxford 1975).

60 Patel, C.H.; North, W.R.S.: Randomised controlled trial of yoga and biofeedback in the management of hypertension. Lancet *ii:* 93–95 (1975).

61 Patel, C.: Biofeedback-aided behavioral methods in the management of hypertension; MD thesis, London (1976).

62 Patel, C.: Reduction of serum cholesterol and blood pressure in hypertensive patients by behaviour modification. J. R. Coll. gen. Pract. *26:* 211–215 (1976).

63 Patel, C.; Carruthers, M.: Coronary risk factor reduction through biofeedback-aided relaxation and meditation. J. R. Coll. gen. Pract. *27:* 401–405 (1977).

64 Patel, C.H.: Biofeedback-aided relaxation and meditation in the management of hypertension. Biofeedback Self-Regul. *2:* 1–41 (1977).

65 Patel, C.; Marmot, M.M.; Terry, D.J.: Controlled trial of biofeedback-aided behavioral methods in reducing mild hypertension. Br. med. J. (in press).

66 Patel, C.H.; Marmot, M.M.; Terry, D.J.; Carruthers, M.; Sever, P.: Coronary risk factor reduction through biofeedback-aided relaxation and meditation. Proc. 52nd Annu. Scientific Meet. of the American Heart Association, Anaheim 1979, Part II. Circulation *60:* Abstract 882, pp. II–226 (1979).

67 The Pooling Project Research Group: Relationship of blood pressure, serum cholesterol, smoking habits, relative weight and ECG abnormalities to incidence of major coronary events: final report of the Pooling Project. J. chron. Dis. *31:* 201 (1978).

68 Puska, P.; Tuomilehto, J.; Salonen, J.; Neitaanmaki, L.; Maki, J.; Virtamo, J.; Nissinen, A.; Koskela, K.; Takalo, T.: Changes in coronary risk factors during comprehensive five-year community programme to control cardiovascular disease (North Karelia Project). Br. med. J. *ii:* 1173–1178 (1979).

69 Ratcliffe, H.L.; Cronin, M.T.I.: Changing frequency of arteriosclerosis in mammals and birds at Philadelphia Zoological Gardens. Review of Autopsy Records. Circulation *18:* 41 (1958).

70 Report of the Committee of Principal Investigators: A co-operative trial in the primary prevention of ischaemic heart disease using clofibrate. Br. Heart J. *40:* 1069–1118 (1978).

71 Research Committee: Low fat diet in myocardial infarction: a controlled trial. Lancet *iii:* 501–504 (1965).

72 Research Committee: Controlled trial of soya-bean oil in myocardial infarction. Lancet *ii:* 693–700 (1968).

73 Rochmis, P.; Blackburn, H.: Exercise tests. A survey of procedures, safety and litigation experience in approximately 170,000 tests. J. Am. med. Ass. *217:* 1061–1066 (1971).

74 Rose, G.: Coronary heart disease: check the 'healthy' patient. Mod. Med. *21:* 6–11 (1976).

75 Rose, G.; Hamilton, P.J.: A randomised controlled trial of the effect of middle-aged men of advice to stop smoking. J. Epidem. Community Hlth *32:* 275–281 (1978).

76 Rose, G.; Heller, R.F.; Pedoe, H.T.; Christie, D.G.S.: Heart disease prevent project: a randomised controlled trial in industry. Br. med. J. *1980:* 1747–1751.

77 Rosenman, R.H.; Brand, R.J.; Jenkins, C.D.; Friedman, M.; Straus, R.; Wurm, M.: Coronary heart disease in Western Collaborative Group Study: Final follow-up of 8½ years. J. Am. med. Ass. *233:* 872 (1975).

78 Rosenman, R.H.; Friedman, M.; Straus, R.; Jenkins, C.D.; Zyzanski, S.J.; Wurm, M.: Coronary heart disease in the Western Collaborative Group Study: a follow-up experience of 4½ years. J. chron. Dis. *23:* 173–190 (1970).

79 Russek, H.I.; Russek, L.G.: Behaviour patterns and emotional stress in the etiology of coronary heart disease: sociological and occupational aspects; in Wheatly, Stress and the hart, pp. 51–32 (Raven Press, New York 1977).

80 Russek, H.I.; Zohman, B.L.: Relative significance of heredity, diet and occupational stress in coronary heart disease of young adults. Am. J. med. Sci. *235:* 266–277 (1958).

81 Salonen, J.T.; Puska, P.; Mustaniemi, H.: Changes in morbidity and mortality during comprehensive community programme to control cardiovascular diseases during 1972–7 in North Karelia. Br. med. J. *ii:* 1178–1183 (1979).

82 Stewart, I. McD. G.: Relation of reduction in pressure to first myocardial infarction in patients receiving treatment for severe hypertension. Lancet *i:* 861–865 (1979).

83 Syme, S.L.; Borhani, N.O.; Buechley, R.W.: Cultural mobility and coronary heart disease in an urban area. Am. J. Epidem. *82:* 334–336 (1965).

84 Syme, S.L.; Hyman, M.M.; Enterline, P.E.: Some social and cultural factors associated with the occurrence of coronary heart disease. J. chron. Dis. *17:* 277–289 (1964).

85 Taggart, P.; Carruthers, M.: Endogenous hyperlipidaemia induced by emotional stress of racing driving. Lancet *i:* 363–366 (1971).

86 Thomas, C.B.; Murphy, E.A.: Further studies on cholesterol levels in the John Hopkins Medical Students. The effect of stress at examinations. J. chron. Dis. *8:* 661 (1958).

87 University Group Diabetes Program: A study of the effects of hypoglycaemic agents on vascular complications in patients with adult-onset diabetes. VI. Supplementary report on non-fatal events in patients treated with tolbutamide. Diabetes *25:* 1129–1153 (1976).

88 Valkonen, T.; Niemi, M.L.: Decline of mortality from cardiovascular disease in North Karelia. Br. med. J. *i:* 46 (1980).

89 Yater, W.M.; Traum, A.H.; Spring, S.; Brown, W.G.; Fitzgerald, R.P.; Geisler, M.A.; Wilcox, B.B.: Coronary artery disease in men 18 to 39 years of age: report of 866 cases, 450 with necropsy examinations. Am. Heart J. *36:* 334 (1948).

90 Vaughan Williams, E.M.; Hassan, M.O.; Floras, J.S.; Sleight, P.; Jones, V.J.: Adaptation of hypertensives to treatment with cardioselective and non-selective beta-blockers. Absence of correlation between bradycardia and blood pressure control and reduction in slope of QT/RR relation. Br. Heart J. *44:* 437–487 (1980).

91 Veterans Administrations Co-operative Study Group on Antihypertensive Agents: Effects

of treatment on morbidity in hypertension. II. Results in patients with diastolic blood pressure averaging 90 through 114 mm Hg. J. Am. med. Ass. *213:* 1143–1152 (1970).

92 Veterans Administration Co-operative Study Group on Antihypertensive Agents: Effects of treatment on morbidity in hypertension. Results in patients with diastolic blood pressures averaging 115 through 129 mm Hg. J. Am. med. Ass. *202:* 1028–1034 (1967).

93 Wallace, R.K.; Benson, H.: The physiology of meditation. Sci. Am. *226:* 84–90 (1972).

94 Wilhelmsson, C.; Vedin, J.A.; Emfeldt, D.; Tibblin, G.; Wilhelmsen, L.: Smoking and myocardial infarction. Lancet *i:* 415–420 (1975).

95 Wolf, S.G.: Cardiovascular reactions to symbolid stimuli. Circulation *18:* 287–292 (1958).

96 Wolpe, J.: Psychotherapy be reciprocal inhibition (Stanford University Press, Stanford 1958).

97 Worth, R.M.; Kato, M.; Rhoads, G.; Kagan, A.; Syme, S.L.: Epidemiologic studies of coronary heart disease and stroke in Japanese men living in Japan, Hawaii and California: mortality. Am. J. Epidem. *102:* 481–490 (1975).

98 World Health Organisation: European Collaborative Group. An International Controlled trial in the multifactorial prevention of coronary heart disease. Int. J. Epidem. *3:* 219–224 (1974).

99 World Health Statistics Annuals 1978, vol. 1 (World Health Organisation, Geneva 1978).

100 Wright, B.M.; Dore, C.F.: A random-zero sphygmomanometer. Lancet *i:* 337–338 (1970).

25 The Relaxation Response: Physiologic Basis, History, and Clinical Usefulness[1]

Herbert Benson

Considerable emphasis has been placed upon the relationship between behavioral factors and the development of coronary artery disease. There is, however, the opposite potential: behavioral processes may lead to the alleviation and reversal of some of the predisposing features of this illness. I shall present evidence that specific behaviors and thought patterns are associated with the elicitation of an innate physiologic capacity: the relaxation response and shall discuss the history of this response, its physiologic basis, clinical usefulness, use in prevention, and our most recent findings concerning the underlying mechanism of its actions.

In the past decade, there has been a growing interest in nonpharmacologic, self-induced altered states of consciousness because of the alleged benefits of better mental and physical health and an increased ability to deal with tension and stress. Many believe that altered states of consciousness represent a normal and natural human desire [7]. Indeed, mood-altering by man has been historically documented in many cultures throughout the world. One such altered state of consciousness has been attained through practices such as meditative prayer, found in virtually all religions, through cultic meditational techniques such as transcendental meditation (TM) and yoga, as well as through secular practices such as autogenic therapy and hypnosis [2, 4].

Despite the diversity of these practices, there appears to be a common denominator. Subjective and objective data exist which support the hypothesis that a physiologic response, termed the *relaxation response,* underlies an altered state of consciousness [4]. The elicitation of the relaxation response results in physiologic changes which are thought to characterize an integrated hypothalamic response [33, 34]. These physiologic changes are consistent with generalized decreased sympathetic nervous system activity. Uniform and significant decreases have been observed in oxygen consumption and carbon dioxide elimination with no change in respiratory quotient. In addi-

[1] Supported in part by Grants HL-22727 and HL-07374 from the National Institutes of Health, United States Public Health Service.

tion, there is a simultaneous lowering of heart rate (HR) and respiratory rate and a marked decrease in arterial blood lactate concentration. The electro-encephalogram shows intensification of slow alpha-wave activity with occasional theta waves. The physiologic changes of the relaxation response are distinctly different from those observed during quiet sitting or sleep and characterize a wakeful, hypometabolic state.

Physiologic changes similar to those constituting the relaxation response were initially termed the *trophotropic response* by *Hess* [15]. He electrically stimulated one hypothalamic area of the cat brain and induced physiologic changes like those later noted during the elicitation of the relaxation response in man. These physiologic changes are opposite to those of a response originally described by *Cannon* [8] in 1914, which he termed the emergency reaction – popularly called the *fight-or-flight response*. The physiology of the fight-or-flight response, correspondingly, consists of generalized increased sympathetic nervous system activity and includes increased catecholamine production with associated increases in blood pressure (BP), HR and respiratory rate, and skeletal muscle blood flow [1, 8]. The relaxation response appears to be a basic bodily response that may have significance in countering overactivity of the sympathetic nervous system in man and other animals [15].

The Subjective Experience

Many of the subjective experiences associated with the elicitation of the relaxation response constitute an altered state of consciousness. These subjective experiences have been described as peace of mind, feeling at ease with the world, and a sense of well-being. Other descriptions have been of an ecstatic, clairvoyant, beautiful, and totally relaxing experience [10].

The concept of altered states of consciousness, in general, has been somewhat unacceptable to Western man. As *Ornstein* [24] asserts, the Western 'impersonal, objective scientific approach, with its exclusive emphasis on logic and analysis, makes it difficult for most of us even to conceive of a psychology which could be based on the existence of another intuitive gestalt mode of thought'. The ultimate aim of practices or techniques used to attain this state has varied – union with God, transcendence from the physical, an inner awareness of one's self. This is not to be interpreted as viewing religion or philosophy in a mechanistic manner, since the purpose of any of these exercises corresponds to the philosophy or religion in which it is used.

Moreover, no one technique can claim uniqueness. *James* [18] expresses this view: 'To find religion is only one out of many ways of reaching unity; and the process of remedying inner discord is a general psychological process.'

Despite the diversity of descriptions of these experiences, however, striking similarities between the techniques used to achieve this altered state strongly suggest the existence of a common physiologic basis, which is hypothesized to be the relaxation response. Further, it appears that this altered state of consciousness has been experienced by man throughout all ages in both Eastern and Western cultures. Four elements seem to be integral to these varied practices and are necessary to evoke the relaxation response: a quiet environment; decreased muscle tone; a mental device, i.e. a sound, word, or phrase repeated silently or audibly; and a passive attitude.

Meditative practices that may bring forth the relaxation response have been an important part of Indian culture for thousands of years. Age-old practices of yoga strive for 'union' of the self with a supreme being or principle. Yogic meditation often involves concentration on a single point to exclude all thoughts that are associated with everyday life [4, 12]. Yoga has evolved into techniques that often place more emphasis upon the physical aspects of achieving an altered state of consciousness. Essential to these forms of yoga are appropriate posture to enhance concentration and regulation of respiration [2, 4].

One of the meditative practices of Zen Buddhism, Zazen, employs a yogic technique of coupling respiration with counting to ten – one on inhaling, two on exhaling, and so on. With time, one stops counting and simply 'follows the breath' [19] in order to achieve a state of no thought, no feeling, to be completely 'in nothing' [17]. Similar experiences have been described in many other Eastern practices, including the Japanese and Chinese religions of Shintoism and Toaism, and Sufism, an Islamic mystical tradition.

In the East, these meditational techniques, which are hypothesized to elicit the relaxation response, were extensively developed and became a major element in religion and everyday life. In the Western world, however, practice of various meditative techniques that are thought to bring forth the relaxation response was limited primarily to religious traditions. Many Christian writers, including St. *Augustine* and *Martin Luther,* wrote descriptions of prayers, often called contemplative exercises, which could be used to transcend the mundane world in order to realize a union with God. One example is the following set of instructions given by *Gregory of Sinai* in the 14th century for the 'Prayer of the Heart', or 'The Prayer of Jesus', a repetitive prayer of early Christian origin:

> 'Sit down alone and in silence. Lower your head, shut your eyes, breathe out gently, and imagine yourself looking into your own heart. Carry your mind, i.e. your thoughts, from your head to your heart. As you breathe out, say: "Lord Jesus Christ, have mercy on me." Say it moving your lips gently, or simply say it in your mind. Try to put all other thoughts aside. Be calm, be patient and repeat the process very frequently' [13].

In the Judaic literature one also finds portrayals of contemplative or meditative exercises. Again, the ultimate purpose is union with God. One of the early forms of mysticism in Judaism is Merkabolism, which dates back to approximately the 1st century BC. The meditative exercises of Merkabolism included placing one's head between one's knees, whispering hymns, and repeating the name of a magic emblem. Repetition of the magic emblem would chase away distractions and cause the 'demons and hostile angels to flight' [29].

Meditative practices may also be found outside of a religious context, and many descriptions of transcendental experiences appear in the secular literature. *Tennyson* experienced visions of ecstasy that were the foundation of his deepest beliefs of the 'unity of all things, the reality of the unseen, and the persistence of life' [30]. For him, transcendence was achieved through the repetition of his own name!

Throughout history many techniques or practices that are similar in nature have been used to achieve an altered state of consciousness. It is proposed that the relaxation response underlies many of the subjective experiences of this altered state. The recently documented physiologic effects of these various practices reflect the commonality of these experiences and thus of the relaxation response.

A Simple Noncultic Technique

Incorporating the four elements common to a multitude of historical techniques, a simple noncultic technique was developed in our laboratory. Use of the technique results in the same physiologic changes that our laboratory first noted using TM as a model. The instructions for this noncultic technique are the following:

(1) Sit quietly in a comfortable position and close your eyes. (2) Deeply relax all your muscles, beginning at your feet and progressing up to your face. Keep them deeply relaxed. (3) Breathe through your nose. Become aware of your breathing. As you breathe out, say the word *one* silently to yourself. For example, breathe in... out, *one;* in... out, *one,* etc. Continue for 20 min. You may open your eyes to check the time, but do not use an alarm. When you finish, sit quietly for several minutes at first with closed eyes and later with opened eyes. (4) Do not worry about whether you are successful in achieving a deep level of relaxation. Maintain a passive attitude and permit relaxation to occur at its own pace. Expect other thoughts. When these distracting thoughts occur, ignore them by thinking 'Oh well' and continue repeating *'one'*. With practice, the response should come with little effort. Practice the technique once or twice daily, but not within 2 h after any meal, since the digestive processes seem to interfere with the subjective changes.

Clinical Usefulness

Humans, like other animals, react in a predictable way to stressful situations [14]. When we are faced with situations that require behavioral adjustment, and involuntary response, the fight-or-flight response, is activated. It is associated with increased sympathetic nervous system activity and thus with increases in BP, HR, respiratory rate, skeletal muscle blood flow, and metabolism, preparing, speaking teleologically, for conflict or escape. The continual stresses of contemporary living, however, have led to the excessive elicitation of the fight-or-flight response. Further, within the constructs of our society, the behavioral features of this response, running or fighting, are often inappropriate. Indeed, the excessive and inappropriate arousal of the fight-or-flight response with its corresponding sympathetic nervous system activation may have a role in the pathogenesis and exacerbation of several disorders. Regular elicitation of the relaxation response may be of preventive and therapeutic value in diseases in which increased sympathetic nervous system activity is implicated.

Several longitudinal investigations have demonstrated that the regular elicitation of the relaxation response lowers BP in both pharmacologically treated and untreated hypertensive patients [5, 6, 9, 25, 26, 31]. In an early investigation done by our laboratory, would-be initiates of TM, who were also hypertensive, volunteered to participate in the study [5, 6]. Baseline measurements of BP were taken weekly for approximately 6 weeks, after which the subjects were taught to bring forth the relaxation response through the practice of TM. Of the 36 patients included in the study, 22 received no medication during the investigation and 14 remained on unaltered antihypertensive medications during both the control and experimental periods. In the 22 nonmedicated subjects, control BP averaging 146.5 mm Hg systolic and 94.6 mm Hg diastolic decreased significantly to 139.5 mm Hg systolic ($p < 0.001$) and 90.8 mm Hg diastolic ($p < 0.002$) after the regular elicitation of the relaxation response through the practice of TM. In the 14 patients who maintained constant antihypertensive medications, mean control BP of 145.6 mm Hg systolic and 91.9 mm Hg diastolic dropped significantly to 135.0 mm Hg systolic ($p < 0.01$) and 87.0 mm Hg diastolic ($p < 0.05$) post-intervention.

Several other researchers report similar findings. *Datey* et al. [9] noted decreases in both systolic BP (SBP) and diastolic BP (DBP) in 47 hypertensive patients who evoked the relaxation response through the practice of another yogic technique, called *shavasan*. In this study, subjects served as their own controls. Information regarding the length of the preintervention control period and the number of control BP measurements made, however, was not reported.

In two well-controlled longitudinal investigations, *Patel* [25, 26] combined yogic relaxation with biofeedback techniques in the treatment of 20 patients with hypertension. The average SBP in these subjects was reduced by 20.4 ± 11.4 mm Hg, while mean DBP was reduced by 14.2 ± 7.5 mm Hg ($p < 0.001$). A hypertensive control group matched for age and sex was employed. Length of testing sessions, number of attendances, and the procedure for measuring the BP of the control group were identical to those of the treatment group. Control patients were not given instruction in the relaxation technique, however, but simply were asked to rest on a couch. No significant changes in BP occurred in the control group.

Further substantiation of the usefulness of the relaxation response in the treatment of hypertension has come from *Stone and DeLeo* [31], who obtained significant decreases in SBP and DBP using a Buddhist meditation exercise. The control group, which received no psychotherapeutic intervention, was matched for BP, age, and race, and exhibited virtually no change in SBP and DBP.

Another example to the clinical usefulness of the relaxation response is that of reducing the number of premature ventricular contractions (PVC) [3]. Participating in a study were 11 nonmedicated ambulatory patients who had proven ischemic heart disease of at least 1 year's duration, with documented relatively stable PVC. Frequent PVC are correlated with an increases mortality in such patients [11, 32]. The frequency of the PVC was measured over 48 consecutive hours, after which the subject was taught to elicit the relaxation response by using the noncultic technique described above. After 4 weeks of regularly practicing the relaxation technique and recording their frequency of practice, the patients returned to repeat the 2 days of monitoring.

A reduced frequency of PVC was observed in 8 of the 11 patients. Before the intervention, the PVC per hour per patient for the total group had averaged 151.5 for the entire monitoring session. 4 weeks after the intervention was instituted, the average PVC per hour per patient dropped to 131.7. The reduction of PVC was even more marked during sleep. Initially, the number of PVC per hour per patient during sleeping hours averaged 125.5, while after 4 weeks of regular elicitation of the relaxation response, the PVC during sleep decreased to 87.9 ($p < 0.05$). When the PVC were expressed per 1,000 heart beats per patient for the entire group, there was a significant decrease during sleeping hours from 29.0 to 21.1 ($p < 0.05$).

The results suggest that the regular elicitation of the relaxation response with its hypothesized decreased sympathetic nervous system activity may have been the mechanism by which PVC were reduced. This finding is consistent with that of *Lown* et al. [21] who, in a recent case study, reported that a patient was able to abolish his arrhythmias by meditation. These results were attributed to lessened sympathetic tone [22], although others [35] implicate increased parasympathetic activity as a mechanism for the reduction of PVC.

Usefulness in Prevention

An experiment conducted at the corporate offices of a manufacturing firm investigated the effects of daily relaxation breaks on five self-reported measures of health, performance, and well-being [27]. For 12 weeks, 126 volunteers filled out daily records and returned bi-weekly for additional measurements. After 4 weeks of baseline monitoring, they were divided randomly into three groups: group A was taught a technique for producing the relaxation response; group B was instructed to sit quietly; group C received no instructions. Groups A and B were asked to take two 15-min relaxation breaks daily. After an 8-week experimental period, the greatest mean improvements on every index occurred in group A; the least improvements occurred in group C; group B was intermediate. Differences between the mean changes in groups A vs C reached statistical significance ($p < 0.05$) on four of the five indices: symptoms, illness days, performance, and sociability-satisfaction. Improvements on the happiness-unhappiness index were not significantly different among the three groups. The relationship between amount of change and rate of practicing the relaxation response was different for the different indices. While less than three practice periods per week produced little change on any index, two daily sessions appeared to be more practice than was necessary for many individuals to achieve positive changes. Somatic symptoms and performance responded with less practice of the relaxation response than did behavioral symptoms and measures of well-being.

During the baseline period, mean SBP were 119.7, 118.4, and 114.2 for groups A, B, and C, respectively; mean DBP were 78.7, 76.8, and 75.7 [28]. Between the first and last measurements, mean changes in SBP were −11.6, −6.5 and +0.4 mm Hg in groups A, B, and C; mean DBP decreased by 7.9, 3.1, and 0.3. Between the 4-week baseline period and last 4 weeks of the experimental period, mean SBP decreased by 6.7, 2.6, and 0.5; while mean DBP decreased by 5.2, 2.0 and 1.2. For both SBP and DBP, mean changes in group A were significantly greater than those in group B ($p < 0.05$) and in group C ($p < 0.001$). The same pattern of changes among the three groups was exhibited by both sexes, all ages, and at all initial levels of BP. However, in general, within group A, the higher the initial BP, the greater the decrease. Thus, BP within the 'normal' range was significantly lowered after regular elicitation of the relaxation response. This lowered BP might ultimately prevent the development of subsequent hypertension.

Recent Findings

Although the physiologic changes of the relaxation response are consistent with decreased sympathetic nervous system activity, the direct measurement of plasma norepinephrine during its elicitation did not reveal significant decreases in the concentration of this hormone [23]. Indeed, some have found increased levels of plasma norepinephrine in subjects who regularly elicit the relaxation response [20].

Our most recent physiologic data resolve this apparent paradox of unchanged or increased plasma norepinephrine levels associated with the elicitation of the relaxation response [16]. Sympathetic nervous system reactivity was assessed in 10 experimental and 9 control subjects who were exposed to graded orthostatic and isometric stress on monthly hospital visits. Between visits, experimental subjects practiced a technique that elicited the relaxation response, whereas control subjects sat quietly for an equivalent time. HR and BP reactions to the graded stresses did not differ between visits in either group. However, in the experimental group, the levels of plasma norepinephrine corresponding to graded stresses were significantly augmented after the elicitation of the relaxation response. No changes in plasma norepinephrine levels were noted in the control group. After completion of this phase, these results were then replicated in the control group in a crossover experiment. That is, HR and BP responses were unchanged, but plasma norepinephrine levels were significantly higher after this group crossed over and elicited the relaxation response. Hence, the repeated elicitation of the relaxation response resulted in greater sympathetic nervous system reactivity that was not reflected in larger HR and BP responses. These observations are most consistent with reduced norepinephrine end-organ responsivity.

Conclusions

Although emphasis has been placed on the processes by which mind and behavioral processes lead to disease states, we should be aware of the beneficial, healthful aspects of other thought processes. Specific behaviors and thought patterns elicit the innate physiologic changes termed the relaxation response. The relaxation response appears to be a valuable adjunct to our current therapies, and it may also be useful as a preventive measure. This response can be elicited by nonreligious or noncultic techniques or by other methods, which a patient may prefer. A religious patient, for example, may select meditative prayer as the most appropriate method for bringing forth the relaxation response. The freedom to choose a technique that conforms to a patient's personal beliefs should enhance compliance. Elicitation of the relaxation response is a simple and natural phenomenon; it does not require complex equipment for monitoring of physiologic events or involve the expense and side effects of drugs.

References

1   Abrahams, V.C.; Hilton, S.M.; Zbrozyna, A.W.: Active muscle vasodilatation produced by stimulation of the brain stem: its significance in the defense reaction. J. Physiol., Lond. *154:* 491–513 (1960).
2   Benson, H.: The relaxation response (Morrow, New York 1975).
3   Benson, H.; Alexander, S.; Feldman, C.L.: Decreased premature ventricular contractions through use of the relaxation response in patients with stable ischemic heart disease. Lancet *ii:* 380–382 (1975).

4   Benson, H.; Beary, J.F.; Carol, M.P.: The relaxation response. Psychiatry *37:* 37–46 (1974).
5   Benson, H.; Rosner, B.A.; Marzetta, B.R.; Klemchuk, H.M.: Decreased blood pressure in borderline hypertensive subjects who practiced meditation. J. chron. Dis. *27:* 163–169 (1974).
6   Benson, H.; Rosner, B.A.; Marzetta, B.R.; Klemchuk, H.M.: Decreased blood pressure in pharmacologically treated hypertensive patients who regularly elicited the relaxation response. Lancet *i:* 289–291 (1974).
7   Brecher, E.M. and editors of *Consumer Reports:* Licit and illicit drugs (Consumers Union, New York 1972).
8   Cannon, W.B.: The emergency function of the adrenal medulla in pain and the major emotions. Am. J. Physiol. *33:* 356–372 (1914).
9   Datey, K.K.; Deshmukh, S.N.; Dalvi, C.P.; Vinekar, S.L.: 'Shavasan': a yogic exercise in the management of hypertension. Angiology *20:* 325–333 (1969).
10   Dean, S.R.: Is there an ultraconscious beyond the unconscious? Can. psychiat. Ass. J. *15:* 57–61 (1970).
11   Desai, D.; Hershberg, P.I.; Alexander, S.: Clinical significance of ventricular premature beats in an out-patient population. Chest *64:* 564 (1973).
12   Eliade, M.: Yoga: immortality and freedom; translation by W.R. Trask (Routledge & Kegan Paul, London 1958).
13   French, R.M. (translator): The way of a pilgrim (Seabury Press, New York 1968).
14   Gutmann, M.C.; Benson, H.: Interaction of environmental factors and systemic arterial blood pressure: a review. Medicine, Baltimore *50:* 543–553 (1971).
15   Hess, W.R.: The functional organization of the diencephalon (Grune & Stratton, New York 1957).
16   Hoffman, J.W.; Arns, P.A.; Stainbrook, G.L.; Landsberg, L.; Young, J.B.; Gill, A.; Benson, H.: Altered sympathetic nervous system reactivity with the relaxation response. Clin. Res. *29:* 207A (1981).
17   Ishiguro, H.: The scientific truth of Zen (Zenrigaku Society, Tokyo 1964).
18   James, W.: The varieties of religious experience (New American Library, New York 1958).
19   Johnston, W.: Christian Zen (Harper & Row, London 1971).
20   Lang, R.; Dehof, K.; Meurer, K.A.; Kaufmann, W.: Sympathetic activity and transcendental meditation. J. neural Transm. *44:* 117–135 (1979).
21   Lown, B.; Temte, J.V.; Reich, P.; Gaughan, C.; Regenstein Q.; Hai, H.: Basis for recurring ventricular fibrillation in the absence of coronary heart disease and its management. New Engl. J. Med. *294:* 623–629 (1976).
22   Lown, B.; Tykocinski, M.; Garfein, A.; Brooks, P.: Sleep and ventricular premature beats. Circulation *48:* 691 (1973).
23   Michaels, R.R.; Haber, M.J.; McCann, D.S.: Evaluation of transcendental meditation as a method of reducing stress. Science *192:* 1242–1244 (1976).
24   Ornstein, R.E.: The psychology of consciousness (Freeman, San Francisco 1972).
25   Patel, C.H.: Yoga and biofeedback in the management of hypertension. Lancet *ii:* 1053–1055 (1973).
26   Patel, C.H.: Twelve-month follow-up of yoga and biofeedback in the management of hypertension. Lancet *i:* 62–64 (1975).
27   Peters, R.K.; Benson, H.; Porter, D.: Daily relaxation response breaks in a working population. I. Effects on self-reported measures of health, performance, and well-being. Am. J. publ. Hlth *67:* 946–953 (1977).

28   Peters, R.K.; Benson, H.; Peters, J.M.: Daily relaxation response breaks in a working population. II. Effects on blood pressure. Am. J. publ. Hlth *67:* 954–959 (1977).

29   Scholem, G.G.: Jewish mysticism (Schocken Books, New York 1967).

30   Spurgeon, C.F.E.: Mysticism in English literature (Kennikat Press, Port Washington 1970).

31   Stone, R.A.; DeLeo, J.: Psychotherapeutic control of hypertension. New Engl. J. Med. *294:* 80–84 (1976).

32   Tominaga, S.; Blackburn, H., and the Coronary Drug Project Research Group: Prognostic importance of premature beats following myocardial infarction. J. Am. med. Ass. *223:* 1116 (1973).

33   Wallace, R.K.; Benson, H.: The physiology of meditation. Sci. Am. *226:* 84–90 (1972).

34   Wallace, R.K.; Benson, H.; Wilson, A.F.: A wakeful hypometabolic physiologic state. Am. J. Physiol. *221:* 795–799 (1971).

35   Weiss, T.; Lattin, G.W.; Engelman, K.: Vagally mediated suppression of premature ventricular contractions in man. Am. Heart J. *89:* 700 (1975).

26 Assessment and Alteration of Physiological Reactivity

Bernard T. Engel

Two major theoretical models about the nature of the organization of physiological responses have existed for many years. These models have considerable relevance for students of type A behavior. The models are important for two reasons: First, because the research findings are important in understanding how autonomic reactivity patterns are organized. Since many investigators believe that the mechanisms by which type A behavior mediates ischemic heart disease operate, in part, through these autonomic response patterns, it is imperative that they be understood clearly. The second reason that these models are important is that it is possible that the statistical model developed by psychophysiologists to characterize autonomic response patterns may also be useful in characterizing other behavior patterns such as those which have been used to define type A behavior.

One of the psychophysiological models is based on so-called activation theory [3, 17]. This theory proposes that there exists a generalized state of physiological arousal ranging from sleep or unconsciousness at one extreme, to excitement or agitation at the other extreme. The alternative model proposes that this continuum does not exist; rather, there are consistent and reliable individual differences in response disposition [5]. Individual responses are organized and patterned: they are determined in part by the eliciting stimulus, and in part by the responding subject. Thus, the responses show both stimulus and individual specificity.

Activation Theory

Activation theories have a long history in physiology. They derive in large measure from conceptual models about the way the autonomic nervous system is organized. Although an extensive analysis of this history is beyond the scope of this paper, a few landmarks are worth noting – the interested reader is referred to *Kuntz* [16] or *Pick* [20] for more detailed reviews. *Johnstone*, the English anatomist, writing in the 18th century, characterized what we call today the sympathetic ganglia as filters. According to him these filters intercepted the will and rendered the motions of the viscera involuntary. Furthermore, these same filters intercepted the sensory inputs from the visceral organs and kept their information from consciousness. *Bichat*, writing 50 years later, argued that the ganglia comprised an autonomous nervous system which was isolated from the brain and spinal cord. His student, *Reil*, correctly identified the white rami as fibres connecting the cord to the ganglia. However, he reasoned that all impulses were carried from the cord to the periphery – that there was not afferent feedback. By the middle of the 19th century *Remak* had corrected *Reil's* error; but he concluded that the communication links between the sympathetic nervous system and the central nervous system were limited to spinal reflexes. By the end of the 19th century and beginning of the 20th century *Gaskell* and *Langley* had developed the modern concept of the autonomic nervous system: they recognized clearly that there were connections between the peripheral autonomic nervous system and the central nervous system, and that these connections not only occurred at the spinal level, but extended into the brain. Having made this discovery, *Langley* then came to the extraordinary conclusion that the visceral, afferent fibres were not part of the autonomic nervous system. Thus, *Langley* defined the autonomic nervous system as a purely motor system. Subsequently, *Cannon* [2] allowed visceral afferent information back into the autonomic nervous system. However, by ascribing consciousness to the cortex, by assigning the highest order projections of the autonomic nervous system to the hypothalamus, and by defining emotion as a release of hypothalamic outflow from cortical inhibition, *Cannon* [2] managed to preserve the remarkable fiction that autonomic responses are non-selective. His conception of the all-or-none character of autonomic reactivity is most vividly expressed in his characterization of the role of the autonomic nervous system in behavior. He believed that the integrity of the autonomic nervous system was essential in the maintenance of survival, and he ascribed to it a primary role as the driving force underlying the basic biological behavior patterns of fight or flight. According to *Cannon* [2], when the cortex perceived the existence of danger, it released the sympathetic nervous system from inhibition. This release from cortical inhibition led to an all-or-none discharge of the sympathetic nervous system, the magnitude of which was determined by the degree and duration of the cortical disinhibition. The all-or-none character of autonomic activity is, of course, a synonym for activation theory.

Another manifestation of activation theory can be found in *Gellhorn's* [10] notion of autonomic tuning: he believed that the balance of the autonomic nervous system was altered ('tuned') by stimulation. Like *Cannon* [2], *Gellhorn* [10] believed that tuning was a property of the brain and that peripheral autonomic responses were reflexive. Contemporary theories about autonomic function clearly reflect this activation point of view. One still can find such phrases as 'massive sympathetic discharge' invoked as a mechanism to characterize the impact of 'stress' on various organisms including man. One still can find frequent references to one or another index used to characterize this massive discharge. The index varies from one report to another, e.g. for some it is electrodermal activity, for others heart rate (HR), blood flow or blood pressure (BP), and for others it is plasma or urinary norepinephrine. It should be clear that no matter how sophisticated the index is, it can be justified only if autonomic reactivity is undifferentiated, and only if autonomically mediated responses are non-specific motor expressions of central neural events.

Specificity Theory

The specificity model has its roots in psychosomatic theories which related specific diseases to specific emotions [1]. This theory has largely been discredited, primarily because the psychoanalytic basis for linking specific, affective, verbal reports with specific diseases has been refuted. However, the experimental evidence of patterning among peripheral autonomic responses remains. The definition of specificity is complex because the concept of specificity recognizes two forms of specificity: stimulus-response (SR) specificity and individual response (IR) specificity. Furthermore, two related features of specificity have been studied, uniqueness and consistency [5, 8]. SR specificity is defined as the tendency for a stimulus to evoke characteristic responses from a group of subjects: SR consistency is defined as the tendency for a single stimulus to elicit a consistent hierarchy of responses from a group of subjects; SR uniqueness is defined as the tendency for different stimuli to elicit different responses from a single group of subjects (table I). Table IIA lists a few examples of concepts which are related to the concept of stimulus specificity. For example, the utility of the notion that stimuli can be emotion-provoking derives from the assumption that it is possible to distinguish among stimuli in terms of their capacities to elicit differentiable responses. If activation theory were true, the only differences one could see among responses elicited by different stimuli would be differences in degree. Stressors are purported to exist because it has been assumed generally that a stim-

Table I. Necessary conditions for demonstrating response specificities

	Subjects	Stimuli	Responses
A. Stimulus specificities			
1 Uniqueness	single group	> 1	≥ 1
2 Consistency	single group	1	> 1
B. Individual specificity			
1 Uniqueness	> 1 group	1	≥ 1
2 Consistency	1	> 1	> 1

Table II. Response specificities and their related concepts

A. Stimulus specificity
  1 Uniqueness
    (a) Stimulus discrimination
    (b) Emotion-provoking stimuli
    (c) In general, any concepts which assert that different stimuli evoke different responses from a group of subjects
  2 Consistency
    (a) Nomothetic traits
    (b) Stressor
    (c) In general, any concepts which assert that a single stimulus evokes similar responses from a group of subjects

B. Individual specificity
  1 Uniqueness
    (a) Organ specificity
    (b) Symptom specificity
    (c) In general, any concepts which assert that one class of subjects responds differently to a single stimulus than does another class
  2 Consistency
    (a) Personality type
    (b) Idiographic trait
    (c) In general, any concepts that assert that a subject emits a consistent pattern of responses irrespective of the stimulus

ulus (qua stressor) will elicit consistent response patterns from all subjects – i.e. a stressor has a property which enables it to override individual differences. Clearly, stimulus consistency is compatible with the activation theoretical formulation.

IR specificity is defined as the tendency for an individual to emit characteristic responses to a group of stimuli: IR consistency is defined as the ten-

dency for a subject to emit a consistent hierarchy of responses to a set of stimuli [6, 7a, 9]; IR uniqueness is defined as the tendency for one group of subjects to respond differently to a given stimulus than does another group of
subjects. A diagnostic test is a striking example of a stimulus which elicits
individual uniqueness. Individual consistency is an interesting concept for
several reasons. First is that it enables one to characterize a single individual
across a range of situations (stimuli); second is that it enables one to characterize not merely a single, idiosyncratic response tendency but also an entire
pattern of responses; finally, individual consistency is a useful concept
because it permits one to characterize not only the pattern of an individual's
responses across situations, but also because it permits one to quantify a particular response as one in which the individual is hyperactive. This last fact
is particularly interesting because it often is the case that the hyperactivity
is pathognomonic [6, 7a, 18, 19]. Specificity research findings are that autonomic response patterns are not all-or-none. Rather, they are highly organized and show both IR and SR specificity. Clearly, the existence of IR specificity is a refutation of the activation theoretical position, at least in its most
simplistic form [21].

There are other lines of evidence which greatly weaken the usefulness
of the activation concept. Perhaps the most relevant to the purposes of this
topic is the evolution of the concept of 'central command' in autonomic
neurophysiology. A number of experimental studies have shown conclusively that complex patterns of autonomic response are organized in the brain
and that these patterns are based on functional considerations, and not on
all-or-none principles or on sympathetic-parasympathetic dichotomies [4,
12, 14]. Furthermore, it is now clear that these central command patterns are
subject to voluntary control [11, 13a]. *Goodwin* et al. [11] have shown that it
is possible to obtain the cardiovascular adjustments to exercise from cooperative subjects even when there is no muscle movement but only an 'intent' to
act. *Eldridge* et al. [4] in an elegant set of experiments showed that direct electrical stimulation of the subthalamic nucleus can elicit the cardiovascular,
pulmonary, and motor components of locomotion in cats which were de-
corticated, had their vagus nerves and sinus nerves cut, and were curarized.
Thus, they were able to show that the peripheral expression of locomotion occurred even though the major afferent pathways for eliciting cardiovascular
or pulmonary responses were sectioned, and the motor behavior (which
could be recorded from the biceps femoris nerves) was blocked pharmacologically. *Joseph and Engel* [13a] trained monkeys to slow and speed HR;
when they stimulated areas of the brain which elicited tachycardia and

pressor responses, they found that the monkeys could consistently overcome the effect of the imperative brain stimulation when they were voluntarily slowing their hearts, but that this effect was not present either when the animal was voluntarily speeding or when it was in a control condition. Also interesting was their finding that the slowing effect was largely limited to HR; BP rose consistently whether HR fell or rose.

Thus, the evidence for a high degree of specificity within the autonomic system is strong. It can be seen in studies in man and in animals; it can be seen in terms of patterned responses to external stimulation and it can be seen in terms of patterned, elicited, central neural responses. These data clearly limit the generality of activation theories. Furthermore, they have profound implications for studies which attempt to assess physiological response patterns in special classes of patients such as those who manifest type A behavior. The data on IR specificity show that individuals emit idiosyncratic physiological response patterns. Although there are only a few studies which have related IR specificity to disease, the findings from them indicate clearly that in many patients there is a correlation between the physiological function in which the patient shows his maximal reactivity and the sign or symptom which characterizes his medical problem. *Malmo and Shagass* [18] showed that patients with head or neck complaints reacted relatively more in muscles from these regions than did patients with cardiac complaints, and that the cardiac complainers reacted more in HR than did the head and neck complainers. *Engel and Bickford* [7a] showed that hypertensive patients relative to normotensive controls were pressor reactors; and furthermore, that the hypertensives emitted response patterns which were more consistent than were the patterns of the normotensive controls.

Response Specificity and Type A Behavior

Usefulness of the Analytic Model
The statistical model used to analyze SR or IR specificity permits one to quantify the degree of consistency that a stimulus elicits or that an individual emits. Furthermore, it permits one to characterize the particular response which is maximally evoked by a stimulus or emitted by a subject. Since behavior pattern A is made up of a set of measurable and specifiable behaviors, and since there are now known to be important individual differences in the dominant behavior [13, 14a], it would be useful to be able to characterize individuals across situations and across behavioral indices. It

would be especially useful to characterize these people both physiologically and behaviorally. Such characterizations would enable one to subclassify individuals on the basis of these two response profiles. It might be possible that one or another behavior tendency interacts especially strongly with one or another autonomic tendency. Clearly there is a great need to characterize more precisely those persons who are most likely to develop coronary artery disease, and to isolate some of the mechanisms which might mediate that process.

Earlier it was noted that the usefulness of specific indices of autonomic function are rational within the framework of activation theory. However, their utility is poor if specificity is true. One needs to demonstrate the validity of his index. In those cases where there is focal reactivity – e.g. hypertensive patients show a strong tendency to be pressor hyperreactors – then the response in which the subject overreacts should be identified and monitored. Otherwise, if one chose his index incorrectly, he could be badly misled. If the index were inappropriately chosen, one could come to the erroneous conclusion that the subjects either did not differ from controls or that they were hyporeactors. The problem with global indices is different, but equally serious. If one were to measure catecholamine responses, he probably would have a valid index of total sympathetic nervous activity. However, he would have no knowledge of the role of the parasympathetic nervous system in the subject's response, nor would he know how the increase in sympathetic activity was mediated – i.e. whether the major source of the norepinephrine release came from vascular, cardiac or other visceral sympathetic fibers, or which compartment within the response system was the major contributor to the total catecholamine response.

Relevance to Intervention Programs

The *Engel and Bickford* [7a] findings showed that hypertensive patients tend to be pressor reactors. These data suggest that if one intervenes in these patients so as to attenuate their pressor responses, he also will reduce their BP levels. In a series of studies [7b, 7c, 10a, 15] we have shown that it is possible to train these patients to control – i.e. to raise or to lower their BP – and that it is possible to achieve clinically significant reductions in BP using these procedures.

The problems in treating coronary-prone patients are much more complicated. There already is evidence that the attributes which comprise type A behavior are present in different people to different degrees [13, 14a]. Therefore, before one can begin to consider a behavioral intervention, he must know with which behavior he is to intervene. Likewise, there may be physiological IR specificity among these patients, and one must know which physiological response is salient for a given patient since that response will become a major outcome measure in assessing the effectiveness of the intervention. This last point is especially important since it may be that the need for intervention – namely the risk of coronary heart disease – is present primarily in those patients who show a particular response pattern.

References

1   Alexander, F.: Psychosomatic medicine, its principles and applications (Norton, New York 1950).
2   Cannon, W.B.: Bodily changes in pain, hunger, fear and rage; 2nd ed. (Appleton, New York 1929).
3   Duffy, E.: Activation; in Greenfield, Sternbach, Handbook of psychophysiology (Holt, Rinehart & Winston, New York 1972).
4   Eldridge, F.L.; Millhorn, D.E.; Waldrop, T.G.: Exercise hyperpnea and locomotion: parallel activation from the hypothalamus. Science *211:* 844–846 (1980).
5   Engel, B.T.: Response specificity; in Greenfield, Sternbach, Handbook of psychophysiology (Holt, Rinehart & Winston, New York 1972).
6   Engel, B.T.: Stimulus-response and individual-response specificity. Archs gen. Psychiat. *2:* 305–313 (1960).
7a Engel, B.T.; Bickford, A.F.: Response specificity: Stimulus-response and individual-response specificity in essential hypertensives. Archs gen. Psychiat. *5:* 478–489 (1961).
7b Engel, B.T.; Gaarder, K.R.; Glasgow, M.S.: Behavioral treatment of high blood pressure. I. Analyses of infra- and intradaily variations of blood pressure during a one-month baseline period. Psychosom. Med. *43:* 255–270 (1981).
7c Engel, B.T.; Glasgow, M.S.; Gaarder, K.R.: Behavioral treatment of high blood pressure. III. Follow-up results and treatment recommendations. Psychosom. Med. (in press).
8   Engel, B.T.; Moos, R.H.: The generality of specificity. Archs gen. Psychiat. *16:* 574–582 (1967).
9   Fahrenberg, J.; Walschburger, P.; Foerster, F.; Myrtek, M.; Muller, W.: Psychophysiologische Aktivierungsforschung. Ein Beitrag zu den Grundlagen der multivariaten Emotions- und Stress-Theorie (Psychologisches Institut, Forschungsgruppe Psychophysiologie, Munich 1979).
10 Gellhorn, E.: Autonomic balance and the hypothalamus (University of Minnesota, Minneapolis 1957).
10a Glasgow, M.S.; Engel, B.T.; Gaarder, K.R.: Behavioral treatment of high blood pressure. II. Acute and sustained effects of relaxation and systolic blood pressure biofeedback. Psychosom. Med. *44:* 155–170 (1982).
11 Goodwin, W.M.; McCloskey, D.I.; Mitchell, J.H.: Cardiovascular and respiratory responses to changes in central command during isometric exercise at constant muscle tension. J. Physiol., Lond. *226:* 173–190 (1972).

12   Hilton, S.M.; Speyer, K.M.: Central nervous regulation of vascular resistance. A. Rev. Physiol. *42:* 399–411 (1980).

13   Jenkins, C.D.: Coronary prone behavior. Primary Cardiol. *April:* 63–72 (1981).

13a   Joseph, J.A.; Engel, B.T.: Instrumental control of cardioacceleration induced by central electrical stimulation. Science *214:* 341–343 (1981).

14   Korner, P.I.: Central nervous control of autonomic cardiovascular function; in Berne, Geiger, Handbook of physiology. The cardiovascular system. I (Waverly Press, Baltimore 1979).

14a   Krantz, D.S.; Glass, D.D.; Schaffer, M.A.; Davia, J.E.: Behavior patterns and coronary disease: A critical evaluation; in Cacioppo, Petty, Perspectives in cardiovascular psychophysiology (Guilford Press, New York 1982).

15   Kristt, D.A.; Engel, B.T.: Learned control of blood pressure in patients with high blood pressure. Circulation *51:* 370–378 (1975).

16   Kuntz, A.: The autonomic nervous system; 3rd ed. (Lea & Febiger, Philadelphia 1945).

17   Lindsley, D.B.: Emotion; in Stevens, Handbook of experimental psychology (Wiley & Sons, New York 1951).

18   Malmo, R.B.; Shagass, C.: Physiologic study of symptom mechanisms in psychiatric patients under stress. Psychosom. Med. *11:* 25–29 (1949).

19   Malmo, R.B.; Shagass, C.; Davis, F.H.: Symptom specificity and bodily reactions during psychiatric interview. Psychosom. Med. *12:* 362–376 (1950).

20   Pick, J.: The autonomic nervous system (Lippincott, Philadelphia 1970).

21   Roessler, R.; Engel, B.T.: The current status of the concepts of physiological response specificity and activation. Int. J. psychiat. Med. *5:* 359–366 (1974).

27 Psychosocial Variables in Relation with Coronary Risk Status Modification

M. Kornitzer, F. Kittel, M. Dramaix, G. De Backer

Psychosocial variables have been studied for different reasons: (1) to find clues to the etiology of coronary heart disease (CHD); (2) to evaluate their relationship to coronary risk factors or the coronary risk profile, and (3) to evaluate their relationship to the modification of coronary risk factors in the setting of prevention projects. This last point is the purpose of this paper, as psychosocial variables have indeed been registered at the entry examination of the Belgian Heart Disease Prevention Project, which is part of the WHO European Collaborative Trial [3].

Material and Methods

The methods and techniques used in the Belgian Heart Disease Prevention Project have been described elsewhere [1], and will only be summarized here. 30 factories were paired off, according to type of industry, and one member of each pair was randomly allocated to the intervention group, with the other serving as a control. 19,390 male subjects 40- to 59-year-old were listed. 83.7% of those took part in the baseline examination. In the intervention group, all subjects were initially screened for risk factors: systolic blood pressure (SBP), body mass index, relative weight, serum cholesterol, and smoking habits. The examination also included questions on social factors, such as marital status, socioprofessional class, educational level and geographic location in Belgium. In connection with the last point, it should be recalled that Belgium includes a Dutch-speaking community in the North (Campine in the North-east and Flanders in the North-west), a French-speaking community in the South (Wallonia), while the capital, Brussels, is composed of a bilingual population. All subjects answered psychological questionnaires such as the SH-EPI [2], on the basis of which scores were calculated for various items: anality (A), obsessionality (B), neuroticism (N), extroversion (E), and social conformism (L). They also received the Jenkins Activity Survey (JAS), a self-administered questionnaire version of the structured interview of *Rosenman and Friedman*, in order to assess type A pattern. Four scores were derived from the JAS: type A pattern or JAS-AB, a score of 'speed and impatience' or JAS-S, one of 'job involvement' or JAS-J, and one of 'hard-driving' or JAS-H.

In the control group, 10% of the subjects in each occupational unit were randomly selected to undergo the same thorough initial examination as all the subjects in the intervention group; the other 90% were subjected only to an ECG at rest. For all the subjects in the intervention group, and for the 10% of the control group that underwent the same thorough initial examinations, risk profiles were established on the basis of the initial results, according to a 'risk score' (table I). The subjects who belonged to the top 21% of the risk score distribution were arbitrarily placed in the high-risk group, and the others in the lower-risk group.

Table I. Belgian Heart Disease Prevention Project: calculation of coronary risk score

Factor	Points to be added to score						
	0	½	1	1½	2	2½	3
Age, years	< 50		50 +				
Job activity	heavy		light		sedentary		
Cigarettes/day	< 5		5 –		20 +		
Systolic blood pressure, mm Hg	< 120		120 –		140 –		160 +
Serum cholesterol, mg/dl	< 210	210 –	220 –	230 –	240 –	250 –	260 +

Intervention Program

The high-risk subjects in the intervention group were given individual counseling twice a year during the first 2 years and annually thereafter, by two physicians in the project. At the start of the project, these subjects were given written information concerning their particular risk factors and they all benefited from the mass counseling program (posters regularly displayed on factory premises, antismoking talks and dietary advice to the factory canteen staff).

The lower-risk group received literature on particular risk factors and benefited from the mass campaign. 1 out of 4 received, at one occasion, individual counseling. The low-risk and high-risk groups could be differentiated in that the former received the intervention program essentially through the mass media whereas the latter received it by individualized counseling.

The subjects' family doctors and the occupational physicians received regular information about the risk factors of each individual, and they played an important part in the intervention program.

The purpose of the program was to lower the following risk factors: serum cholesterol, cigarette smoking, hypertension, obesity and sedentary habit.

Serum Cholesterol. All of the subjects were considered at risk. Individual advice or literature was given concerning the reduction of total fat intake and of dietary cholesterol and the partial replacement of saturated by polyunsaturated fats.

Cigarette Smoking. Subjects who smoked five or more cigarettes a day were encouraged to quit.

Hypertension. Subjects with a mean SBP (mean of four readings on the same day) of 160 mm Hg or more were given preventive advice – to lose weight if they were obese, not to add salt to prepared foods, and to consult their family doctors, who should consider drug prescription. These doctors had already received information and instructions on the treatment of hypertension, with emphasis on the importance of regular follow-up and continuous treatment.

Final Examination

For two thirds of the factories, the final examination took place 6 years after the initial one, whereas for one third it took place 5.5 years after the start of the project. All subjects still at work

Table II. Belgian Heart Disease Prevention Project: intervention group. Incidence of smoking habits in those who smoked cigarettes at baseline – final screening

	Low-risk group % (n = 2,025)		High-risk group % (n = 721)	
Ex-cigarette smokers – actual non-smokers	14.9	19.9	15.4	25.2
Ex-cigarette smokers – actual pipe and/or cigar smokers	5.0		9.8	
Actual cigarette smokers	80.1		74.8	
Decreasing	23.5		34.3	
Stable or increasing	76.5		65.7	

were invited for the final screening and 70% responded favorably. 4,759 subjects of the intervention group participated in the final examination, 3,768 of which were initially low-risk and 919 high-risk subjects.

Hereafter, we will present the relationship between psychosocial variables and prevalence and modification of two major coronary risk factors: cigarette smoking and serum cholesterol.

Ex-Smokers. (a) Prevalence: subjects who were ex-cigarette smokers at entry, whether they were cigar and/or pipe smokers or not. (b) Incidence: subjects who were cigarette smokers at entry and reported, at the final screening, having stopped, whether they switched to cigar and/or pipe or not.

Serum Cholesterol. (a) Prevalence: value at base-line screening. (b) Modification or Δ cholesterol: end-screening cholesterol minus baseline cholesterol, hence a negative value meaning a decrease of serum cholesterol between initial and final screening.

Results

Smoking Habits

In the low-risk group, 19.9% of initial cigarette smokers had stopped, 14.9% of them completely, whereas 5.0% switched to pipe and/or cigar. In the high-risk group, 25.2% had stopped at the time of the final examination, 15.4% of them completely, whereas 9.8% were still smoking cigar and/or pipe (table II). Six sociocultural variables showed a significant relationship with the prevalence of ex-smokers in the low-risk group at baseline. They were older, of a higher socioprofessional and educational level, more often married, speaking French and located in the Southern part of Belgium (table III).

At the final screening, the status of those who had become ex-smokers was somewhat related to age: 28.4% of subjects initially aged 55–59 had stopped as compared to 20% of those aged 40–44. Again, significantly more

Table III. Belgian Heart Disease Prevention Project: intervention group. Smoking habits – ex-cigarette smokers

Sociocultural variables	Low-risk group				High-risk group			
	baseline[1] (n = 3,784)		final screening[2] (n = 2,025)		baseline[1] (n = 939)		final screening[2] (n = 721)	
	%	p	%	p	%	p	%	p
Age								
40–44	19.6		20.0		6.2		22.4	
45–49	21.7	< 0.0001	18.5	< 0.09	5.1	< 0.0008	27.2	n.s.
50–54	26.1		19.7		12.1		24.6	
55–59	29.3		28.4		15.3		27.8	
Social class								
Executives	31.2		22.1		11.9		25.8	
White-collar	24.2	< 0.0001	22.4	n.s.	13.8	< 0.001	23.7	n.s.
Blue-collar	20.6		19.1		6.2		25.8	
Study level								
Primary	20.2		18.8		5.9		23.1	
Secondary	25.4	< 0.0001	21.8	n.s.	13.7	< 0.0006	27.0	n.s.
University	36.4		19.4		10.2		22.0	
Marital status								
Married	22.8	< 0.02	20.8	< 0.01	9.6	n.s.	25.3	n.s.
Alone[3]	16.2		11.2		4.5		25.0	
Language								
Dutch	21.5	< 0.0004	19.9	n.s.	8.6	n.s.	25.3	n.s.
French	30.0		20.5		13.8		25.0	
Geographic region								
Campine	19.8		20.5		5.4		28.2	
Flanders	24.1	< 0.002	20.1	n.s.	11.6	< 0.001	22.0	n.s.
Brussels	23.9		18.8		15.7		24.1	
Wallonia	29.4		13.5		5.9		28.2	

[1] Prevalence. [2] 6-year incidence. [3] Bachelors, widowers, divorced.

married subjects reported being ex-smokers at the final examination compared to subjects qualified as 'alone' (bachelors, widowers or divorced, table III).

For the high-risk group, a similar relationship was observed for all six sociocultural variables with the prevalence of ex-smokers at baseline, even though this relationship was significant for only four variables: age, social

Table IV. Belgian Heart Disease Prevention Project: intervention group. Smoking habits – ex-cigarette smokers

Psycholog- ical and behavioral variables	Median	Low-risk group				High-risk group			
		baseline[1] (n = 3,784)		final screening[2] (n = 2,025)		baseline[1] (n = 939)		final screening[2] (n = 721)	
		%	p	%	p	%	p	%	p
JAS									
AB	<	19.9	< 0.001	19.2	n.s.	6.7	< 0.02	26.3	n.s.
	≥	25.5		21.4		11.8		25.2	
S	<	19.7	< 0.0001	20.4	n.s.	7.7	n.s.	26.9	n.s.
	≥	25.6		20.1		11.0		24.7	
J	<	21.1	< 0.03	19.0	n.s.	10.3	n.s.	26.5	n.s.
	≥	24.2		21.5		8.8		25.1	
H	<	21.6	n.s.	20.3	n.s.	9.8	n.s.	24.4	n.s.
	≥	31.0		18.7		8.1		32.7	
SH-EPI									
A score	<	24.4	n.s.	19.3	n.s.	9.8	n.s.	23.7	n.s.
	≥	23.4		19.0		10.3		27.1	
B score	<	20.3	< 0.0001	19.9	n.s.	9.8	n.s.	27.7	n.s.
	≥	26.2		20.4		10.3		25.7	
N score	<	20.2	< 0.0004	18.9	n.s.	7.6	n.s.	26.2	n.s.
	≥	25.6		21.4		11.0		26.4	
E score	<	25.9	< 0.0001	22.6	< 0.02	9.5	n.s.	27.7	n.s.
	≥	19.4		18.0		9.0		22.9	
L score	<	24.6		19.4	n.s.	9.0	n.s.	27.5	n.s.
	≥	20.4		20.3		9.5		23.0	

[1] Prevalence. [2] 6-year incidence.

class, study level, and geographic region. For the latter, no specific geographic gradient was observed; subjects living in or around Brussels showed the highest ex-smokers' rate. None of the sociocultural variables showed a significant correlation with the incidence of ex-smokers' status (table III).

Nine psychological variables were dichotomized at the median. Except for JAS-H (Hard-driving), score A (anality), and score L (social conformity) all variables showed a significant correlation with the prevalence of ex-smokers in the low-risk group: subjects scoring high on JAS-AB (type A direction), JAS-S (speed and impatience), JAS-J (job-involved), score B (obsessionality), and score N (neuroticism) were significantly more often ex-smokers. The

Table V. Belgian Heart Disease Prevention Project: intervention group. Smoking habits (ex-smokers) – multiple stepwise discriminant function analysis in the low-risk group

Sociocultural variables	Retrospective (n = 2,818) prevalence, p	Sociocultural variables	Prospective (n = 1,892) incidence, p
Study level (primary, secondary, university)	< 0.001	Marital status (married, alone)[1]	< 0.01
Age (40–44, 45–49, 50–54, 55–59)	< 0.001		
Geographic region (Campine, Flanders, Brussels, Wallonia)	< 0.001		
Social class (executives, white-collar, blue-collar)[1]	< 0.001		
n.s.: Marital status		n.s.: Age, social class, study level, geographic region, language	
Prediction of ex-smokers: 50.5%		Prediction of ex-smokers: 58.6%	
Prediction of smokers: 64.2%		Prediction of smokers: 48.9%	

[1] Negatively related to the other variables.

same holds true for those scoring low on score E (extroversion) and L (social conformism) (table IV). Except for the low scores on the extroversion scale, not one single variable showed a significant correlation with the incidence of ex-smokers' status. Only JAS-AB was significantly related to ex-smokers' status at entry in the high-risk group. However, for incidence of ex-smokers, no relation with any psychological or behavioral variable could be observed in univariate analysis (table IV).

In a multiple stepwise discriminant analysis for low-risk subjects including five sociocultural variables, four variables came out as significant discriminators of the prevalence of ex-smokers versus all other smoking categories: study level, age groups, geographic region and socioprofessional class. Marital status was the only significant discriminator for the incidence of low-risk ex-smokers (table V).

When psychological variables are added, introvertion, JAS-S and neuroticism turn out as significant discriminators for the prevalence of ex-smokers, whereas, for incidence, only marital status and introversion discriminate between ex-smokers and other smoking categories (table VI).

In the high-risk group, age and study level are significant discriminators for prevalence of ex-smokers, whereas no variable is significantly related to

Table VI. Belgian Heart Disease Prevention Project: intervention group. Smoking habits (ex-smokers) – multiple stepwise discriminant function analysis in the low-risk group

Sociocultural and psychological variables	Retrospective (n = 2,157) prevalence, p	Sociocultural and psychological variables	Prospective (n = 1,736) incidence, p
E score [1]	< 0.0001	E score [1]	< 0.05
JAS-S	< 0.0001		
Study level (primary, secondary, university)	< 0.001	Marital status (married, alone)	< 0.01
N score	< 0.001		
Geographic region (Campine, Flanders, Brussels, Wallonia)	< 0.01		
Age (40–44, 45–49, 50–54, 55–59)	< 0.05		

n.s.: Marital status, social-class, JAS-AB, JAS-J, JAS-H, A score, B score, L score		n.s.: Age, language, geographic region, social class, study level, marital status, JAS-AB, JAS-S, JAS-J, JAS-H, A score, B score, N score, L score
Prediction of ex-smokers: 54.6%		Prediction of ex-smokers: 55.9%
Prediction of smokers: 62.7%		Prediction of smokers: 59.6%

[1] Negatively related to the other variables.

Table VII. Belgian Heart Disease Prevention Project: intervention group. Smoking habits (ex-smokers) – multiple stepwise discriminant function analysis in the high-risk group

Sociocultural variables	Retrospective (n = 827) prevalence, p	Sociocultural variables	Prospective (n = 672) incidence
Age (40–44, 45–49, 50–54, 55–59)	< 0.001	No variable entered	
Study level (primary, secondary, university)	< 0.01		

n.s.: Social class, geographic region, marital status, language		
Prediction of ex-smokers: 69%		Prediction of ex-smokers: –
Prediction of smokers: 62.3%		Prediction of smokers: –

Table VIII. Belgian Heart Disease Prevention Project: intervention group. Smoking habits (ex-smokers) – multiple stepwise discriminant function analysis in the high-risk group

Sociocultural and psychological variables	Retrospective (n = 606) prevalence, p	Sociocultural and psychological variables	Prospective (n = 545) incidence
Age (40–44, 45–49, 50–54, 55–59)	< 0.001	All variables: n.s.	
Study level (primary, secondary, university)	< 0.001		
JAS-J[1]	< 0.05		
Social class (executives, white-collar, blue-collar)[1]	< 0.05		

n.s.: Language, geographic region, marital status, JAS-AB, JAS-S, JAS-H, A score, B score, E score, L score

Prediction of ex-smokers: 68.0%	Prediction of ex-smokers: 52.2%
Prediction of smokers: 67.5%	Prediction of smokers: 56.3%

[1] Negatively related to the other variables.

incidence of ex-smokers when five sociocultural variables are introduced (table VII). When the JAS and SH-EPI scores are also introduced, JAS-J (job involvement) score came out as being a significant discriminator for the prevalence of ex-smokers. Again, no single variable appeared to be a significant predictor of ex-smokers' status (table VIII).

Comments. Most of the correlations between sociocultural and psychological variables, and prevalence of ex-smokers in low-risk subjects disappeared when incidence of ex-smokers was examined. Three correlations with prevalence remained: age, marital status, and scale of extroversion. It seems that 'soft' intervention techniques directed at the low-risk subjects by means of mass media were able to wipe out initial socioprofessional education or cultural differences in ex-smokers' rate, whereas they had no effect on age differences, nor on those differences due to marital status. For the high-risk group, the picture is quite different. Whereas four sociocultural and one psychological (JAS-AB) variables were related to baseline ex-smokers' status, none showed any significant correlation with the incidence of ex-smokers'

Table IX. Belgian Heart Disease Prevention Project: intervention group. Final screening – serum cholesterol (mg/dl)

Sociocultural variables	Low-risk group		High-risk group	
	baseline (n = 3,818)	Δ cholesterol[1] (n = 3,768)	baseline (n = 941)	Δ cholesterol[1] (n = 919)
	p	p	p	p
Age				
40–44	222 ⎫	2.6 ⎫	266 ⎫	−15.0 ⎫
45–49	224 ⎬ < 0.05	0.9 ⎬ < 0.05	267 ⎬ < 0.01	−16.8 ⎬ < 0.01
50–54	221 ⎪	3.6 ⎪	262 ⎪	−13.8 ⎪
55–59	224 ⎭	6.1 ⎭	258 ⎭	− 6.4 ⎭
Social class				
Executives	230 ⎫	2.4 ⎫	264 ⎫	−12.1 ⎫
White-collar	223 ⎬ < 0.001	2.8 ⎬ n.s.	261 ⎬ n.s.	−10.8 ⎬ < 0.06
Blue-collar	222 ⎭	2.7 ⎭	265 ⎭	−15.7 ⎭
Study level				
Primary	222 ⎫	2.6 ⎫	264 ⎫	−14.1 ⎫
Secondary	225 ⎬ < 0.01	2.3 ⎬ n.s.	265 ⎬ n.s.	−13.7 ⎬ n.s.
University	230 ⎭	−0.6 ⎭	263 ⎭	− 9.1 ⎭
Marital status				
Married	223 ⎫ n.s.	2.3 ⎫ n.s.	263 ⎫ n.s.	−13.6 ⎫ n.s.
Alone	221 ⎭	4.7 ⎭	267 ⎭	−15.2 ⎭
Language				
Dutch	221 ⎫ < 0.0001	2.9 ⎫ < 0.01	262 ⎫ < 0.001	−13.7 ⎫ n.s.
French	241 ⎭	−2.3 ⎭	271 ⎭	−13.7 ⎭
Geographic region				
Campine	217 ⎫	2.6 ⎫	262 ⎫	−16.4 ⎫
Flanders	225 ⎬ < 0.0001	3.2 ⎬ < 0.01	262 ⎬ < 0.001	−11.8 ⎬ n.s.
Brussels	232 ⎪	2.5 ⎪	271 ⎪	−12.0 ⎪
Wallonia	241 ⎭	−4.9 ⎭	273 ⎭	−11.6 ⎭

[1] Δ Cholesterol = final cholesterol – baseline cholesterol.

rate. It seems, that face-to-face counseling had a major impact on sociocultural differences with respect to ex-smokers' status. Our physicians equally influenced smoking habits of blue-collars and executives, married subjects and those living 'alone', and French-and Dutch-speaking Belgians. Bridging those sociocultural differences seems to us a major achievement.

Table X. Belgian Heart Disease Prevention Project: intervention group. Final screening – serum cholesterol (mg/dl)

Psychological and behavioral variables	Median	Low-risk group				High-risk group			
		baseline (n = 3,818)	p	Δ cholesterol (n = 3,768)	p	baseline (n = 941)	p	Δ cholesterol (n = 919)	p
JAS									
AB	<	223	n.s.	2.1	n.s.	263	n.s.	−14.9	n.s.
	≥	223		3.0		265		−13.4	
S	<	222	n.s.	2.4	n.s.	263	n.s.	−15.3	n.s.
	≥	224		2.7		265		−12.8	
J	<	223	n.s.	2.2	n.s.	264	n.s.	−16.2	<0.05
	≥	223		2.8		264		−12.2	
H	<	223	n.s.	2.2	n.s.	264	n.s.	−14.4	n.s.
	≥	223		2.8		264		−14.0	
SH-EPI									
A score	<	224	n.s.	2.2	n.s.	263	n.s.	−12.9	n.s.
	≥	224		1.0		265		−14.2	
B score	<	223	n.s.	1.5	n.s.	264	n.s	−14.6	n.s.
	≥	224		2.2		263		−12.3	
N score	<	223	n.s.	1.5	n.s.	263	n.s.	−14.9	n.s.
	≥	223		2.8		265		−12.8	
E score	<	224	n.s.	2.1	n.s.	263	n.s.	−13.6	n.s.
	≥	223		1.4		266		−15.1	
L score	<	223	n.s.	2.7	<0.05	263	n.s.	−13.5	n.s.
	≥	224		0.6		264		−13.4	

Serum Cholesterol

Baseline cholesterol was related to five sociocultural variables in low-risk subjects: age, socioprofessional and study level, with executives and university graduates showing the highest mean serum cholesterol; language and geographic location, with French-speaking subjects and those living in Brussels or Wallonia showing the highest values. As for Δ cholesterol, we noticed that younger subjects, those speaking French, and those living in Wallonia showed the smallest increase or greatest decrease over time (table IX). For high-risk subjects, out of the three variables showing a correlation with baseline cholesterol (language, geographic location and age), only age remains

Table XI. Belgian Heart Disease Prevention Project: intervention group. Serum cholesterol –
multivariate analysis in the low-risk group

Sociocultural variables	Retrospective (n = 3,506) prevalence		Sociocultural variables	Prospective (Δ chol.) (n = 3,465) incidence	
	f	p		f	p
Geographic region (Campine, Flanders, Brussels, Wallonia)	143	< 0.001	Baseline cholesterol	1210.1	< 0.001
Language (Dutch/French)	12	< 0.001	Geographic region (Campine, Flanders, Brussels, Wallonia)[1]	18.3	< 0.001
Social class (executives, white-collar, blue-collar)[1]	5.8	< 0.002			

n.s.: Age, study level, marital status	n.s.: Study level, social class, marital status, age, language
$r^2 = 4.5\%$	$r^2 = 26.5\%$

[1] Negatively related to the other variables.

significantly related to cholesterol modification over time with younger subjects showing the greatest decrease over time. Also, blue-collars showed a significantly greater decrease than executives and white-collars (table IX).

Not a single psychological variable showed any significant correlation
with baseline cholesterol in either low-risk or high-risk subjects. A lesser
increase over time is observed in socially conforming low-risk subjects,
whereas a greater decrease is observed in less job-involved high-risk subjects
(table X).When a multivariate analysis is performed for the low-risk group,
entering six sociocultural variables, three of them are independently related
to baseline cholesterol: geographic region, language and socioprofessional
class, the latter negatively. All variables together explain a trivial 4.5% of the
variance of serum cholesterol (table XI). The modification of cholesterol over
time is independently related to two variables, baseline cholesterol and geographic region. The former means that regression towards the mean plays an
important role, whereas in the latter we see what is maybe a greater acceptance of our prevention program in subjects living in the Campine, something

Table XII. Belgian Heart Disease Prevention Project: intervention group. Serum cholesterol –
multivariate analysis in the low-risk group

Sociocultural and psychological variables	Retrospective (n = 2,431) prevalence		Sociocultural and psychological variables	Prospective (Δ chol.) (n = 2,400) incidence	
	f	p		f	p
Geographic region (Campine, Flanders, Brussels, Wallonia)	103.5	< 0.001	Baseline cholesterol Geographic region (Campine, Flanders, Brussels, Wallonia)[1]	885 16.4	< 0.001 < 0.001
Language (Dutch/French)	9.6	< 0.002			

n.s.: Age, social class, study level, marital status, JAS-AB, JAS-S, JAS-J, JAS-H, A score, B score, N score, E score, L score $r^2 = 4.7\%$	n.s.: Age, social class, study level, marital status, language, JAS-AB, JAS-S, JAS-J, JAS-H, A score, B score, N score, E score, L score $r^2 = 27.9\%$

[1] Negatively related to the other variables.

Table XIII. Belgian Heart Disease Prevention Project: intervention group. Serum cholesterol –
multivariate analysis in the high-risk group

Sociocultural variables	Retrospective (n = 881) prevalence		Sociocultural variables	Prospective (Δ chol.) (n = 861) incidence	
	f	p		f	p
Geographic region (Campine, Flanders, Brussels, Wallonia)	27	< 0.001	Baseline cholesterol Geographic region (Campine, Flanders, Brussels, Wallonia)[1]	126.5 12.9	< 0.001 < 0.001
Age (40–44, 45–49, 50–54, 55–59)[1]	18.5	< 0.001			

n.s.: Language, social class, study level, marital status $r^2 = 5.6\%$	n.s.: Age, language, social class, study level, marital status $r^2 = 14.8\%$

[1] Negatively related to the other variables.

Table XIV. Belgian Heart Disease Prevention Project: intervention group. Serum cholesterol – multivariate analysis in the high-risk group

Sociocultural and psychological variables	Retrospective (n = 646) prevalence		Sociocultural and psychological variables	Prospective (Δ chol.) (n = 631) incidence	
	f	p		f	p
Language (Dutch/French)	23.7	< 0.001	Baseline cholesterol	60.5	< 0.001
Age (40–44, 45–49, 50–54, 55–59)[1]	12.6	< 0.001	Geographic region (Campine, Flanders, Brussels, Wallonia)[1]	12.9	< 0.001
Geographic region (Campine, Flanders, Brussels, Wallonia)	5.8	< 0.02			

n.s.: Social class, study level, marital status, JAS-AB, JAS-S, JAS-J, JAS-H, A score, B score, N score, E score, L score

$r^2 = 8.3\%$

n.s.: Age, language, social class, study level, marital status, JAS-AB, JAS-S, JAS-J, JAS-H, A score, B score, N score, E score, L score

$r^2 = 12.6\%$

[1] Negatively related to the other variables.

not seen in the univariate analysis. The whole accounts for 26.5% of the total variance (table XI).

When psychological variables are also introduced, none of them significantly adds up to the total variance of baseline cholesterol, whereas baseline cholesterol and geographic region correlate independently with Δ cholesterol. The whole accounts for 27.9% of the variance of Δ cholesterol (table XII). For the high-risk group, two sociocultural variables correlate independently with baseline cholesterol: geographic region and age. All six sociocultural variables account for 5.6% of the baseline cholesterol variance (table XIII).

Modification of cholesterol over time in high-risk subjects is related to baseline cholesterol and geographic region. The former is explained by regression towards the mean whereas in the latter we see that subjects living in the Campine reacted better to the individualized intervention package (table XIII). When psychological variables are also introduced, three variables are significantly and independently correlated with baseline cholesterol: language, age, and geographic region (in that order). All 15 variables account for 8.3% of the total variance (table XIV). Modification of cholesterol over time is again related to baseline cholesterol and geographic region. All 15 variables account for 12.6% of the total variance of Δ cholesterol (table XIV).

Comments. Five sociocultural variables are significantly correlated with baseline cholesterol, of which three in the low-risk group correlate independently: French-speaking subjects living in Wallonia and executives having the highest cholesterol baseline levels. After the 6-year intervention, modification of serum cholesterol is correlated with baseline level and geographic region. Whereas regression towards the mean is part of the explanation, one has to take into account the possibility that both subjects and their physicians (who received communication of the cholesterol entry level), reacted more strongly to the prevention program when the baseline level was rather high. Taking into account that subjects living in the Campine on the average had the lowest cholesterol levels, their cholesterol modification over time was the most favorable. The same holds true for high-risk subjects. Whereas the Walloons showed the highest cholesterol entry levels, both in univariate and multivariate analyses, subjects living in the Campine showed the greatest decrease over time. Here, the individualized prevention package had greater impact on those subjects in whom the French 'good cuisine' is less culturally imbedded, this last point being only a working hypothesis.

References

1   De Backer, G.; Kornitzer, M.; Thilly, C.; Depoorter, A.M.: The Belgian multifactor preventive trial in CVD. I. Design and methodology. Heart Bull. *6:* 143–146 (1977).
2   Rustin, R.-M.; Kittel, F.; Dramaix, M.; Kornitzer, M.; De Backer, G.: Smoking habits and psycho-socio-biological factors. J. psychosom. Res. *22:* 89–99 (1978).
3   World Health Organization European Collaborative Group: Multifactorial trial in the prevention of coronary heart disease. 1. Recruitment and initial findings. Eur. Heart J. *1:* 73–80 (1980).

Subject Index

Adrenal cortical system
    effect on immune response 375
    hormones 373–376
    psychosocial factors arousing 91
    response to effort with and without
        distress 93
    responses to controllable and
        noncontrollable situations 92
    selective response to different psychologic
        conditions 94
    sex differences in responses 97–103
Adrenal function in psychologic stress 253
Adrenaline 366–368, 370, 377
    excretion
        sex differences during stress 98–103
        type A vs. type B subjects 96
    secretion
        hypothalamic defense reaction 142
        low and high control tasks 95
Adrenergic receptors, concepts 306, 307
Adrenocortical hormone 52, 251, 366, 375,
    376
Alcohol abuse, effect on heart 264, 265
Angina pectoris 20, 23, 29, 30, 33, 34, 108,
    239
    clinical diagnosis 220
    coronary atherosclerosis and 320
    emotional behavior and 315
    Framingham Type A Scale, utility 71
    Israeli Heart Study, anxiety scores and
        reactivity to environmental stress 70
    psychophysiological stress tests
        exercise-induced ischemia,
            predictor 218
        intensity of attacks, predicting 218
    psychosocial stress and 420, 421
    sequence of coronary heart disease 244

Angiography
    coronary artery disease and behavioral
        correlates 44–47, 208, 243, 251, 370
    diagnostic 49, 175, 176
    radionuclide 49
Angiotensin-aldosterone, hypothalamic
    defense reaction 142
Antihypertensive drugs, mechanisms of
    action 309, *see also* Clonidine
Anxiety 186, 188, 369, 377
    angina and 370
    effect on platelet adhesiveness 262
Arousal patterns
    environmental stimuli causing 51
Arrhythmias, cardiac 342–348, 374
    animal studies 343–347
    behavioral and emotional factors 305,
        315, 343
    catecholamines and 243
    induction 343
    myocardial ischemia and 342
    stress and 251
    sudden cardiac death 257
Arteriography, coronary 44
Arteriosclerosis
    animal behavior studies 333–338
    corticosterone and 375
    physiological basis 248–254
    stress and 333–335
    type A coronary-prone behavior and 337
Atheroarteriosclerosis, adrenal cortical
    hormones and 373
Atherogenesis, *see also* coronary artery
    disease
    cortisol hyperresponsiveness 52
    type A behavior, role in
        development 39–48